Colonizing the Body

State Medicine
and Epidemic Disease
in Nineteenth-Century India

David Arnold

Colonizing the Body

Colonizing the Body

State Medicine
and Epidemic Disease
in Nineteenth-Century
India

DAVID ARNOLD

University of California Press

BERKELEY   LOS ANGELES   LONDON

University of California Press
Berkeley and Los Angeles, California

University of California Press, Ltd.
London, England

© 1993 by
The Regents of the University of California

Library of Congress Cataloging-in-Publication Data
Arnold, David, 1946–
    Colonizing the body: state medicine and epidemic disease in
nineteenth-century India / David Arnold.
      p. cm.
    Includes bibliographical references and index.
    ISBN 0-520-08124-2 (alk. paper); ISBN 0-520-08295-8 (pbk.:
alk. paper)
      1. Medicine—India—History—19th century. 2. Medicine—
Political aspects—India. 3. Social medicine—India—History.
4. Public health—Political aspects—India. 5. Smallpox—
Government policy—India. 6. Cholera—Government policy—
India. 7. Plague—Government policy—India. 8. Imperialism.
I. Title.
R606.A75   1993
362.1′0954′09034—dc20   92-25623
                                         CIP

Printed in the United States of America
9 8 7 6 5 4 3 2 1

Contents

List of Figures and Tables

Acknowledgments

The field of medical history has expanded rapidly in recent years, and South Asia is playing an important part in widening the thematic and theoretical, as well as purely geographical, parameters of a discipline that once seemed all too firmly rooted in the societies of Europe and North America. The formidable task of recovering and interpreting India's medical history is, however, the work of many minds. I have benefited greatly over the several years of research and writing that have gone into this book from the advice, comments, and criticisms of many fellow toilers in the field of medical and colonial history. I would particularly like to express my grateful thanks to Padma Anagol, Poonam Bala, Jane Buckingham, Ian Catanach, Nigel Crook, Tim Dyson, Paul Greenough, Mark Harrison, Roger Jeffery, Indira Chowdhury Sengupta, Elizabeth Whitcombe, and Michael Worboys. I am especially grateful to Bill Bynum at the Wellcome Institute, to Shula Marks at the Institute of Commonwealth Studies, and to colleagues in the history departments at Lancaster and the School of Oriental and African Studies, London, for their help and encouragement. A word of thanks, too, to the staff at the Hospital for Tropical Diseases in London for curing me of amoebic dysentery in 1982 and so, in a rather substantial way, making this study possible: they must, however, be exonerated from any responsibility for the use to which medicine has been put in the pages that follow.

I am greatly indebted to the Nuffield Foundation for funding initial work on this project in India in 1984 and to the Wellcome Trust for its generous support, which enabled me to conduct further research in 1988–90. I wish to thank the staff of the India Office Library, the SOAS Library, the libraries of the Wellcome Institute and the School of Hygiene and Tropical Medicine in London, the National Archives of India and the Nehru Memorial Library in Delhi, the West Bengal State Archives and the National Library in Calcutta, the Maharashtra State Archives in Bombay, and the Tamil Nadu Archives and Corporation Record Room in Madras for their help over many years.

I owe a continuing debt, too, to the enthusiasm and labors of my subalternist colleagues, Shahid Amin, Gautam Bhadra, Dipesh Chakrabarty, Partha Chatterjee, Ranajit Guha, David Hardiman, Gyan Pandey, and Sumit Sarkar, who have seen and heard many of these chapters at various stages in their evolution. This book owes more to their suggestions and inspiration than they could reasonably be expected to acknowledge. A word of sincere thanks, too, to Lynne Withey at the University of California Press for seeing me through the later stages of this work. My final and greatest debt is to Juliet Miller, whose love has always been the best medicine.

List of Abbreviations

Asst	Assistant
BC	Board's Collections
Bmb	Bombay
Bngl	Bengal
BoR	Board of Revenue
CoD	Court of Directors
Colr	Collector
Cons	Consultations
Comr	Commissioner
Cs	Chief Secretary
DFAR	*Dufferin Fund Annual Report*
Div	Division
Dt	District
Dy	Deputy
Gen	General
GO	Government Order
GoI	Government of India
HCAR	*Health Commissioner's Annual Report*
ICS	Indian Civil Service
IMG	*Indian Medical Gazette*
IMS	Indian Medical Service
IOL	India Office Library and Records
Jud	Judicial
KW	Keep-With
Legis	Legislative
LMS	London Missionary Society

MARCD	Madras Annual Report on Civil Dispensaries
MARCH	Madras Annual Returns of Civil Hospitals and Dispensaries
Md	Madras
Med	Medical
Mgt	Magistrate
Mil	Military
MSA	Maharashtra State Archives
Mun	Municipal
NAI	National Archives of India
NNR	Native Newspaper Reports
NWP	North-Western Provinces
Pnjb	Punjab
Pol	Political
Procs	Proceedings
Pub	Public
Resol	Resolution
Rev	Revenue
San	Sanitary
SC	Sanitary Commissioner
SCAR	Sanitary Commissioner's Annual Report
Sec	Secretary
SoS	Secretary of State (for India)
Supt	Superintendent
TMPSB	Transactions of the Medical and Physical Society, Bombay
TMPSC	Transactions of the Medical and Physical Society, Calcutta
TNA	Tamil Nadu Archives
UP	United Provinces
VR	Vaccination Report
WBSA	West Bengal State Archives

Introduction

A GHASTLY INCIDENT IN BURRA BAZAAR

On June 30, 1908, the following item appeared in Calcutta's European-owned newspaper, the *Statesman*, under the headline "A Mendicant's Ghastly Method: Burra Bazar Incident."

> On Sunday evening Burra Bazar was the scene of some excitement, due to the strange adventure of a low class native, who had formerly been employed as a dome in the Medical College Hospital. It appears that the man, having contrived to secure a human arm and skull from the Hospital with the aid of some of his comrades, went about the streets carrying them in his hands and soliciting alms from passers-by. A crowd collected and followed him asking him to show them the lump of human flesh which he carried; and the man, who was peculiarly dirty and shabbily dressed, responded by tearing it to pieces with his teeth, and at times he bit the almost decomposed arm for the sole object of extorting money. He entered a shop and began holding up the dead arm to the gaze of the crowd, and he was sent away with a small money dole by the shopkeeper, whose religious sentiments must have been shocked by the antics of the man. Eventually the police appeared on the scene and arrested him. He was subsequently sent up by Superintendent Merriman on a charge of having extorted money. The accused is awaiting trial.[1]

Subsequent investigation revealed that the 'dome' (or Dom), whose name was Paltoo, had not in fact been employed at the Medical College Hospital in Calcutta but had somehow acquired the arm and skull from the private medical school of the late Dr. Fernandez in Circular Road. Proof that the arm and skull had not come from the College Hospital was provided by Harilal Basu, assistant surgeon and senior demonstrator of anatomy at the college. He found that the skull had been severed from the rest of the head in such a crude and unprofessional manner that the scalp and much of the hair remained attached to it. The arm, too, showed evidence of having been "irregularly dissected." Such ineptitude, Basu reported, made it clear that this could not have been the result of a dissection carried out at Calcutta's Medical College.[2]

Paltoo had inadvertently brought to light evidence—which the European medical establishment in Calcutta was quick to seize upon—of the inadequate standards of teaching and administration at the private medical schools that had sprung up in the city over the previous twenty-five years. The oldest such institution dated back to 1884, but the grandly titled College of Physicians and Surgeons of India, founded by Dr. Fernandez and his colleague Dr. N. Das, had been in existence only since 1897. Several of these private medical colleges proudly boasted among their directors and teaching staff former members of the Indian Medical Service, the state medical service of colonial India, and other surgeons and physicians with an impressive string of medical qualifications after their names. Thus, the National Hospital and College of Physicians and Surgeons of India, located at 30 Cornwallis Street, Calcutta, and founded in 1905, listed among its staff Lieutenant-Colonel Nandi, MB, CM, IMS; Major N. P. Sinha, MRCP, MRCS, IMS; and Major B. K. Basu, MD, CM, IMS.

As far as the principal of Calcutta's Medical College, C. P. Lukis (soon to be Sir Pardy Lukis and director-general of the IMS), was concerned, the issue brought to prominence by Paltoo's grisly antics in the Burra Bazaar was how such "self-constituted" colleges were to be regulated to ensure that only properly trained and duly qualified doctors and surgeons were given degrees and allowed to practice in India.[3] This revived the old, but increasingly pressing, issue (dating back to the 1880s) of whether there should be a medical registration act for India as there had long been in Britain. Lukis was among those who argued that registration was essential if the standards of Western medicine in India were to be maintained. Bogus degrees issued by unregulated colleges would not only produce poorly qualified doctors and surgeons who would be a danger to their patients and the community among whom they practiced, but they would also by their incompetence and malpractice bring Western medicine as a whole into disrepute. But, others objected, should not every encouragement be given to private medical colleges as a way of facilitating the spread of an independent Western medical profession in India, which had so far found it difficult to establish itself outside the major cities? And what of the practitioners of the various Indian systems of medicine—Ayurveda, Yunani, and Siddha? Were they to be included in a system of state registration or omitted on the grounds that their practice was, to Western minds at least, "irrational" and "unscientific"?[4]

The vexing question of medical registration brought to the fore many of the underlying contradictions and dilemmas in the checkered career of Western medicine in nineteenth-century India. After one hundred and fifty years of British rule, Western medicine was still struggling to establish itself among the people of India. Medicine had been far less successful in this regard than the legal profession which, with a minimum of state sponsorship and regulation, had flourished like a hothouse plant in the steamily litigious atmosphere of colonial India. Why had Western medicine, comparatively speaking, been left out in the cold? One explanation was that it had remained too closely identified with the requirements of the colonial state and so was remote from the needs of the people. It had failed to make the transition from state medicine to public health. Another explanation was that the mass of the population remained content with the innumerable and readily accessible practitioners of indigenous medicine—the *kaviraja*s, the *vaidya*s, and the *hakim*s—and either saw no reason to seek out the few Western-trained practitioners who were available or could not afford their fees.[5] In 1900 even Calcutta, second city of the British Empire and a colonial metropolis of a million people, could support barely a hundred practitioners of Western medicine.[6] Despite the influential patronage of the colonial state, despite its own scientific claims and monopolistic aspirations, Western medicine had singularly failed to displace its indigenous rivals. Indeed, by 1914 the cohorts of a reformed and revitalized Ayurvedic and Yunani medicine were mounting a fresh assault on the privileged status of Western medicine in India, and even homeopathy, despite its European origins, seemed to be winning more adherents, especially in Bengal, than orthodox allopathic medicine. It is not surprising, then, that

Western medicine is often seen as having had only a superficial impact on India, confined to the small "enclaves" of the army and the European community in India and, even as late as the 1940s and 1950s, as having made little impression upon the beliefs and practices of the great majority of the Indian population.[7]

And yet—such is the contradictory nature of the claims presented—Western medicine is also sometimes seen as one of the most powerful and penetrative parts of the entire colonizing process, one of the most enduring and, indeed, destructive or distorting legacies of colonial rule in India as in many other parts of Asia, Africa, and Latin America.[8] From this perspective, the rise of independent medical colleges, like that of Drs. Fernandez and Das in Calcutta in the 1890s and 1900s, can be seen as but one sign among many—growing attendance at hospitals and dispensaries, mass immunization campaigns, even Indian nationalists' critical rhetoric of official neglect of indigenous health care—that Western medicine had already taken off in India, that even before 1914 it was ceasing to be merely the white man's medicine or just state medicine, had already begun to infiltrate the lives of an influential section of the Indian population, and had become part of a new cultural hegemony and incipient political order.

LOATHING AND DESIRE

In the renewed debate over medical registration, Paltoo the Dom was quickly lost sight of. But before he disappears into the jostling crowds and narrow back-streets of Burra Bazaar, we should pursue him a moment longer.

The community to which he belonged, the Doms, were (and are) widespread in many parts of India, particularly in Bengal and Bihar. They were among the lowest of all castes in India, despised even by many Untouchables. Traditionally, they not only filled the customary role of sweepers and scavengers but also performed such polluting and defiling tasks as removing the carcasses of dead animals and carrying the bodies of the human dead to burning grounds, or *ghat*s. They served as menial servants at Hindu cremations, providing the fuel for funeral pyres. Sometimes they were employed as executioners. Dom women worked as *dai*s, or midwives, another lowly occupation, which again brought them close to the body in its most polluting states. Abbé Dubois, writing of South India in the early years of the nineteenth century, called the Doms, or "Dumbars," a "dissolute body," and numbered them among the "class of mountebanks, buffoons, posture-masters, tumblers, [and] dancers."[9]

Perhaps this combination of carnival and carrion goes some way toward explaining Paltoo's curious way of trying to earn a living. But there are two other points about the Doms that add meaning to the scene enacted in Burra Bazaar. As if to put its own imprimatur upon the already miserable and "degraded" status of the Doms, the colonial authorities designated some of their number a "criminal tribe" and so subject to some of the most stringent penalties and restraints the colonial state ever devised.[10] But, in addition, the Doms also served the British in the dissecting rooms of hospitals and medical colleges—like those where Paltoo worked in Calcutta in the early 1900s.

Although valued and approved in early works of Hindu Ayurvedic medicine, dissection and the study of anatomy had not been part of Hindu (or indeed Muslim) medical practice in recent centuries. Helping with human dissections was not a customary task for the Doms, but it was clearly one for which their association with the disposal of the dead peculiarly fitted them. This, then, might be taken as an example of the way in which Western medicine, for all its novelty, might find a certain compatibility with existing social forms and cultural norms in India. So closely did Paltoo and his caste become associated with mortuary work that those who assisted at dissections became known indiscriminately as "doms" or "domes," without even a capital letter to honor their presence. But the presence of the Doms in the dissecting rooms had a curious double resonance. It is indicative of the deep repugnance Indians of almost every caste and creed had for the Western practice of dissection that only the lowest and most despised of Hindu castes could be recruited to assist in this polluting and defiling work. It was as if Western medicine itself bore the taint, the stigma, of the pariah, and there was much about Western medicine (as we will see subsequently) that seemed to situate its practitioners among the outcaste and the defiled.

But in a not uncharacteristic conflict or inversion of cultural values, dissection was seen to be a necessary, even exemplary, part of nineteenth-century Western medical practice. Particularly before the effective development of microscopy and bacteriology late in the nineteenth century, it was largely through interrogation of the dead that doctors aspired to know the diseases of the living. Thus, Indian opposition to postmortems (though certainly it had its parallels in contemporary Britain) was seen as irrational, perversely obstructive to the legitimate needs of medical science. When in January 1836 at the newly established Medical College in Calcutta a Brahmin instructor, Pandit Madhusudan Gupta, and four Indian students performed a human dissection for the first time, it was hailed as a major victory for Western civilization. It was said to mark the day when "Indians rose superior to the prejudices of their earlier education and thus boldly flung open the gates of modern medical science to their countrymen." The momentous event was duly celebrated, in rather militaristic fashion, by firing a fifty-round salute from the guns of Calcutta's Fort William.[11]

But a deep loathing of dissection persisted and fed a widespread belief that Western medicine was more about cutting up bodies than healing them. This was a contributory element in the general atmosphere of suspicion, doubt, and resistance that haunted Western medicine in India for much of the nineteenth century and reached its climax in the rumors and riots against government plague measures in the late 1890s. Opposition to the performance of postmortems on likely plague victims was one reason among many for this upsurge of public anger and defiance. There were, significantly, even circumstances in which Doms themselves dissented from dissection. In 1898 a Dom called Budri, who had been assisting with dissections at Calcutta's Medical College Hospital for fifteen years, scratched his finger on a piece of bone while helping to dissect a suspected plague victim. He developed a high temperature and died two weeks later, presumably from plague. But his fellow Doms, though long associated with the grim work of the dissecting room—or perhaps because they knew it all too well—refused to allow Budri to be dissected in turn. "Budri," recorded the city's health officer, J. Neild Cook,

> was a drunkard and a very popular character among the domes, and though it was their business in life to cut up others, they absolutely refused to let their friend be cut up. They came down [to the hospital at Manicktolla] in considerable numbers and carried him off to the burning-ghat.[12]

Thus, even the most menial servants of Western medicine kept one of its most emblematic practices at a discreet cultural distance. Budri's body belonged to them and to the cremation ground, not to the dissecting table of the colonizers.

This mixture of dissent and desire, the hateful and the hegemonic, in Indian responses to Western medicine is one of the paradoxical elements this book attempts to explore. It is an essay in the political and cultural problematics of the body in a colonized society as reflected and refracted in medical discourse and practice and as manifested in the varying perceptions of, and responses to, epidemic disease. It is a study of a colonizing process, rather than a history of Western medicine in India.

COLONIZING THE BODY

Anyone who sets out to try to write a history of the body is inevitably indebted to Michel Foucault, and anyone familiar with his seminal work will find the influence of *Discipline and Punish*, *The Birth of the Clinic*, and *Power/Knowledge* inscribed, however artlessly, in these pages.[13] But this book is not intended to be an imitative or uncritical reading of Foucault. To an extent unparalleled in his work, it is concerned with the creation of a state-centered system of scientific knowledge and power, rather than the more diffused and generalized forms of knowledge and power he described. It attempts, too, in a further departure from the main body of Foucault's work, to see resistance as an essential element in the evolution and articulation of a particular system of medical thought and action. Indeed, the problematic interdependence of discourse and praxis, and the constant tension between them as represented in a complex colonial situation, lies at the center of the more empirical discussions that follow.

Nineteenth-century India presents us with a medical system that attempted not just to function for the benefit of the colonial rulers themselves (though that was undoubtedly one of its priorities) but also, often ineffectually, to straddle the vastness of a peculiarly colonial divide. The notion of resistance, of an ineradicable otherness, at times opposing from without, at times resurfacing within, the discursive domain of Western medicine itself, often condemned but repeatedly summoned up as an active and not altogether unwelcome principle of negation, has thus to be constantly reckoned with as a central element in the dialectics of power and knowledge in colonial India. It is partly for this reason—to emphasize the importance of the body as a site of colonizing power and of contestation between the colonized and the colonizers—but also in order to stress the corporality of colonialism in India (rather in contrast with those whose primary emphasis has been upon colonialism as a "psychological state") that this study speaks of the "colonization of the body."[14]

The ambiguities and complexities of that phrase, and the multiple compulsions and constraints that lie behind it, are worked out more fully in the chapters that follow. But it should be stressed here that medicine was only one—albeit a particularly critical—example of a colonizing process. Its equivalents are to be found across a whole range of interlocking colonial discourses, sites, and practices: from penology to anthropology, from the army to the plantation and the factory. But to attempt to describe them all would be too vast an undertaking for a single work and would inevitably blur what can more effectively be revealed by concentrating upon a single exemplary form. Nonetheless, it is important to recognize at the outset that medicine did not stand alone but occupied a place within a more expansive ideological order and a wider empirical domain.

But before we proceed further it will be as well to identify some of the principal features of the colonization of the body as it is discussed here. First, there is the nature of colonialism itself. Colonial rule built up an enormous battery of texts and discursive practices that concerned themselves with the physical being of the colonized (and, no less critically, though the interconnection is too seldom recognized, of the colonizers implanted in their midst). Colonialism used—or attempted to use—the body as a site for the construction of its own authority, legitimacy, and control. In part, therefore, the history of colonial medicine, and of the epidemic diseases with which it was so closely entwined, serves to illustrate the more general nature of colonial power and knowledge and to illuminate its hegemonic as well as its coercive processes.[15] Over the long period of British rule in India, the accumulation of medical knowledge about the body contributed to the political evolution and ideological articulation of the colonial system. Thus, medicine cannot be regarded as merely a matter of scientific interest. It cannot meaningfully be abstracted from the broader character of the colonial order. On the contrary, even in its moments of criticism and dissent, it remained integral to colonialism's political concerns, its economic intents, and its cultural preoccupations. While Foucault justifiably warned against too narrow a concentration upon the state and the systems of power that fed directly into it,[16] it is critical in speaking of India under colonial rule to recognize that there, until 1914 and arguably much beyond that date, Western medicine was intimately bound up with the nature and aspirations of the colonial state itself.

It would be pointless to deny that much of what is described here in a colonial context has its precedents and parallels in nineteenth-century Europe, particularly in Britain itself, and was by no means unique to India. Indeed, the second element of what this book seeks to describe under the rubric of the colonization of the body is the diverse array of ideological and administrative mechanisms by which an emerging system of knowledge and power extended itself into and over India's indigenous society, a process in many respects characteristic of bourgeois societies and modern states elsewhere in the world. Bodies were being counted and categorized, they were being disciplined, discoursed upon, and dissected, in India much as they were in Britain, France, or the United States at the time. There is, indeed, a sense in which all modern medicine is engaged in a colonizing process. The history of medicine in European and North American societies over the past two hundred years has been a history of growing intervention and a quest for monopolistic rights over the body. It can be seen in the increasing professionalization of medicine and the exclusion of "folk" practitioners, in the close and often symbiotic relationship between medicine and the modern state, in the far-reaching claims made by medical science for its ability to prevent, control, and even eradicate human diseases. It has aptly been said that the position of medicine today is "akin to that of state religions yesterday." It has acquired an "officially approved monopoly of the right to define health and illness and to treat illness."[17]

But colonial India either showed these developments in an exceptionally raw and accentuated form (in which the Indian experience was as much contrasted with, as compared to, the European) or demonstrated, in a manner largely unparalleled in Western societies, the exceptional importance of medicine in the cultural and political construction of its subjects. Moreover, Western medicine in India was a colonial science and not simply an extension or transference of Western science to a colonial outpost. Without being wrenched free of its metropolitan roots, it nonetheless had grafted onto it ideas and concerns that had their origins in India or in Europe's Orientalizing of India. Western medicine in India was Western medicine for India in a way that Europe-based experts and observers often found distressing or bizarre.

And finally, to a degree unrecognized in Foucault, the career of Western medicine in India showed the importance of different and often opposing "readings" of the body, just as disease stood not for one but for a multiplicity of metaphors and meanings.[18] As the history of epidemic disease in nineteenth-century India—here represented by the deadly trinity of smallpox, cholera, and plague—makes plain, the body formed a site of contestation and not simply of colonial appropriation. The question—Who speaks for the body of the people?—constantly recurred, informing political thought and social action on both sides of the colonial divide. The forms that contestation took were many and varied and shifted substantially over the momentous period of this study, from 1800 to 1914. The search for authority and control was not simply the stark European/Indian dichotomy it is sometimes taken to be. The idea of Orientalism is one which it is useful to invoke and echo in these pages,[19] but its historical limitations do much to test its theoretical boldness. Part of the task of this study is to utilize the history of epidemic disease and medical intervention to uncover different forms of Indian responses, to peel apart the onion layers of resistance, accommodation, participation, and appropriation. It is thus not only an account of colonial power and knowledge but also, of necessity, an essay on internal differentiation within Indian society, on subaltern politics and middle-class hegemony. Medicine was too powerful, too authoritative, a species of discourse and praxis to be left to the colonizers alone.

1 Occidental Therapeutics and Oriental Bodies

At the close of the eighteenth century, India was still, medically speaking, a largely unknown land to Europeans. The Portuguese, pioneers of European trade and dominion in the Indian Ocean and established at Goa in western India since the early sixteenth century, were responsible for some preliminary investigations into medicine and disease. The trading companies of other European powers were active around the shores of the subcontinent for nearly two hundred years, and Dutch, British, and French doctors and surgeons visited India and occasionally practiced among Indians. But little was known—and still less, systematically recorded—about the diseases of India or the manner of their treatment by Indian physicians. Before 1800 Western medicine had made few inroads into India and was largely confined to European enclaves and ports like Madras and Pondicherry in the south; Bombay, Surat, and Goa in the west; and Calcutta and Dhaka (Dacca) to the east. The various forms of indigenous medical practice remained largely unaffected in their character and content by Western contact. Indeed, far from home and the assistance of their own physicians, Europeans sometimes turned for help to India's *hakim*s and *vaidya*s (Muslim and Hindu doctors respectively), and their readiness to seek Indian assistance was encouraged by a belief that local doctors would be more familiar with the diseases of the climate and with the locally occurring medicines an obliging nature had provided for their treatment.[1]

A hundred years later, at the end of the nineteenth century, a dramatic transformation had occurred in both the character and the relative position of Western and indigenous medicine in India. To be sure, there was still much that Western medicine did not know about the diseases of India, and many areas, especially of village India, where its writ did not run. But it had broken out of its earlier enclavism to become one of the most confident expressions of British political and cultural hegemony in India. While the practitioners of Western medicine—Indian and European—remained a distinct minority among the half-million medical practitioners listed in the census returns, the Western system of medicine had come by 1900 to enjoy a formidable degree of authority over British India, within the councils of government, and over the lives of its 300 million subjects. While the indigenous systems of medicine were slowly emerging from a long period of stagnation and decline and were being rejuvenated (partly through emulation of Western medicine, partly in conscious rivalry with it), Western medicine had become far more than an exclusively European preserve and proudly proclaimed its universality. Although it might meet with little more than passive acceptance from the large majority of Indians whose lives it affected, Western medicine was gaining in prestige and popularity among the Western-educated middle classes. Whatever its actual achievements in containing or curing disease—and about these there were many doubts and trenchant criticisms—its dominance within the realm of state medicine and public health was assured.

But there was nothing inevitable about this process of medical colonization, nor was it uncontested. How and why this singular transformation occurred—how Western medicine was able to establish itself in India and claim authority over Indians and Europeans alike—is the subject of this chapter and those that follow.

In attempting to examine the reasons behind this change and the manner of the transformation, we encounter a series of interrelated issues. There is, first of all, a question of chronology and continuity. How rapidly and by what stages did Western medicine establish itself in India? On this point there is singularly little agreement. Some writers, such as Radhika Ramasubban, have suggested that until 1900, or even later, Western medicine exercised—and indeed sought—very little influence over the mass of the Indian population. Closely tied to the military requisites and commercial priorities of the colonial state, it almost entirely ignored the needs of the Indian people and remained largely confined to a small enclave of white residents and soldiers.[2] Some writers have gone so far as to argue that Western medicine has never really broken away from its enclavist origins and still remains remote and exotic, beyond the reach of the vast majority of the Indian people. Thus, the social anthropologist McKim Marriott asserted in 1955 that Western medical facilities had "hardly touched" the villages of rural Uttar Pradesh in northern India. Clinics and dispensaries were at best, he wrote, "momentary stopping places on the sick man's pilgrimage from one indigenous practitioner to another." "Western medicine sits outside the door of the village," he continued, "dependent upon governmental subsidy and foreign alms for its slim existence."[3]

But many other writers have assigned to Western medicine a more active and interventionist role dating back to some point during the nineteenth century. One of the critical moments in the expansionist career of Western medicine in India has been identified with the mid 1830s, when the triumph of the "Anglicists" over the "Orientalists" is seen to have ended colonial patronage of indigenous medicine and marked the confident assertion of the Western system as the only legitimate form of medical practice. Another possible break came in the 1860s, when the report of the Royal Commission on the Sanitary State of the Army and the appointment of provincial sanitary commissioners pointed the way toward a broader and more pervasive system of state medicine and public health for India. But arguably, the moment of transition from enclavism to public health came only in the 1890s with the establishment of a new "tropical medicine," based on the germ theory of disease, and a corresponding intensification in state medical intervention in India as in many other parts of the colonial world, epitomized by the measures taken during the Indian plague epidemic of the 1890s and 1900s.[4] That there is no ready consensus as to when Western medicine departed from its "enclavist" origins and began to serve an expanded notion of public health is perhaps indicative of the gradual nature of the changes affecting Western medicine in nineteenth-century India, the strength of its continuities, and—for reasons that require investigation—the relative weakness of its moments of transformation.

A second, and closely connected, issue concerns the nature of the relationship between what for convenience we call "indigenous" and "Western" medicine (as if they were totally independent and internally homogeneous systems of thought and practice).[5] The history of this interaction goes back to the first European encounters with Indian medicine in the sixteenth and seventeenth centuries (or much further back, to the early exchanges between ancient Greece and India); but we still know relatively little about how the Indian medical systems were interpreted and utilized by Europeans, and how those systems in turn responded to the advent of so formidable an adversary as Western medicine had become by the late nineteenth century.

It has often been assumed that Western medicine (like other branches of European science and technology), once introduced to India by the colonial power, enjoyed an almost automatic ascendency over its rivals, a medical manifest destiny which no indigenous system or systems could possibly gainsay. Only a most partisan or uncritical reading of the history of Western medicine in nineteenth- and twentieth-century India could possibly support this view. No more convincing are those accounts of Ayurvedic and Yunani (respectively Hindu and Muslim) medicine which suggest that they retained their pristine purity throughout the colonial period or that Western medicine never exercised a more than peripheral influence on Indian society and on Indians' understanding of healing and disease.[6] The relationship between Western and Indian medicine needs to be looked at in more pluralistic and dialectical terms, terms that allow for a continuing interaction between the two during the long history of colonial rule in India or that express the relationship as a protracted epistemological struggle which says more about the nature of political and economic power under colonial rule than about the abstract merits of two contrasting, competing, but not wholly incompatible, medical systems. It is important in this connection to move away from a purely metropolitan view of an expansionist science and to appreciate the extent to which Western medicine in India was not merely a projection of the medicine taught and practiced in Britain but was constantly engaged in a dialogue with India or, at least, with an "Orientalist" version of what India—its climate, its peoples, its cultures—represented.

Third, as this last comment suggests, medicine cannot be considered in isolation from the political, economic, and cultural forces at work in British India. It is necessary to assess the various compulsions that lay behind attempts to propagate Western medicine in India, the agencies involved in this work of medical evangelization, and the various constraints—political and cultural, financial and technical— which operated in the reverse direction. The colonial context within which Western medicine was required to function and the contradictions—many of them remarkably deep-seated and pervasive—that beset its diverse operations also require investigation. Medicine involved ideas and practices which need to be understood as part of the exploratory and regulatory mechanisms of colonial rule. Medicine, to echo Daniel R. Headrick's rather mechanistic analysis, might be a "tool of empire," a technological boon to an expansionist Western power.[7] But it could also, no less significant in a conquered territory, be an important element in the unfolding ideology of empire and, later, in the emergence of anticolonial discourse and an aspirant counterhegemony.

COLONIAL SCIENCE
AND COLONIAL MEDICINE

In an article entitled "The Spread of Western Science," published in 1967, George Basalla asked how it was that "modern science" came to be diffused from its homeland in Western Europe and established throughout the rest of the world. Dissatisfied with conventional explanations about the dissemination of Western science purely through European expansion and conquest, he wanted to know who were the carriers of Western science, which fields of science they took with them, what changes took place within Western science during the period of transplantation, and hence the means by which a flourishing scientific tradition was re-created within societies outside Western Europe.

His response to these questions—pertinent to our own investigation into medicine in nineteenth-century India—was to propose that Western science spread in three main phases. In the first phase the "non-scientific society" served Europe as a source of scientific ideas and observations. In the course of their exploration of the globe, Europeans visited new territories, drew maps, conducted surveys, collected samples, and gathered specimens. Although trade and the prospects for European settlement were important stimuli to this scientific reconnaissance, Basalla saw its main significance in the development of Europe's own scientific culture. European investigators were heirs to the Scientific Revolution, that "unique series of events" which taught the civilization of the West that "the physical universe was to be understood and subdued not through unbridled speculation or mystical contemplation but through a direct, active confrontation of natural phenomenon." The observations and materials gathered during this initial phase informed Europe's evolving scientific knowledge and understanding and fueled further theorization. "Exotic" material from the rest of the world enabled European science to undergo a process of learning and development at the same time that it was being globally disseminated.

Basalla labeled the second phase of his typology "colonial science," by which he meant "dependent," rather than inferior, science. The term "colonial" was intended to be descriptive, not pejorative, and not to imply "the existence of some sort of scientific imperialism whereby science in the non-European nation is suppressed or maintained in a servile state." The range of scientific disciplines involved was greater than in the initial, exploratory, phase, but colonial scientists remained dependent upon an external scientific culture based in Europe without being able to become full participants in it. Their training directed them to fields and problems not of their own choosing but already delineated by scientists in Europe. It was difficult for them to enter its leading scientific societies, to gain access to the "invisible colleges" in which the latest scientific ideas were debated and exchanged.

Basalla's third and final phase saw the apparent completion of the transplantation process, marked by a struggle to achieve an "independent scientific tradition." Spurred on, as in the United States or the infant republics of South America, by the drive for national independence and self-reliance, this phase was aided by the creation of local institutions, traditions, and honors. A political, educational, and technological infrastructure emerged which allowed modern scientific research to be established and sustained within national boundaries. The process of transference was now complete.[8]

The value of Basalla's model for the purpose of the present discussion is that it provides a broad typology within which to locate the history of India's colonial medicine. Escaping from an earlier historiography of science, constructed around great men and great discoveries, it encourages us to see developments in a wider context and to confront such basic questions as what might be meant by a term like "colonial science," or, by extension, "colonial medicine." But by its assumptions and omissions, Basalla's model also raises a number of issues not pursued or left unresolved in his essay.

There is, for instance, no clear periodization. Basalla suggests that the scale and duration of each phase might vary from country to country according to the historical circumstances. But Phase One is unmanageably elastic and takes little account of the enormous changes that occurred in the character of the science projected by Europe onto the rest of the world between the first voyages of discovery and the penetration of Africa four hundred years later. Clearly, the kind of medical science reaching India from Europe on the eve of World War I was very different from that a century earlier at the end of the Napoleonic Wars—not only in its technical aspects but also in its political authority. Despite passing reference to the needs of commerce and settlement in Phase One, the relationship between science and the political and economic imperatives of European states is largely ignored in Phase Two, leaving "colonial science" peculiarly detached from the specific requirements of the colonial regimes that sustained it. Although it would be needlessly reductionist to see science as only the tool of commercial and political enterprise, it would be equally unrealistic to deny the practical value which colonial regimes and imperial paymasters saw in such scientific fields as botany, geology, and medicine. Again, while Basalla strives to incorporate into his model societies as diverse as China, Japan, and India on the one hand and the Americas on the other, he fails to create a suitable niche for the "traditional" sciences of Asia and their relationship with a dominant West. The model merely assumes the simple displacement of the former by the latter, whereas the situation—in practice if not always in theory—was far more equivocal. Basalla's model is diffusionist, rather than interactive or dialectical. More immediately, Basalla does not discuss medical science, a curious omission in view of the prominence of medicine among European sciences abroad and the contribution which physicians made to botany, geology, and other scientific disciplines as well as their own.

The history of Western medicine in nineteenth-century India demonstrates the limitations (though certainly not the irrelevance) of a Eurocentric, diffusionist model and illustrates the need to relate the history of scientific ideas and practices not only to forces emanating from the metropolis but also to local constraints and imperatives, to political and professional influences, as much as to the evolution of scientific theory and technique. While Western medicine in India was in essence the same medicine as that practiced in Europe at the time and followed or participated in many of its critical developments, it would be a mistake to imagine that it therefore lacked a distinctive identity and history of its own or that it was impervious to the physical, social, and political milieu in which it operated. On the contrary, as will be argued here, Western medicine in India was always involved in a dialectical relationship, caught between the thrust of metropolitan science on the one hand and the gravitational pull of India's perceived needs, constraints, and potentialities on the other. It was this intermediate relationship, this need to serve two masters simultaneously, which helped to create the almost unresolvable tensions and contradictions that beset both the theory and the practice of colonial medicine in India.

Even if the reach and efficacy of Western medicine was strictly limited in the period up to the 1860s and, as Radhika Ramasubban contends, barely extended beyond a small European enclave, it was nonetheless important in laying the foundation for later developments and in establishing the claims of Western medicine, and of Western authority more generally, over India and its colonial subjects. It built up a corpus of colonial knowledge which sought to comprehend and encompass India's material world as well as the health of those who inhabited it.

Part of the power of the colonial medical discourse of the period lay in the manner in which medicine self-consciously conceived of itself as a science, based on careful local observation and eschewing the ill-informed "speculation" of the past and the rank "superstition" associated with Indian concepts of disease and healing. In a characteristic expression of this scientific attitude, William Twining, one of the most original and influential medical writers of early nineteenth-century India, began his *Clinical Illustrations of the More Important Diseases of Bengal* in 1832 with the observation that

> The spirit and philosophy of medical science, in the present day, require a diligent investigation of the foundation on which opinions are advanced; and such foundation is only to be established by the laborious and accurate observation of facts: a system of late years happily substituted for the vague conjectures of former ages.[9]

Almost every medical textbook and treatise of the period began with a declaration that the work was based on clinical observation. James Johnson, a Royal Navy surgeon whose work had a profound influence on the next fifty years of medical thought and practice in

India despite the brevity of his own sojourn in that country, was scathing about medical authorities who pronounced from Europe on the diseases of the tropics without ever having been there. His book, he declared in 1813, was "not the mere offspring of a fertile imagination, or a good library"; it was based on fifteen years' "observation and experience, in a vast variety of climates," including that of India.[10] James Annesley, a former surgeon at the Madras General Hospital, similarly presented his *Researches* into the diseases of "warm climates" in 1828 as the product of twenty-five years' service in India and other "inter-tropical" locations.[11] Such repeated emphasis upon local experience and observation was essential to the emerging character of colonial medical science, for (as in the long-running controversy over the etiology of cholera) it repeatedly pitted the expertise and understanding of the old India hand against the brash universalizing of metropolitan science. The argument was repeatedly made that only those who knew India from long experience could possibly pronounce upon the nature of its diseases and its medical or public health requirements, or were in a position to understand how cultural and environmental factors might affect the practical application of Western medical science. This was, moreover, a line of argument that the colonial government in India often found politically or financially expedient to endorse.

Annesley and Twining were among the many nineteenth-century physicians who saw themselves as contributing through their "patient industry" to a wider scientific community beyond India as well as providing more immediate practical guidance for colleagues newly arrived from "home." For some doctors a career in India might be a poor, but unavoidable, substitute for employment in Britain. Others, however, clearly saw India not as a form of professional exile but as a unique opportunity for observing and investigating disease and the many influences affecting human health. In the first issue of the *Transactions of the Medical and Physical Society of Bombay*, published in 1838, the society's secretary, Charles Morehead, himself a product of medical training in Edinburgh and Paris, remarked on the great "variety of circumstances" in which disease could be observed in India. Among these were

> Europeans from infancy to middle age, the newly arrived, the long resident, the temperate, the intemperate, the exposed to, and the protected from injurious circumstances, the habituated

to one climate, and to many; all the variety of native
population, with their different pursuits, habits, and modes of
life, in regard to food, clothing, and habitation.[12]

The Preface to the first volume of the *Transactions* of a sister
society—the Medical and Physical Society of Calcutta—in 1825 contained a similar prospectus, revealing the wide ambitions and scientific aspirations of at least some British doctors in India at the time.
The anonymous author began by remarking that "the great outlines
of disease" were likely to be "much the same in all countries." India
was not, in his opinion, "an unexplored region" where new diseases
and cures were likely to be discovered (a curiously complacent claim
when "Asiatic cholera" was about to burst upon the world). But, like
Morehead a decade later, he saw enormous opportunities for medical
research and observation in India. He remarked that

> habit, food, and climate, exercise indisputable influence upon
> the human system, both in a healthy and diseased state; and it is
> equally important to pathology and physiology, to determine
> the modifications which they induce, and the varieties that may
> be attributed to their operation, in a country so different as
> India, both in its physical and social relations, from those
> regions in which medical observation has been hitherto most
> extensively engaged.[13]

If few original contributions to nosology—the classification of
diseases—could be expected, the East (with India as its gateway) had
a vast, but still largely unexplored, materia medica which might yet
make useful additions to European pharmacology. If little of practical
value was to be expected from the "imperfect science" of India's
vaidyas and *hakims*, "still," continued the *Transactions*' Preface, "to
liberal and cultivated minds, the progress and condition of science in
all ages, and in all climes, must be objects of interest." The Calcutta
Society would, therefore, "gladly welcome" the light that might be
"thrown upon the past or present existence of Oriental medicine, by
information gathered from authentic sources, or derived from actual
observation." The medicine of the Hindus, even more than that of
the Muslims, with which Europe already had some partial acquaintance, might, the writer thought, repay investigation. It would at least
be "novel . . . and perhaps not wholly uninstructive."[14]

But the value of the Calcutta Society and its journal was seen to lie not only in the benefits which "our brethren" in Europe might derive from medical investigations in India but also from the stimulus it would give members of the medical profession in India to sustain their perhaps otherwise flagging scientific interests. Medical men in the country, explained the writer as if to emphasize that this was, indeed, "colonial science" conducted at the periphery, labor under many difficulties. Apart from a fortunate few, who reside in the main cities and civil stations, they are

> scattered far apart from each other, over a vast extent of country; they hear and see nothing of the stir of science, and catch but indistinct and partial glimpses of the advancement of knowledge. Their limited means and frequent removals [from one post to another], put it out of their power to provide themselves with regular and expensive supplies of books, and there are no public libraries beyond the limits of the Presidencies [here meaning the provincial capitals of Calcutta, Bombay, and Madras rather than, as usually, the provinces themselves]: they can derive, therefore, little benefit from the recorded experience of others, and they have rarely any opportunity of confirming or correcting their own, by that of an associate, a rival, or a friend:—their scene of action is too restricted, and too entirely their own, to admit of emulation or ambition; and the official reports, in which alone their practice is commemorated, are too much matters of form and routine, to merit or attract animadversion.

In such circumstances, they need to be rescued by a learned society before "their zeal dies within them."[15]

These remarks, echoed in many other scientific publications of the period, highlight some of the leading characteristics of colonial medicine in nineteenth-century India: the self-conscious adherence to science as a rational pursuit based upon close and objective observation, a commitment to its active pursuit and propagation, an awareness of the "modifications" imposed upon Western medicine by the local influences of climate, custom, and diet, and the skeptical but not altogether scornful attitude toward indigenous medicine.

Until about the 1850s, when science split into a number of more specialized fields, medicine was the master narrative of scientific discourse in India, the disciplinary core and professional base around which other "exploratory" sciences were clustered. As D. G. Crawford has shown, many of the pioneers of botany, zoology, geology, meteorology, ethnography, and philology in late eighteenth- and early nineteenth-century India were medical practitioners, nearly all of them surgeons (meaning, in this context, doctors generally) in the service of the East India Company. Whether from personal interest (nurtured by their broad scientific training in medical schools like Edinburgh's and the "gentlemanly" fashion for science at the time) or in furtherance of their official duties and responsibilities, a great number of them wrote accounts of the plants, animals, rocks, climate, and inhabitants of the regions of India and its neighboring territories.[16] The proceedings (as well as the names and declared aims) of such organizations as the Medical and Physical Society of Calcutta testify to the breadth of their intellectual curiosity and professional pursuits. Thus, the first, and not unrepresentative, volume of the Calcutta *Transactions* included articles by H. H. Wilson on leprosy "as known to the Hindus" and N. Wallich on "the tree which produces the Nipal [Nepal] camphor wood and sassafras bark," several articles on Indian plants and drugs, including George Playfair on "Madar, and its medicinal uses," as well as essays on such diverse topics as the locusts of the Doab, snakebites and leeches, cholera in China, and the "luminous appearance of the ocean."[17] "The preliminary education of medical men," declared Sir James Outram in 1860,

> places them on a level, in respect of intellectual accomplishments, with the *average* of those with whom it is our good fortune to recruit covenanted Civil Service—and above the average of our purely military officers; and their professional education gives them special qualifications for aiding in developing the resources of the country, and in ameliorating the conditions of its inhabitants. They are necessarily acquainted, to a greater or less extent, with Geology, Botany, and other branches of Natural History. To *their* researches do we owe most, if not all, the economic discoveries in Natural History by which the East has of late enriched the industrial resources of the world.[18]

It needs to be stressed, too, in partial contradiction of Basalla's understanding of "colonial science," and despite the scientific and professional isolation many Company surgeons undoubtedly felt, that the flow of medical ideas, practices, and personnel was not simply one way, from metropolis to periphery. The value of India as a tropical observatory, where diseases as varied as cholera, dysentery, leprosy, and malaria could be more practically or effectively investigated than in Europe, was widely acknowledged. The results of this work, widely reported in British and European medical journals and textbooks, passed rapidly into the mainstream of nineteenth-century medical science. Particularly before the 1860s, a significant number of doctors from India retired to Britain to continue their medical careers there. Some took up important teaching posts, notably at the Army Medical School at Netley, "the mother of all tropical and service [medical] schools," whose significance has been greatly (and perhaps unreasonably) overshadowed by the establishment of the London and Liverpool schools of tropical medicine nearly half a century later.[19] Others became important figures in the history of sanitary reform and medical education in Britain, often while continuing to contribute to debates about medical and sanitary affairs in India. As the careers of Sir James Ranald Martin and Edmund A. Parkes in the mid nineteenth century attest, the links between British Indian and metropolitan medicine were not only strong but also mutually influential.[20]

THE RISE OF TROPICAL MEDICINE

Medicine stood at the center of the Company surgeons' scientific understanding of the material world, just as their knowledge of medicine was in turn informed by their acquaintance with several kindred sciences. Their inability to identify the precise causes of ill health (a failure to which many freely admitted) encouraged them to situate disease, especially epidemic disease, within a wider physical and cultural landscape. Their observations and speculations ranged much more widely than if (like a later generation of medical researchers and practitioners) they had narrowly identified disease as the product of certain invading microorganisms and ignored its social and environmental context. The broad and interrelated nature of their scientific concerns, exemplified by the "medico-topographical" surveys produced from the 1820s onward, raised Western medicine in India beyond a simple preoccupation with European health and survival and brought it within the play of wider environmental, economic, and social forces. It also established a "topographical" or "environmentalist" tradition in India's colonial medicine which stubbornly persisted throughout the nineteenth century and beyond.

The medical discourse of the period was clearly linked not only to the ideas and methodologies of contemporary science in Europe but also to the political expedients and economic imperatives of colonial rule and to the accumulation and classification of colonial knowledge about India. It became possible and meaningful for Company surgeons to address the problems of disease and medicine as they affected Indians as well as Europeans only when British power had increased to such an extent that India and Indians were being brought under colonial scrutiny and control, when the nature and durability of British rule had become an urgent practical issue, and when the medical establishment had expanded in line with growing military and civilian requirements.

Leaving aside some earlier European investigations into Indian disease, and at the risk of some oversimplification, we can see a thematic progression in British medical works relating to India produced between the 1770s and 1850s. John Clark's *Observations on the Diseases in Long Voyages to Hot Countries*, published in 1773, was concerned exclusively with the health of Europeans (especially sailors), a narrow and external view also shared by Charles Curtis's 1802 monograph, *An Account of the Diseases of India, as They Appeared in the English Fleet, and in the Naval Hospital at Madras, in 1782 and 1783*. In William Hunter's *Essay on the Diseases Incident to Indian Seamen, or Lascars, on Long Voyages*, dated 1804, the focus was wider in as much as Indians were the object of medical attention, but still only as seagoing servants of the Company. James Johnson's important book on *The Influence of Tropical Climates, More Especially the Climate of India, on European Constitutions*, which first appeared in 1813 but was reissued in an extensively revised edition by J. R. Martin as late as 1856, marked a significant shift to the problems of European survival not at sea, but on land in an alien and hostile environment. Shortly after Johnson, two major texts, James Annesley's *Sketches of the Most Prevalent Diseases of India* (1825) and William Twining's *Clinical Illustrations of the More Important Diseases of Bengal*, first published in 1832, provided detailed accounts of disease among Indians while still giving priority to European health. Charles Morehead's two-volume *Clinical Researches on Disease in India*, published in 1856, went beyond earlier works both in its encyclopedic range and in its integration of European and Indian health within a single framework of analysis.

Significantly, Clark, Hunter, and Johnson were naval surgeons and thus representative of the still-maritime orientation—or, at most, amphibian nature—of British power in South Asia. In Clark, Curtis, and Hunter, the need to protect Britain's trade and maritime forces against French attacks and to preserve the health of soldiers and sailors during lengthy periods of naval warfare continued to inform medical attitudes and responsibilities. In keeping with this practical outlook, Hunter explained the importance of his subject—the health of Indian seamen—not just in terms of the "cause of humanity" but also of "the interest of a great commercial nation, which derives advantage from the labours of this class of men."[21] By contrast, Annesley in Madras, Twining at Calcutta's General Hospital, and Morehead, who before he retired from India in 1859 was principal and professor of clinical medicine at Grant Medical College in Bombay, were all accustomed to the idea of Britain as a territorial power firmly established in India, with obligations toward the Indian as well as European inhabitants. Clark, Johnson, and, to some extent, Hunter situated their discussion of disease within a well-established genre of maritime health and the diseases of "warm climates," a term that occasionally included the Mediterranean but usually signified a broad belt of the globe from the West Indies and the shores of West Africa through India to island Southeast Asia and the China Seas. Twining, by contrast, was one of the first medical writers to produce a manual of medicine and disease specific to a single region of colonial India. Medically speaking, British rule had announced its intention to stay.

From early in the nineteenth century, medicine and disease also began to figure prominently not only in specialized medical literature but also in wide-ranging surveys of the Company's territories. In September 1807 the East India Company invited the surgeon Francis Buchanan to conduct a survey of eastern India. He was directed to report on the physical condition of the people, their diet, the diseases to which they were subject, and the modes of treatment used, as well as to provide information about the region's topography, the religion and customs of the people, their systems of land tenure and husbandry, and the natural resources, commerce, and manufacturing of the country. Buchanan's reports, compiled over the following seven years, duly reflected his medical training and scientific interests.[22]

The *Transactions* of the Calcutta and Bombay Medical and Physical societies contain a large number of "medico-topographical" surveys, most of them compiled in the course of official tours of medical and military duty. In his *Sketches of the Most Prevalent Diseases of India*, published in 1825, and his *Researches into the Causes, Nature, and Treatment of the Most Prevalent Diseases of India, and of Warm Climates Generally*, three years later, James Annesley also addressed himself to the study of the medical topography, climate, and seasons of India. Medicine, he believed, could be put on a "rational footing" only if due attention were first given to the influence of the climate, the seasons, and the geographical distribution of disease. His own "topographical and statistical reports" for the Madras Presidency were a preliminary attempt to put this idea into action.[23]

More influentially, in 1835 James Ranald Martin in Calcutta persuaded the Government of India to authorize a series of medico-topographical reports by medical officers on the various stations and districts where they were located. His *Notes on the Medical Topography of Calcutta*, published in 1837, was warmly received by William Farr, the celebrated medical statistician and nosologist in London, and was closely followed in India by such works as John M'Cosh's *Topography of Assam* and Robert Rankine's *Notes on the Medical Topography of the District of Sarun*. The genre continued well into the second half of the century, when it was partly superseded by the more comprehensive imperial and district gazetteers.[24] The breadth of the approach of the medico-topographical surveys reflected the broad range of the surgeons' scientific interests and the centrality of medicine in their understanding and investigation of the Indian environment.

The surveys also demonstrated the perceived utility of medicine to the security and material interests of the regime they served. Medical topography epitomized the colonial order's practical and political need to know, as much as any intellectual curiosity the scientifically minded surgeons might themselves bring to their subject. They were state servants quite as much as they were scientists. In Martin's expansive formulation, enunciated in 1856, the medical topographer was required to

> investigate all the circumstances which tend to deteriorate the
> human race, and to lower its vigour and vitality; all that relates
> to the external causes of disease, their propagation, and their
> prevention; all plans for improving the physical, and through it,
> the moral condition of the people.[25]

Reflecting the interventionist and sanitary-minded 1850s and Farr's work as registrar-general in England, rather than the earlier and more cautious vision of the Company's directions to Buchanan, Martin continued:

> The natural features and peculiarities of every locality affect materially the life and health of the inhabitants. Any general system of sanitary inquiry should, therefore, embrace information respecting the surface and elevation of the ground, the stratification and composition of the soil, the supply and quality of the water, the extent of marshes and wet ground, the progress of drainage; the nature and amount of the products of the land; the condition, increase or decrease, and prevalent diseases of the animals maintained thereon; together with periodical reports of the temperature, pressure, humidity, motion, and electricity of the atmosphere. Without a knowledge of these facts it is impossible to draw satisfactory conclusions with respect to the occurrence of epidemic diseases, and variations in the rate of mortality and reproduction.[26]

Disease and medicine thus entered centrally into the exploratory and classificatory discourses of the early nineteenth century, and did so for materialistic as well as scientific or avowedly humanitarian reasons. Disease, especially epidemic disease, was too potent a factor in the viability and profitability of empire for the Company and its servants to ignore. It was not only the health and survival of Europeans that was at stake. Epidemics, especially when they occurred in conjunction with famine, depopulated villages and drastically depleted state revenues from agriculture and trade. If disease had to be entered in the debit column of empire, then medicine might be (or, in the reckoning of doctors, ought to be) counted among its redeeming assets. An "increased security of life and property" was one of the rewards Martin anticipated from a more systematic and scientific "state medicine" for India.[27]

C. Macnamara, a surgeon at Calcutta's Ophthalmic Hospital, also emphasized the material value of disease control to the colonial state. He remarked in 1866 that British rule had "doubtless done a vast deal for India." Having found the country in "a state of anarchy and ruin," it had secured peace and protection for all classes. But "beneficial work" still needed to be done in overcoming "the ravages which

epidemic and endemic diseases annually commit among the people."
Cholera, in his view, stood in the forefront of these destructive
diseases. It needed to be combated because of the "untold misery" it caused the population as a whole, but also because, by its
destructiveness,

> the State loses a vast store of force, which was never created to
> be squandered in this way. Taking, therefore, the lowest and
> most sordid view of the matter, Government is bound to do all
> in its power to improve the health of the lower classes, because
> the fearful mortality at present existing among them is a direct
> and positive loss to the State.[28]

As medical servants of the state, surgeons like Macnamara and
Martin were inevitably concerned with the practical contributions
their knowledge and skill could make to the welfare of India and to
the security and prosperity of its colonial regime. At times (as Macnamara's remarks about "lowest and most sordid view of the matter"
suggest) doctors doubtless found it necessary to stress the material
benefits of medical and sanitary intervention in order to coax and
cajole a reluctant state into action. Medical practitioners sometimes
showed clear signs of frustration at government indifference and inertia; but, in the main, most of them seem to have seen no sharp contradiction or divergence of interest between serving the state and
serving science.

THE ENVIRONMENTALIST PARADIGM

Colonial medicine appraised India through a series of exploratory and
classificatory "grids." One of the most important of these was spatial.
In a narrowly defined sense, this spatial element was represented by
the hospital, the jail, and the army barracks, institutions that were to
a great degree colonial innovations and that were small enough to
allow for close observation and for strict regulation of diet and other
presumed influences on disease. The institutional arenas of the barracks and the jails are discussed in chapter 2.

At a more general level, colonial medicine, through its topographical surveys and its discourse on the physiological and pathological effects of "warm climates," defined India as an exotic space, a
dangerous and unfamiliar environment. Diseases, while still obliged
to obey the same "universal" laws as in Europe, functioned in an un-
accustomed or accentuated manner, and medicine, correspondingly,

had to undergo certain "modifications" dictated by a different climate and appropriate to different human constitutions. A geographical and perceptual space—"the tropics"—had to be constructed before the terms on which Western medicine could operate within this novel environment could be fully determined and before Europeans and Indians alike could be effectively brought within its operational parameters.

The idea that physical environment exercised a potent influence on human health and disease was an ancient one. It could be traced in European thought at least as far back as Hippocrates and his *Airs, Waters and Places*. It was also, as Francis Zimmermann has recently demonstrated, a well-established theme in Ayurvedic medical thought.[29] Although there is little evidence to show that nineteenth-century British medical writers were aware of this indigenous literary tradition, they sometimes cited local Indian opinion in partial confirmation of their own observations about the unhealthiness of certain localities or regions. Environmentalist ideas enjoyed a marked revival in eighteenth-century Europe, stimulated by the publication of Montesquieu's *De l'esprit des lois* in 1748, and in turn had a seminal influence on early colonial ideology and administration in India in matters as diverse as the Permanent Settlement of 1793 and the prospects for European colonization. As late as 1856 J. R. Martin quoted, with evident approval, Montesquieu's views on the physical lethargy produced by hot climates and the consequent disposition toward barbarous and despotic institutions.[30] Encouraged by neo-Hippocratic ideas in Europe, but also responding to the novelty and intensity of the climate and disease environment they confronted in India, Company surgeons drew upon a wealth of German and French as well as English topographical surveys, going back to the mid eighteenth century, and, more immediately, upon the literature generated by European encounters with disease in the West Indies and West Africa, to guide them in their attempts to relate ill health to physical environment.[31]

Not all of India's diseases fell within this environmentalist paradigm.[32] Leprosy, for instance, though widely observed in nineteenth-century India and the subject of erratic state control, was seldom seen to be determined by climate or environment; indeed, such a connection was often expressly denied.[33] Smallpox, as chapter 3 shows, was also understood to be largely independent of environmental influences. But the great majority of diseases, the "fluxes" and "fevers" which formed the staple of nineteenth-century medical works and the stock-in-trade of most medical practice, were seen to be in various degrees affected by the nature of India's environment. This perceived relationship between environment and disease lay at the heart of the claim made by Charles Morehead, among others, that "disease in India is not disease in England."[34]

There was a large measure of consensus among medical authors as to which were the most characteristic or widely "prevalent" diseases of India. Fevers (mainly signifying what we now call malaria) along with liver and bowel diseases made up the reigning trinity, though individual writers might give priority to one or another of these. Nonepidemic diseases—such as leprosy, beriberi, and tetanus—were seldom discussed in any detail nor, until toward the end of this period, was tuberculosis, despite the considerable medical attention it commanded in Europe.[35] Kala-azar, tropical sprue, even typhoid ("enteric fever") were not identified until relatively late in the nineteenth century. Writing from their maritime perspective, Hunter and Clark included scurvy among the major diseases of the region, but the more emphatically land-based British power in South Asia became, and the better the cause of scurvy was understood, the less relevant scurvy became, except to prison doctors. Johnson in 1813 dwelt extensively on "bilious fever," the "grand epidemic," as he saw it, of warm climates, but also on hepatitis, "the endemic of India" (hepatitis, it should be noted, was a term broadly assigned to various disorders of the liver, including the effects of chronic amoebic dysentery). In 1818 George Ballingall, an army surgeon in Madras, concentrated on liver complaints and dysentery (and was one of the first medical observers to make a distinction between what we now know as amoebic and bacillary dysentery). He argued, rather exceptionally, that fever, though a major cause of invaliding, did not "occupy the most prominent part in the sick returns of the Indian army."[36] Annesley, writing in the immediate aftermath of the 1817–21 cholera epidemic, ranked that disease (which had been only summarily discussed by most earlier writers) first among the "most prevalent diseases of India," and this view was shared by many subsequent medical writers.[37] Twining, a few years after Annesley, confined his *Clinical Illustrations* to dysentery and diarrhea, diseases of the liver and spleen, cholera, and fevers. W. L. MacGregor, an army surgeon, in 1843 identified three "great" diseases in his study of army health in northern India: fever, cholera, and dysentery. Five years later, Kenneth Mackinnon described fever, dysentery, and cholera as "the great staples of mortality" among the population of northern and eastern India, while Martin in 1856, echoing Johnson, regarded fevers, bowel complaints, and liver diseases as the prime causes of ill health and mortality in India.[38] In the range of diseases he chose to survey, Charles Morehead in Bombay represented a significant departure from most earlier writers. "I have aimed," he wrote in the introduction to his *Clinical Researches* of 1856,

> not merely to increase practical knowledge of the diseases usually termed tropical—malarious fever, hepatitis and dysentery; but also to show that affections—pneumonia, phthisis pulmonalis, pericarditis, Bright's disease—familiar to European observers, are sufficiently common in India, more particularly in some classes of the native community.

But even Morehead, keen though he was to expand the parameters of Western medicine in India beyond the conventional run of diseases, had to confess that he was guilty of another common lacuna: he had almost nothing to say about the diseases of women and children.[39]

Despite a tendency to designate fevers by the particular regions in which they occurred—"Gujarat fever," "the putrid fever of Bengal," and so forth—most of the diseases and conditions discussed by British physicians in India (with the partial exception of "Asiatic cholera") were already familiar from Europe's own epidemiological experience or from medical encounters with other parts of the globe. The work of military and naval surgeons in Europe was often cited (not surprisingly, given the professional background of most medical men in India). Sir John Pringle's mid–eighteenth-century work, *Observations on the Diseases of the Army*, was frequently quoted in discussions of the causes and treatment of India's fevers, as were medical accounts of the disastrous, fever-fated Walcheren expedition of 1809. The other major reference point was the literature relating to other "warm climates," notably the West Indies. At the time when James Johnson was writing, the West Indies had generated a much larger and more authoritative medical literature than India. This was an indication of the greater economic and political importance previously attached to the Caribbean and the joint stimulus to medical inquiry there of intensive military and naval activity and a class of resident white planters.[40] By the 1820s and 1830s, with the consolidation of British power in South Asia and the economic decline of the West Indies, the latter ceased to be such a prominent and pertinent source of reference for medical writers in India. The absence of yellow fever from India—the most life-threatening disease of Europeans in the West Indies—and, conversely, the Indian origins of cholera, also made the example of the other Indies appear of diminishing significance to South Asia.

The unfamiliarity of the Indian environment and its extreme and deleterious effects on the human body were repeatedly stressed. Charles Curtis, drawing upon the experience of his brief stay in Madras in the 1780s, wrote that he realized soon after arriving in India that "European nosology and definitions" would there "prove but uncertain or fallacious guides." A "stranger" like himself had "a good deal to unlearn" from his European training and experience and needed in his medical practice "to feel and trace out for himself" every step of the way.

> Nor [Curtis added] is this perplexity, and the difficulties which we have to encounter, to be wondered at . . . in a country, where scarce a single production, whether of the animal or vegetable kingdom, is to be met with, bearing a true resemblance to its prototype in Europe; where, except for one or two weeks about the shifting of the monsoons . . . a shower of rain, or a breeze of wind, are almost unknown; where scarce ever a haze or cloud appears upon the horizon, to mitigate the dazzling ardour of an almost vertical sun; and where the thermometer through the whole 24 hours, seldom or never points under 80° of Fahrenheit, but generally far above it.[41]

The perceived strangeness of India and the malevolence of its climate were no doubt accentuated by the physical discomfort Europeans themselves experienced and the high levels of mortality they witnessed among their compatriots. In describing prickly heat as "one of the miseries of a tropical life," Johnson was generalizing from his own ordeals as well as drawing upon observation of his fellow Europeans.[42] The medical commentators and topographers of the period began to build up a medical representation of India's pathogenic climate and landscape that was very different from the romantic vistas shown in the Daniells' picturesque aquatints of the period or from the long-standing idea of India as an alluring "land of desire," filled with all the "treasures of Nature."[43] When the soldier, Orientalist, and adventurer Richard Burton wrote in 1851 of his welcome escape from "pestiferous Scinde and pestilential Gujarat," he was articulating a view of India that had become commonplace among the military and civilian, as well as medical, servants of the Company by mid-century.[44] A growing awareness of the prevalence of disease did not inhibit colonial attempts to exploit India's wealth and resources, but it did emphasize nature's bondage rather than nature's bounty, a bondage which might be broken only by the rigorous application of medical science.

Most early medical texts were based upon experience of Bengal (and, to a lesser extent, maritime Madras), where the East India Company's commercial and administrative involvement was greatest, and where climate, vegetation, and topography were furthest from the norms—the "prototypes" as Curtis described them—of northwestern Europe. For John Clark in the 1760s, as for many other doctors during the next century or more, Bengal stood out as a singularly unhealthy and hazardous region. This unhealthiness could be recognized not just by its physiological and pathological effects upon the body (especially the unacclimatized European body) but also by the extreme nature of the climate and topography. Since it was the lethal combination of heat and humidity and the hot, moist air's capacity to hold poisonous, disease-generating "miasma" in suspension that appeared to make tropical regions so deadly, Bengal's jungles, creeks, and marshes, its hot and humid climate, and the great variations in temperature between and within seasons seemed to provide an almost archetypal example of the savage effects a hostile environment could have on the human constitution. Small wonder (it was reasoned) that severe and malignant fevers, acute liver complaints, dysentery, and diarrhea were to be found everywhere in Bengal and in such deadly profusion.

Some writers understood the effects of climate to be indirect, providing the preconditions for disease or intensifying the effect of poisonous emanations from rotting vegetation, animal matter, or the dank soil. Although the "miasma" or "malaria" ("bad air") which were thought to cause or transmit disease could not be precisely identified or traced to a specific source, the conviction remained firm that they must surely flourish in such uncongenial surroundings. F. P. Strong, a Calcutta surgeon, was most emphatic on this point. "However malaria may be generated," he wrote in the 1830s, "there can be no doubt that it is produced most abundantly in all those parts of Bengal which are not cleared of jangal [jungle], drained, and kept clean." In the environs of Calcutta, chief city of the province, one had only to look around to see the "essentials necessary for the formation of malaria—jangals, lakes, marshes, gardens crowded with trees, and woods of every description, and weeds, stagnant water, filthy pools, and low grass jangals of every kind." In these there existed "ample means for a constant supply of the poison, assisted. . . by the natural heat and moisture of the climate." When to these were added "unnatural or meteoric changes of climate" or "unnatural inundations of seas, or river water," then "disease and death scourge[d] the land."[45]

In his topographical survey of Dhaka, surgeon James Taylor identified similar environmental influences which made the countryside "abound with malaria" and left its inhabitants "in a state of perpetual fever." The most sickly time of year came as the annual river floods began to subside in late September. From then until late November, Taylor declared, was the season of malaria, when "the elements of decomposition or the proportions of water and dead vegetable matter, and a certain degree of temperature appear to be in the most favourable adaptation for the production of this agent." The miasma produced by the thick and stinking layer of decaying vegetable matter brought down by the rivers combined with the heat and "a state of atmospheric quiescence" to produce fevers of a particularly malignant kind.[46]

Even where the physical environment could not be implicated as an "exciting cause" of ill health and disease, its influence could still be invoked as a "predisposing" factor in making people susceptible to ailments of almost every conceivable kind. In relating remitting and intermitting fevers universally to "vegeto-animal miasmata or marsh exhalation," James Johnson observed:

> These miasms arise from the wide-extended bosom of the earth, wherever animal and vegetable substances are lying in a state of decomposition; but in a tropical climate, where heat and moisture give, not only activity to the *agent*, but a predisposition for its reception to the *subject*, their united efforts are tremendous![47]

Annesley, too, argued that the diseases of warm climates were essentially the same as those which prevailed in summer in temperate countries, but they were "rendered more intense by more powerful causes," such as climate, were "more continued in their action, and much more prolonged, and hence their effects become more marked than elsewhere."[48] The violence of the climate and the extreme effects of heat and humidity were held largely to blame for this tropical aggravation of disease. Twining, like Ballingall and others, identified dysentery in India as a more severe disease—more rapid in its progress and more frequently fatal in its outcome—than the condition designated by the same name in England. He attributed this difference primarily to the effects of a tropical climate. "Considerable and abrupt diurnal changes of temperature, great heat with humidity, and the transition from the hot to the cold season" appeared to him to be the main "exciting causes" of dysentery as observed in Bengal.[49] Twining held much the same view of intermittent fever, which he was inclined (unlike many of his contemporaries) to attribute directly to the effects of climate rather than to intervening miasma:

> Malaria has been generally acknowledged the efficient cause of intermittent fevers; but it is abundantly evident to every medical man in Bengal, the very first year that he witnesses the results of the change of season and the temperature, between the 20th October and 1st December, that intermittents are intimately connected with the diurnal changes of temperature, which take place at the commencement of the cold season. At that time the evaporation is infinitely less than it had been for the six weeks previously; and the frequency of intermittents is augmented beyond all proportion, after the cold nights and foggy mornings commence, and when the heat of the days is much decreased. The state of the human constitution induced in Bengal by the previous hot-weather and rains, doubtless paves the way for the influence of the commencement of the cold weather, in the production of many diseases which then prevail. To these causes, and to disorders of internal organs, and principally to a disordered condition of the abdominal viscera, I ascribe the intermittent fevers, which occur more frequently in November and December than in all the rest of the year.[50]

The importance attached to climate and topography as determinants of disease, a theme so elaborately worked out and so authoritatively stated in the medical texts of the early nineteenth century, remained a remarkably powerful force in medical ideas in India for the rest of the century. Even when challenged by a new paradigm, the germ theory of disease, many old India hands still clung resolutely to climatic or environmental determinism or hastened to explain that microbes and germs provided no more than a partial explanation for the incidence and etiology of specific diseases.[51]

CLIMATES AND CONSTITUTIONS

The "tropical medicine" of the late eighteenth and early nineteenth centuries was a study not only of environmental forces, of tropical landscapes and warm climates, but also of the effects these had upon the "constitutions" of Europeans and indigenes. The language of constitutions was, of course, common enough in Europe in the late eighteenth and early nineteenth centuries, but it assumed added significance in India in that it provided an index of Europeans' "exoticism" in tropical climates and an expression of inherent differences between Europeans and Indians.

Extremes of climate, it was often argued, had a powerful effect upon the vital organs, especially the liver, still (as in an earlier pathology) seen as the seat of most bodily disorders. "In hot climates," Clark informed his readers in 1773, "of all the viscera in the human body, the liver is most subject to disease."[52] "From *heat*," declared Johnson forty years later with his customary passion, "spring all those effects which originally *predispose* to the reception or operation of other morbific causes," and in support of this theory he advanced an elaborate argument, explaining how, by sympathetic or analogous action ("a consent of parts"), tropical conditions stimulated the flow of biliary secretions inside the body in much the same way as they caused profuse perspiration on the outside. When this secretion was checked, as by the abrupt fall in nighttime temperature, various ailments were bound to result—from impaired appetite and constipation to severe liver disorders and "hepatitis." Indians, by virtue of the color of their skin and other forms of physical and cultural adaptation to the heat and humidity, were far less likely than Europeans to be affected by these changes. But in white men and women, the body's organs and vessels were "more violently stimulated than in Europe," and in this lay the root cause of their greater susceptibility to tropical disorders.[53]

But there was no agreement as to the precise effects of a tropical climate on European constitutions and, in particular, whether its effects were inflammatory and congestive or enervating and asthenic. According to Clark, a warm climate "relaxes the solids, dissolves the blood, and predisposes to putrefaction." He found the effects most evident among European women, whose "lively bloom and ruddy complexions" were rapidly "converted into a languid paleness; they become supine and enervated, and suffer many circumstances of ill-health peculiar to the sex, from mere heat of climate and relaxation of system."[54] Others maintained that the effect of heat was to inflame or congest the organs and overheat the blood. "Many of the diseases prevalent in warm climates as well as tropical ones," wrote MacGregor in 1843, "are the effect of increased irritability." He went on to explain that the "irritating effects of heat on the human system render it more liable to febrile disorders" and saw this as the reason why Europeans seldom escaped an attack of fever when they first landed in India. It was not only the "general system" of the body that suffered: "the constant exposure to a high temperature acts on the circulation of the various organs causing congestion," with the liver again the organ most likely to be affected.[55] In thus seeking to locate the effects of climate in disorders of the blood, bile, and other bodily fluids, the medical authors of the period combined environmentalism with elements of a humoral pathology which still influenced early nineteenth-century medical thought in Europe.

The idea that disease in a tropical environment was more acute than in temperate climes nurtured a belief that Western medicine, to be effective, had to be "modified" accordingly. The antiphlogistic therapies so widely favored in the first half of the nineteenth century—bleeding and the administration of large doses of calomel and other mercurials—were prescribed to combat the supposedly inflammatory effects of a tropical climate. In a country where the onset of disease occurred with alarming rapidity and gave rise to such violent symptoms, where apparently healthy people might die in agony from cholera within hours of its first symptoms appearing, it seemed imperative to act promptly and decisively. "The rapidity with which morbid actions run their course in warm climates," warned Annesley in his *Researches*, "calls for the most decided treatment." He anticipated that the "boldness" with which many of the cases in his book were treated would "surprise the practitioner in more temperate countries," where diseases advanced more slowly, assumed a milder form, and responded to more moderate therapies.[56]

Again, it was Johnson who most emphatically expressed the need for drastic and vigorous medical intervention in the tropics. He pronounced on the basis of his own (somewhat slender) experience that the "Peruvian bark" (cinchona), recommended by John Clark, James Lind, and others, was ineffectual in the treatment of Bengal's "endemic fever." He turned instead to venesection and found that copious bleeding (repeated whenever the symptoms of fever recurred) gave his patients decisive relief, and he followed this with large doses of calomel to purify the blood and free the bowels. Johnson believed that considerable quantities of blood needed to be drawn—as much as forty ounces at a time—and that anything less drastic would fail to have the required therapeutic effect. He quoted with enthusiasm a naval surgeon who had himself bled for fever in the desperate hope that this treatment might save his life. The effect of opening the vein was "astonishing," the surgeon reported with sanguinary zest. "The blood gushed from the orifice, with an impetuosity I have never before witnessed: the bulkhead, and beams of the deck above, were instantly covered with it." His assistant was "so alarmed that he would have checked the effusion," but the surgeon "insisted on the contrary" until twenty ounces of blood had spurted from his arm. "He is now a living instance," concluded Johnson magisterially, "of the good effects resulting from bold venesection, purgatives, and mercurials."[57] Such recourse to heavy bleeding, which was extensively used against cholera as well as malarial fevers, could only have contributed to patients' debility, while calomel was administered in such large and repeated doses that it not only produced the desired "salivation" but also rotted the gums, caused teeth to drop out, and attacked the jawbones of the hapless patients.

Many later practitioners viewed the punitive ferocity of these antiphlogistic therapeutics with understandable revulsion or, like Morehead, argued that they made matters worse by accentuating the asthenic effects of a tropical climate on European constitutions, which required strengthening tonics rather than violent bleedings and enervating purges. But for thirty years or more after Johnson, venesection and mercurials enjoyed a remarkable (and deadly) vogue in India. This reflected in part the powerful influence of Johnson's work and personality, as well as the desperation of physicians who could find no more effective way of combating malaria and cholera. But it was also a demonstration of the underlying belief that such "heroic" treatments were necessary to counter the exceptional virulence of disease in the tropics and the "inflammatory" effects on Europeans of the Indian climate.[58]

Before the 1830s, when informed observation about disease among the Indian population was still scant and statistical data almost nonexistent, Europeans saw themselves as susceptible to a host of fevers, fluxes, and hepatic diseases from which Indians were apparently largely immune. "It is singular how infinitely more Europeans are disposed to liver disease and dysentery than the natives," Annesley remarked in 1825. To support this claim, he produced figures from the Madras Army to show that more than 21 percent of white soldiers were affected by liver disease, compared to only 0.1 percent of Indians, and that Europeans were fifteen times more likely than Indians to suffer from dysentery.[59]

This common perception of European vulnerability to the diseases of a tropical climate was based in part upon observation, albeit of a restricted kind. There were, no doubt, reasons why in the army rates of sickness and mortality from certain diseases were so high among Europeans. But a belief in their general vulnerability also reflected the conviction that Europeans were by nature "exotics" in India and so exposed to the effects of an environment to which indigenes must, by contrast, be well "assimilated." Johnson, whose book addressed the problems of European survival in the tropics generally, adopted the familiar argument of the time that human beings, like plants and animals, did not adapt easily to unfamiliar climates. Transplanted from their native soil they tended to droop, lose their accustomed vigor, and "gradually decline." He, like other British physicians of the time, cited the fate of the Portuguese in the East as evidence of Europeans' inability to maintain their health and vitality in the tropics, and doubted whether whites could reproduce themselves in India beyond two or at most three generations. In his view, they were subject, too, to "depressing passions," to the fears and anxieties which possessed those far from home and left them mentally as well as physically vulnerable to the inroads of disease.[60] Annesley thought along similar lines. Man, he wrote, was best suited to the circumstances and vicissitudes of the country in which Providence has ordained him to exist. . . . The European is constituted in a manner the best suited to the climate which he inhabits; and a similar conformation of the system of man to the circumstances of the country, may be traced in every part of the globe. When, however, man migrates from the climate which contributed to generate the peculiarities of his frame, to one which is remarkably different from that to which he is assimilated, then disorders of various kinds and grades may be expected.[61]

But the extreme hazards to which Europeans, as exotics, were exposed in a tropical environment were not seen as an absolute bar to their presence, or even to their temporary residence. Some writers claimed that with time Europeans became "seasoned" to the effects of climate and disease, but this assertion was a subject of continuing dispute in India, as later in Africa, and in any case offered scant reassurance for the health of newly arrived soldiers and civilians.[62] More generally, it was seen as the physician's task to devise ways of protecting or rescuing Europeans' health from the deadly climate in which they found themselves. This belief gave rise to a variety of medical and sanitary responses—from topographical surveys to establish which localities were more salubrious than others and so might provide safe sites for barracks and sanatoriums, to the temporary evacuation of troops and prisoners to avoid an outbreak of cholera, or the condemnation of aspects of European diet, dress, and social behavior believed inimical to health in the tropics. Many of these responses were of greatest relevance to the army (and as such are taken up for discussion in chapter 2), but others were of more general significance.

One of the consequences of this understanding of the "modifications" imposed upon European health and therapeutics by India's tropical environment was that it made medicine into a comparative, and not an exclusively European, exercise. Physicians wanted to know whether Indians were indeed less subject to certain diseases than themselves and why this might be so. They were curious whether Indians possessed, in their medical practices, in their understanding of disease, and in their diet and dress, attributes that might also serve the interests of European health.

Johnson was a strong advocate of European adaptation to Indian ways. His views, based upon a passing acquaintance with Bengal in the early years of the nineteenth century, reflected a more liberal approach to racial and cultural relations between Europeans and Indians than is found in a later generation of more imperially minded and racially aloof writers. Although he dismissed much Indian medical practice as "a strange medley of ludicrous and ridiculous customs," he commended Indians for their "cold treatment" or "refrigerating principle" in the treatment of fevers and praised the effectiveness of some of their purgatives and tonics. He deplored European indulgence in great quantities of "heating" foods and alcoholic drink, contrasting it with Indians' apparent moderation and temperance. He regarded their light and flowing clothes as far more appropriate to the climate than heavy European dress; he defended the "Asiatic effeminacy" of Europeans in India, with their palanquins, servants, and languid lifestyle, as a sensible adaptation to a torrid climate; and he thought favorably of the European soldier who married or cohabited with an Indian woman, who cooked, washed, and performed "every menial drudgery for *massa* in health, besides becoming an invaluable nurse when he is overtaken by sickness."[63]

Twining, too, believed that there was much that sensible and sober Europeans could do to mitigate the effects of India's "great heat" and thereby preserve their health. But he also held that there were significant constitutional as well as cultural differences between Europeans and Indians to be taken into account. He accordingly concluded each section of his *Clinical Illustrations* with remarks on "the modifications of disease to which the Natives of the country are liable" and, in a revised edition of his book published in 1835, devoted an entire section to "the constitutions of the Natives of India." In his opinion, maladies "which may be reasonably ascribed to high temperature, and the result of inflammation" were "generally much slighter" among Indians than Europeans, "probably in a great degree owing to the peculiarities of their constitutions, adapted to the climate." But he also suggested that the difference was "in some measure dependent on the simplicity of their habits with respect to food and drink, which must be acknowledged in many respects more reasonable than our own." He believed that with "protracted exposure to malaria, with much fatigue, and privations," their constitutions were soon subdued by "malignant fevers of the most destructive description."[64] Equally, the remedies the physician employed had to be adapted to the nature of Indians' constitutions, to their customary diets and cultural practices. The strong medicines and fearsome therapies used on Europeans, the venesections and heavy doses of calomel, might be unnecessary in the treatment of Indians—because, Twining explained, of the "habitual temperance of these people, and the peculiarities of their constitution"—or would prove too drastic for Indians' weaker constitutions to endure. Even a convalescent diet of sago and rice water, "a low diet" for a European, was likely to be "stimulant and injurious to Asiatics, while any degree of acute disease exists."[65]

Europeans might appear most vulnerable by reason of their lack of acclimatization, medical opinion held, but they were better able to avoid, or even resist, the worst effects of climate and disease. Indians were more likely to die from the effects of disease because of their weaker constitutions but also (as British attitudes toward Indian culture and society grew more critical) because of their fatalism and inertia or the oppressive weight of their poverty, customs, and superstition. Vulnerability to disease was thus also and increasingly seen to be a moral and cultural problem as much as an environmental one, and moral and cultural advantage was more and more seen to favor Europeans over Indians. Mackinnon summed up prevailing medical attitudes in the 1840s when he wrote that disease depended only partly upon "general climate, the range of the thermometer, its sudden alteration, the prevailing winds, the fall of rain, the level of the lands, the quality of soil, etc."; it was also dependent on "local causes, and on the social condition, habits, and morals, of the population."[66] From explaining ill health and disease almost exclusively in terms of India's physical environment, medical writers by mid-century were moving toward explanations which gave greater prominence to the peculiar characteristics of Indian society, morality, and culture. India's pathogenic environment had been stretched to include social and cultural idiosyncrasies as well as climatic and topographical phenomena, though the distinction between the two was often blurred.

As a sense of extreme European vulnerability began to fade, Indians were increasingly held responsible for their own ill health and mortality. Their physical weakness and vegetarian diets, their ignorance and indolence, their crowded homes and insanitary cities, their religious practices and social institutions from child marriage to the caste system ("an enormous injury to public health," J. R. Martin averred, because "prejudicial to public happiness"),[67] were all cited singly or cumulatively as evidence that Indians were the authors of their own misery. In his topographical account of Saran district in Bihar, published in 1839, Robert Rankine identified a number of causes for disease, many of which demonstrated the growing propensity to blame Indians for their own ill health. The towns he found wanting in proper ventilation (stagnant air being associated with a concentration of miasma) and held that it would be the "greatest improvement that could be made" to widen the streets and let in more air. This, he believed, "would tend greatly to promote the general health of the inhabitants, renew and purify the confined atmosphere . . . and check the generation of those myriads of insects, which constantly annoy the inhabitants."[68] In rural Champaran (then part of Saran district) he attributed the extreme poverty and unhealthiness of the laboring classes to the exploitation of their zamindars, or landlords, to the nature of the caste system, and the laborers' fondness for drink, as well as to the miasma generated by marshes, wastelands, and jungles.

> When we reflect [he wrote] on the poor diet in common use amongst the great mass of the natives of Chumparun, their wretched clothing, habit of reposing on the ground in their damp abodes, with scarcely a mat under them, we can be at no loss to account for their predisposition to disease of every kind.[69]

If social conditions, the habits and morals of the people, came more and more to bear the burden of responsibility for disease, it was easier for Europeans to believe that they need not wilt in Indian soil, but could rather, by observing certain basic precautions, survive and prosper. Disease was not predicated on climate alone (and even when it was, its effects could be partly mitigated). It also reflected cultural and social practices, moral as well as physical well-being. Medicine thus began to provide arguments for European superiority even in an environment which had but recently appeared most inimical to European health and to show that European medicine had the authority to speak for Indian as well as European constitutions.

ENCOUNTERS WITH INDIAN MEDICINE

In freeing itself from its specifically European origins and coming to terms with its "tropical," "Asiatic," or "Oriental" context, Western medicine in India was forced to interact not only with the diseases of the region but also with its medical ideas and practices. Early attitudes were tentative and, as often as not, appreciative. This was partly because in their understanding of disease, as in their therapeutic practices, Indian and European medicine had much in common. As newcomers to India, the British felt they might usefully learn much that was of value to them that had been accumulated through centuries of "empirical" trial and observation.

To some extent Western physicians were engaged in a typically Orientalist exercise. With the rapid growth of British territorial power in South Asia and the rise of Orientalist scholarship in the late eighteenth century, Company physicians looked both to texts and to "native informants" to provide them with insights into the nature of Indian, especially Hindu, medicine. Part of the stimulus for this investigation came directly from the East India Company and its Court of Directors in London. In a dispatch dated June 3, 1814, the court expressed its interest in encouraging Orientalist learning and instruction in India. It understood (on the basis of reports already received from India) that there existed in Sanskrit "many tracts of merit . . . on the virtues of plants and drugs, and on the applications of them in medicine, the knowledge of which might prove desirable to the European practitioner."[70]

The practical utility of discovering Indian drugs and incorporating them into the Western system of medicine was thus the primary official motivation behind the investigation of Indian medical texts, but it would be a mistake to imagine that material advantage was the only incentive. The growing tendency (mainly, but not exclusively, within the medical profession itself) to see medicine as a demonstration of the superiority of the civilization of the West over that of the East also had a powerful effect on the way Indian medicine was perceived and its relationship with Western medicine was understood. Medicine was one of the fields of inquiry through which Orientalist scholarship sought to represent and capture the essence of Indian (especially Hindu) civilization, just as through their topographical exercises medical writers sought to define the nature of India's physical environment.

In fact, the early Orientalists, despite the prominence among them of Company surgeons such as John B. Gilchrist, William Hunter, and John Leyden, did not give much time to reading and translating Indian medical texts. Sir William Jones, the leading British Orientalist of the late eighteenth century and the founder of the Asiatic Society in 1784, was trained in law, not in medicine, and showed no more than a passing interest in the subject. On one occasion he remarked that what was contained in the "old books" of the Hindus relating to medicine and disease, "we ought certainly to discover." The aphorisms culled from Ayurvedic medical works by the seventeenth-century French traveler François Bernier appeared to him to be "judicious and rational." But in general he took a somewhat skeptical view of the benefits to be derived from such a laborious inquiry. He frankly doubted that there existed in any of the languages of Asia a single "original treatise on medicine considered as a science," and, apart from "a mere empirical history of diseases and remedies," thought it unlikely that the East had much to contribute to Europe's existing store of medical knowledge.[71]

It was not until a generation after Jones, between about 1810 and 1830, that Benjamin Heyne and Whitelaw Ainslie in Madras and H. H. Wilson in Bengal began the scholar-surgeons' investigations of Ayurveda. Their work was followed up by J. F. Royle's *Antiquity of Hindu Medicine* in 1838 and by T. A. Wise's *Commentary on the Hindu System of Medicine* in 1845. A critical attitude toward Hindu medicine was evident in all of these works. Ainslie, although greatly impressed by the range and practical value of India's materia medica and by the skills of the physicians he encountered in Madras, found two grounds for reproaching Hindu medicine. From the standpoint of rationality and secularism common to Company surgeons at the time, Ainslie deplored the way in which medicine had become mixed up with religion, so that Ayurveda was revered as the gift of the gods, "a circumstance which has been an insurmountable obstacle to improvement" and a reason why medicine in India was "still sunk in such a state of empirical darkness." He equally regretted that the ancient practice of dissection, clearly referred to in early Ayurvedic texts, had been abandoned and forgotten, for without the study of human anatomy the physician was inevitably left in profound ignorance of the body's internal functions and disorders.[72]

The readiness shown by Ainslie to contrast the early achievements of Hindu science and civilization with its later degeneracy was even more pronounced in Wise's *Commentary*. He praised the "advanced state of power and learning" in ancient India and acknowledged Ayurveda as a scientific system of medicine in its own right. But he contrasted its initial accomplishments with the complacency of later Hindu physicians, who were "satisfied with the knowledge and power...acquired at a very early period." The decline of Hindu medicine was further precipitated, in his view, by the invasions of the Muslims and their hostility to Hindu medicine. With Ayurveda in decline, the people of India fell back on "superstition and quackery." "The native practice of medicine may now be said to be in this lamentable state of depression over all Hindustan," Wise wrote in a typically Orientalist comparison between past glories and current squalor, "but it was far otherwise, as cultivated by the ancient Hindus."[73] He recognized much common ground between the humoral pathology of ancient India and that until recently followed in Europe—much as Buchanan and others acknowledged in Hippocrates and Galen a shared origin for the Yunani and European systems of medicine. But while Western medicine had made enormous advances, Ayurveda and Yunani had, Wise believed, stood still or declined. Western medicine represented progress; the medicine of the Hindus and Muslims stood for an inert, tradition-bound India. Wise declared his aim to be to resuscitate the worthwhile elements of Ayurveda (mainly its diagnostics and prescriptions) but also to overturn "that blind reverence which an imperfect knowledge of the Medical Shastras is so liable to engender among the Native physicians, and which has operated most perniciously in retarding the advancement of knowledge."[74]

Early nineteenth-century European physicians also looked to their Indian counterparts for practical guidance in the identification, classification, and treatment of diseases, especially diseases unfamiliar to the West or resistant to their own drugs and therapies. Just as climate and environment imposed certain "modifications" upon Western medicine in India, so too did the influence of Indian medical practice and knowledge. In this way the "tropical" or "colonial" medicine that emerged in the first half of the nineteenth century was not an exclusively Western product, simply shipped out from London and Leyden, Edinburgh and Paris, and propagated unchanged in Calcutta, Madras, and Bombay. It also bore some traces of its interaction with the cultural as well as material environment into which it was introduced. It was increasingly clear, however, that this was not to be a free and open exchange between equals, but largely a case of Europe taking from India whatever appeared useful to its own understanding and practice and discarding the rest as worthless or irrelevant junk.

The most conspicuous aspect of this colonizing epistomology was the investigation and partial incorporation of India's rich materia medica. This was not an entirely new process. For centuries the Portuguese, the Dutch, and other Europeans had noted the value of certain drugs employed in India but unfamiliar to Europe. The use of indigenous drugs was encouraged by the expense and difficulty of obtaining "Europe" medicines in the East Indies and by a belief that a country which produced the diseases ought also, by the harmonizing laws of nature, to produce its own antidotes and cures. But the quest for useful drugs (which paralleled the description and classification of other "useful plants"[75]) was undertaken far more systematically in the early nineteenth century than ever before. Ainslie's *Materia Indica* of 1826 (which had appeared in an earlier form in 1813) was one of the first attempts to establish "a kind of combining link betwixt the materia medica of Europe and that of Asia."[76] His effort was sustained through articles in learned journals like the *Transactions* of the Calcutta Medical and Physical Society, by translations and compilations of Ayurvedic and Yunani works like George Playfair's *Taleef Shereef*, and by W. B. O'Shaughnessy's *Bengal Pharmacopoeia* of 1844, which aimed to provide a guide to locally available substitutes for such drugs as belladonna, cinchona, and strychnine and to facilitate the search for new remedies in India.[77]

The investigation of Indian medicine advanced along two different, sometimes complementary, sometimes opposing, routes: through the translation and critical examination of texts and through the observation and interrogation of the *vaidya*s and other practitioners. George Playfair's "translation" of the *Taleef Shereef, or Indian Materia Medica*, published in 1833 by the Calcutta Medical and Physical Society, is a strangely hybrid work, indicative of the unresolved tension then existing between Western physicians and Indian medical texts. In introducing his book to a European audience, Playfair explained that in twenty-six years as a doctor in India he had often regretted not having a published guide that would allow him "to become acquainted with the properties of native medicines." As used by Indian practitioners, they were frequently "productive of the most beneficial effects in many diseases, for the cure of which our pharmacopoeia supplied no adequate remedy." He hoped that the publication of the *Taleef Shereef* in English would encourage other European doctors to take due note of "native medicines" and their uses.[78] But the manner of the book's presentation is as bizarre as many of its entries. It is said to be "translated from the original, with additions," but nowhere is the nature of the original text discussed or the name of its author given. Playfair moves in and out of his text like a slippery eel. Sometimes "I" represents the unnamed author; at other times it heralds Playfair's own editorial interventions. Thus, on a purgative called "Aak" (identified by Playfair as *Asclepias gigantea*) he comments, "Many and wonderful virtues are ascribed to this plant; but I must refer those who have faith in charms to the original *Taleef Shereef*, where their curiosity will be amply gratified." Playfair then gives his own assessment of its properties: "useful in swellings, promotes suppuration in indolent tumors, and cures eruptions of the skin." "W.T." (presumably the initials of William Twining), who supervised publication for the Calcutta Medical and Physical Society, was apparently even more censorious, explaining in tiny print at the end of the book that "a few articles contained in the original work, viz. medicines principally used in sorcery and incantation, have been omitted with the translator's permission."[79]

The *Taleef Shereef* is permeated with the humoral pathology of Yunani medicine, but (partly because the same tradition still lingered on in European medical thought) Playfair does little to qualify or contradict it. Nor does he entirely disguise or reprove the very different preoccupations of the original author from those that were coming to govern Western medicine in India—later works of materia medica had no room for the elixirs and aphrodisiacs to be found here. Pleasure, like superstition, was soon to be exiled from colonialism's physic garden. The properties of "Arvie," the original author is permitted to explain, "are in a small degree cool; and it is useful in giving strength to the system; prevents the involuntary emission of semen; it produces wind, and is heavy and hurtful to the throat." Likewise, "Baraykund" is "sweet, bitter, pungent, and increases the powers of manhood, and generally strengthens the system; it increases bile, but removes a superabundance of phlegm or wind." It, too, is "useful in seminal weakness."[80]

The reluctance (even in Playfair's "translation") to allow an Indian text to speak for itself was not uncommon. But more frequently, textual investigations were reported in the form of a critical commentary

or summary of the "useful" parts that could be extracted from otherwise unhelpful or obscure Yunani or Ayurvedic works. H. H. Wilson,
who arrived in India in 1808 as a Company surgeon but soon became
the leading Sanskritist of his generation, was one of the first to write
about Indian medicine on the basis of a close acquaintance with
Ayurvedic texts. In 1823 he published an article on "The Medical and
Surgical Science of the Hindus" and apparently intended to write a
comprehensive account, which he never completed, of the subject.[81]
But he did publish articles in the *Transactions* of the Calcutta Medical
and Physical Society on leprosy and cholera as they appeared in
Ayurvedic literature. In the second of these, "On the Native Practice
in Cholera," Wilson relied on information from Bengali informants,
notably his protégé, Ramcomul Sen, a Vaidya by caste and one of the
patrons of the Native Medical Institution in Calcutta.[82] But in the
earlier essay on "Kushta, or Leprosy, as Known to the Hindus," his
sources were the Sanskrit texts of Caraka and Susruta. Wilson began
by remarking that "upon first exploring a spot, with which we are but
imperfectly acquainted, it is the most obvious course of proceeding to
direct our path by the information of native guides." With a disease
like leprosy, about which a great deal of uncertainty persisted in
Europe, Indian sources might give guidance based on "long experience and accumulated observation." But Wilson also made it clear
that he was proceeding from the superior vantage point of Western
medicine, trusting to the "sufficient security" of Europe's "advanced
. . . medical knowledge" to ensure that any "errors" in the Hindu
texts would not lead him too far "astray."

On first looking into the works of Caraka and Susruta, Wilson
professed great disappointment. The causes attributed to leprosy he
found "very miscellaneous and unmeaning," though patient scrutiny
revealed some of them to be "less wild and unmethodical" than they
at first appeared. He was willing to entertain the possibility that leprosy was a contagious or hereditary disease but quickly dismissed the
suggestion that it was a divine punishment for human sins. He found
Ayurvedic texts even less helpful when it came to the treatment of
the disease. "It is in this part of their system that the Hindu writers
are essentially deficient," he wrote. The idea of "augmenting efficacy
by multiplying ingredients disfigures their work with a prodigious
number of the most preposterous and ridiculous compounds." But
while he thought it essential to be aware of the many and consider-

able "defects" of Hindu medicine, Wilson still believed it worthwhile
for Western medical science to investigate the various ingredients
prescribed in the hope of finding "some substances of real utility"
amidst such apparent "chaos." If even one of the substances tested
"should furnish even but a palliative of the disease," he concluded,
"the result of the inquiry will be its own sufficient reward."[83]

BEYOND TEXTS

Indian medical texts were often hard for Europeans to obtain and difficult, even with the requisite linguistic skills, to render into intelligible English. Much was simply discarded as "worthless" or as impos-
sibly corrupted by later interpolation.[84] Benjamin Heyne attempted a
literal translation of a medical compendium known as *Kalpastanum*
but "after many trials" gave up the task as "beyond my power." He
next tried to "make an extract" from it, but "the aphoretical style of
the author" made this equally difficult. It was impossible, he claimed,
to make direct translations of Oriental works because they were written in a "poetical style," abounded in "similes, metaphors, and all
kinds of figures," and were "replete with allusions to . . . customs,
propensities, and religious ceremonies, unintelligible to an European." In the end Heyne simply decided to omit such passages as
appeared to him "useless to an European reader." He then embarked
on a second text but again abandoned his attempt to translate it when
this "extraordinary treatise" turned out to be "a banquet of absurdity
sufficient to satisfy the most voracious guests."[85]

Frustration with the nature and content of Ayurvedic and Yunani
texts and the inability to render them into a form suitable for use by
Western medicine was one reason for turning away from literary
sources to living informants. Even the reading of texts was seldom
performed unaided. Wise was helped in compiling his *Commentary*
on Hindu medicine by Abhaycharan Tarkapanchanan, superintendent of the Bengali Department at Muhammad Mohsin's Hughli College at Chinsurah, and by Madhusudan Gupta, formerly a teacher at
the Native Medical Institution in Calcutta and later a lecturer in Anatomy at the city's new Medical College. Gupta was valuable to Wise
as a man with a foot in both medical camps, a pandit "whose accurate
knowledge of the medical shastras" was combined with "an extensive
knowledge of the sciences of Europe."[86]

But Europeans also turned away from texts because they considered them unreliable as guides to contemporary medical practice. Heyne sweepingly dismissed the majority of medical practitioners in India as "illiterate pretenders to knowledge," most of whom were "quacks, possessors and vendors of nostrums."[87] Buchanan, too, identified many up-country practitioners as low caste, illiterate, and "destitute of science."[88] There seemed little point, then, in looking into Sanskrit or Persian works to find a guide or explanation for their practices. But the shift away from texts was also indicative of a growing disparagement of Indian medicine, a tendency to see it as a form of folk practice, founded on superstition and "empiricism" rather than professional training and a literate tradition. In part, this was the extension to India of the attack on folk medicine already under way in Europe and the jealous defense of medicine as the monopoly of qualified professionals.

But, in the early decades of the century at least, there was some willingness to learn from direct observation, from conversations with *hakims*, *kavirajas*, and other "native informants" knowledgeable about Indian drugs and medical practices. William Twining, who made a special study of the malaria-related "spleen diseases" of Bengal, noted the various drugs and therapies employed by local doctors in treating this condition. He claimed to have tried "with benefit" some of the medicines they prescribed and thought them especially suitable for use on Indians, whether because they preferred their own medicines and shunned European therapies or because their constitutions called for different remedies from Europeans'. Following local practice, he experimented with the use of long iron needles to puncture swollen spleens. He thought this unlikely to have much beneficial effect, but remarked that:

> The natives of this country generally use remedies in disease, from practical knowledge of their efficacy, without much reasoning; therefore I would not reject any of their therapeutical expedients as despicable, without an enquiry into their modus operandi, and an experimental investigation of their utility.[89]

Twining also turned to local physicians for advice or for confirmation that the therapies he employed to treat fevers or dysentery were likely to be effective. Through "frequent communication on this subject with hakeems or native physicians," he ascertained that they followed broadly similar therapies with regard to dysentery, and he wrote with approval of their use of "coee munda" (a gruel made from parched rice boiled in water) as a restorative for patients recovering from bowel diseases.[90]

Twining was writing in the 1820s and 1830s when many Western doctors were still interested in learning what they could from Indian physicians. They were broadly sympathetic toward the modes of diagnosis and treatment used by the *hakim*s and *kaviraja*s, partly because they had much in common with their own, even if they remained critical of their religious outlook and their woeful neglect of surgery and anatomy. But by the 1850s and 1860s attitudes, never universally enthusiastic, had hardened. As Western medicine grew in confidence and political authority, as it freed itself from the humoral pathology which had earlier kept it in touch with the principles of Ayurvedic and Yunani medicine, and as it began to take upon itself responsibility for Indian as well as European health and thus to see indigenous medicine more clearly as its rival, it also exhibited a growing tendency to dismiss indigenous medicine and its practitioners, almost without qualification. Whereas the Calcutta Medical and Physical Society in 1825 was prepared to consider Indian medicine an "imperfect science" but one still worthy of investigation, increasingly it was scorned as no science at all, but rather a fraud and a danger to those among whom it was practiced. Martin in 1837 rebuked Indian physicians for what he called their "shameless impostures."[91] Morehead a few years later saw it as one of the foremost objectives of the new Grant Medical College in Bombay to counter the "demoralizing effects of the irrational, superstitious, and, too often, criminal empiricism" of Indian practitioners. Their practice, he declared, was "wholly unscientific." It was devoid of even a knowledge of their own *sastra*s and consisted mainly of "charms, amulets, and incantations."[92] In 1867 the *Indian Medical Gazette* referred to the "stargazing, divining native *baed*s [*vaidya*s] or *hakeem*s . . . with their nostrums and Grecian [i.e., Hippocratic] lore." It published, with apparent approval, an extract from a newspaper article which called on the government to suppress the "evils" of indigenous medicine much as it had earlier suppressed the notorious crime of *thagi*:

> The two evils which we have pointed out, *viz.*, the unlicensed practice of Native Hakeems, and the unrestricted sale of poisonous drugs, are fraught with the direst consequences. Life is daily jeopardized, and the door to crime and knavery thrown

wide open . . . we urge upon Government the necessity of taking action in the matter, and of putting an end to this barbarous state of things by legislative enactment.[93]

There were exceptions to this condemnatory trend, such as the attempts in the Punjab and North-Western provinces to train *hakims* and their sons in the basic skills of Western medicine[94] or the continuing interest in certain Indian drugs and therapies.[95] But, in the main, indigenous medicine and its practitioners were being deliberately pushed aside and denied authority over even the Indian body. Far from being a source of comfort and healing to the sick, Indian medicine was represented as confused, dangerous, and anachronistic, even, like *thagi*, a barbarous crime against the individuals on whom it was practiced.

There was one other way in which indigenous texts and "native" testimony could be bypassed, and that was by direct observation and physical examination of the body. Western medicine in early nineteenth-century India attached great importance to clinical observations, and a prominent element in these was the use of postmortems. It was a practice that characterized the much-boasted rationality and clinical objectivity of Western medicine, just as its neglect among Indian physicians was held to be a primary reason for their medical ignorance. The clinical "observations" and "illustrations" of Annesley, Morehead, Parkes, and other writers of the period derived their claims to scientific objectivity and authority largely from their studies of morbid anatomy and their attempts to relate the state of diseased internal organs examined after death to the symptoms manifested externally during life. If Indians of almost every caste and class vehemently opposed postmortems (which, to be fair, were also less than popular in the Britain of Burke and Hare) and viewed the practice as representative of the vile nature of Western medicine, then European physicians saw their opposition as a demonstration of Indian superstition and an obstacle to the advancement of medical science in India.[96]

Another illustration of the importance attached to a direct and physical interrogation of the body arose from investigations into malaria in northern India in the 1840s. T. E. Dempster was a member of a committee appointed to examine the possible connection between canal irrigation and the incidence of malaria. In order to establish this relationship in statistical terms and to assess whether the expansion of irrigation works had led to an increase in malaria, Dempster tried at first to gather information orally from the local population. This proved largely unsuccessful: villagers were suspicious of his motives or could not accurately recall previous epidemics and attacks of fever. Despairing of oral testimony, Dempster made use instead of the by then well-known connection between fever and enlarged spleens to devise a "spleen test" for malaria. This was done by examining villagers individually, feeling for a swollen spleen, and recording the resulting distribution of abnormal spleens over an extended territory as an index of the range and intensity of malaria itself. In 1843–44 some twelve thousand individuals were tested in this way. As Dempster himself put it, the inhabitants of malarious tracts carried "in their own persons a record of past suffering, which can at all times be easily read, and which no one can either falsify or suppress."[97] "Reading" the body in this direct manner, a practice which had its parallels in many other colonial medical practices discussed in later chapters, thus came to displace the reading of texts or the eliciting of information from "native informants."

ORIENTALISM AND ANGLICISM

The dual nature of Western approaches to Indian medicine in the early part of the nineteenth century—the utilitarian and the hegemonic—was further exemplified by attitudes toward medical education for Indians. One impetus behind official involvement with Indian medicine was the need to recruit and train "native doctors" for the subordinate medical service in India. They were required as trained medical assistants (compounders, apothecaries, dressers, and so forth) to help European doctors and surgeons with their routine work and to save the Company the expense of employing more Europeans. By the early nineteenth century, it was no longer considered safe to entrust the lives of Company servants to indigenous practitioners who had no acquaintance with Western medicine.[98]

In response to a proposal from the provincial Medical Board in May 1822, the Government of Bengal authorized the training of up to twenty Indian medical recruits for the army or civilian government service. One outcome of this decision was the creation of a Native Medical Institution in Calcutta to provide them with medical instruction. Teaching was conducted in the vernaculars, and a number of medical texts (including a version of Twining's work on the diseases of Bengal) were translated for the purpose. Around 1827 classes were also started in Yunani medicine at the Calcutta Madrasa and in Ayurveda at the Sanskrit College, where the texts used included the works of Caraka and Susruta.[99]

This official "patronage" for India's medical systems and its subsequent withdrawal in 1835 have been the subject of some misinterpretation. It has been assumed that in 1835 a sympathetic "Orientalist" policy of supporting and encouraging indigenous medicine was abruptly overturned and replaced by an intolerant "Anglicist" one, that this change had disastrous consequences for the indigenous medical systems and brought to an end an era of "peaceful coexistence."[100] In fact, official policy seems all along to have been directed toward the ultimate triumph of European medicine. The intention was not to promote indigenous medicine as an equal or alternative to the Western system but (as with Indian materia medica) to draw upon what was "useful" from indigenous therapeutics while encouraging students (by teaching the Western and Indian systems side by side) to discover for themselves the superiority of European medicine. Instruction in Ayurvedic and Yunani medicine might also have been a tactical concession to the many students who came from the Vaidya caste, traditionally a caste of Hindu physicians, and possibly from other Hindu and Muslim families with roots in the Indian systems.[101] Teaching one system of medicine alongside the other was thus a way not so much of "engrafting" Western scientific knowledge onto Indian classical culture as of preparing for the gradual displacement of the latter by the former. Dr. John Tytler, the Superintendent of the Native Medical Institution and a leading figure in the Orientalist camp, explained this strategy in April 1834:

> European science like the Christian religion has by far the best chance of succeeding among the nations of Hindoostan by our avoiding even the appearance of coercion and allowing and even encouraging them to study their own system and ours together and quietly make the comparison themselves. We thus prove that we have no jealousy of their knowledge, we incline all their national feeling in our favour and give their understanding full room to act. . . .
> Coercion always produces the direct contrary effect to what is intended. The outward profession of a belief in any system of science like that of a belief in religion is of no value unless

attended with an inward conviction. Almost nothing is gained
by getting a student to repeat in College our systems of science
unless he can be convinced of their truth and brought to act in
the world according to their principles.[102]

The question at issue was not, therefore, whether the medical systems of East and West were equally valid—a claim that even the
most fervent Orientalist was likely to eschew—but rather the means
by which Western medicine could most successfully be propagated in
India, while also, more practically, supplying the state with the
trained medical personnel it required. By the 1830s, however, the Native Medical Institution had become a target for a growing European
reaction against state support for Indian learning and in favor of a far
more overt (and in Tytler's sense, "coercive") strategy of teaching
Western science solely through the medium of English language and
texts. In October 1833 the governor-general, Lord Bentinck, appointed a committee for the purpose of "improving the constitution
and extending the benefits of the Native Medical Institution, and
digesting a system of management and education calculated to give
effect in both of these respects to the wishes of Government." There
followed a heated and wide-ranging debate about the relative merits
of English and vernacular instruction and the best means of preserving links between Britain and India. In its report in October 1834, the
committee found that the Native Medical Institution was poorly organized, student attendance was lax, and the teaching was deficient,
especially in failing to provide practical instruction in human anatomy. It advised the abolition of the institution, along with the medical classes at the Madrasa and Sanskrit college, and the establishment
of a new college to teach Western medicine exclusively, with English
as the sole medium of instruction. Bentinck approved these recommendations in January 1835, and Calcutta's Medical College came
into existence shortly afterward.[103]

Although the degree of divergence between the Anglicists and
Orientalists has been exaggerated, at least as far as the teaching of
medicine was concerned, the demise of the Native Medical Institution
and the classes in Ayurvedic and Yunani medicine was an important
symbolic shift. Official support for indigenous medicine had hardly
been wholehearted before 1835, though there continued to be an interest in the practical uses of India's materia medica, but a clear and
public declaration had now been made of the superiority of Western

medicine and of official disdain for the indigenous medical systems. Any impression that Western medicine might be considered suitable for Europeans alone, or might happily coexist alongside other medical ideas and practices, had now been dispelled, even though, in theory, a decision had been made only with regard to the narrow realm of higher education and training for government service.

Even more than previously, Western medicine after 1835 was taken as the hallmark of a higher civilization, as a sign of the moral purpose and legitimacy of colonial rule in India, just as indigenous medical ideas and practices could be casually equated with ignorance and barbarism. It was in this latter vein that T. B. Macaulay, in the course of his celebrated "Minute on Education," unleashed his Anglicist diatribe against Indian civilization and learning. For him it was axiomatic that the "dialects" commonly spoken in India bore "neither literary nor scientific information" and contained "no books on any subject which deserve to be compared to our own." The British government in India could hardly countenance, at public expense,

> medical doctrines which would disgrace an English farrier, astronomy which would move laughter in girls at an English boarding school, history abounding with kings thirty feet high and reigns thirty thousand years long, and geography, made up of seas of treacle and seas of butter.

By contrast, one of the many virtues Macaulay saw in the English language was that it abounded

> with just and lively representations of human life and nature; with the most profound speculations on metaphysics, morals, government, jurisprudence, and trade; with full and correct information respecting every experimental science which tends to preserve the health, to increase the comfort, or to expand the intellect of man.[104]

J. R. Martin, writing in somewhat more temperate tones shortly after the establishment of the Calcutta Medical College, compared it to Bentinck's other, much-lauded act: the abolition of *sati* (the immolation of a Hindu widow on her husband's funeral pyre) in 1829. Indeed, he considered that in the long term it would prove

> of far greater importance, in as much as the diffusion of European medical science, with its collateral branches, must prove one of the most direct and impressive modes of demonstrating

to the natives, the superiority of European knowledge in general, and that they must cultivate it actively if they would rise in the scale of nations.[105]

A few years later, Charles Morehead, whose hostility to Indian medicine and its practitioners has already been noted, told the first generation of graduates from Grant Medical College in Bombay that they were "the first approved and accredited agents in a great work of national amelioration." They were "to go forth armed with great powers of conferring inestimable benefits on others, not only in mitigating their physical suffering and soothing their mental anxieties, but also in enlightening and elevating their minds." If they failed in this "great mission," he said, they had only themselves to blame.[106] Medicine was thus seen to be more than liberation from disease. It was also viewed as a means by which Indian society might be liberated from its ignorance and superstition.

One incident more than any other symbolized the evangelizing zeal of Western medicine in India by the 1830s and 1840s. On January 10, 1836, Pandit Madhusudan Gupta, himself of the Vaidya caste and a former teacher of medicine at the Sanskrit College, became the first Indian in modern times to perform a human dissection. At the Native Medical Institution, dissections had never, for reasons of religion and caste, been performed on human corpses, only on sheep and other animals. Since one of the principal indictments of Indian medicine was its ignorance of anatomy, the dissection epitomized the growing ascendancy of Western medicine over its Indian rivals. "This day," declared one exuberant commentator, "will ever be marked in the annals of Western medicine in India" as the moment when "Indians rose superior to the prejudices of their earlier education and thus boldly flung open the gates of modern medical science to their countrymen."[107]

CONCLUSION

During the early years of colonial rule in India there emerged a system of colonial medicine which was more than a simple replication of Western medicine in Britain at the time. The great significance attached to environmental factors—climate, topography, vegetation —in the causation and transmission of disease, together with the supposed effects of heat and humidity on European constitutions, meant that the practitioners of Western medicine saw an imperative need to adapt and modify their practice to physical circumstances that were very different from those found in Europe. Once established, this environmentalist paradigm remained the dominant one in epidemiological thought in India almost throughout the nineteenth century, even after it had been effectively deposed in Europe by the germ theory of disease. Moreover, environmentalism evolved and expanded during the first half of the century to include a variety of social and cultural characteristics, which were also thought to contribute to the idiosyncratic nature of disease in India. Thus, the environmentalist paradigm was also an Orientalist one (in the sense in which the term *Orientalism* has been employed by Said and others), embodying and projecting Western ideas of how India was intrinsically different from the West, even in the nature of its diseases and the therapeutics appropriate for their treatment and cure. As chapters 3 to 5 show, in the more detailed discussions of smallpox, cholera, and plague, as Western medicine developed into a system of public health from the 1860s onward, so the environmentalist and Orientalist perceptions of the early nineteenth-century medical writers informed state policy on a grand scale and became intimately bound up with the perceived limits and practicalities of Western medicine in India.

The development of colonial medicine in nineteenth-century India was also informed by interaction with indigenous medical systems. The extent of this hybridization was, to be sure, limited, constrained by metropolitan ties and by a strong and growing sense of the innate superiority of Western medical ideas and techniques. Indigenous drugs attracted more lasting interest than native therapies, but even the appropriation of India's materia medica was a plundering of parts, not a wholesale incorporation. Appropriation, subordination, and denigration were the processes by which Western medicine marked its conquest over indigenous medicine.

From the position of an outsider, concerned mainly with the health of white "exotics," Western medicine rapidly assumed a position of clear authority over Indian medicine and Indian bodies. Its attitude was monopolistic, not pluralistic, and by the 1860s the medical profession was calling for the regulation, even the outlawing, of its Indian rivals. However, although it had begun to speak with an authoritative voice, Western medicine was clearly constrained from exercising as much actual power as its expansive rhetoric seemed to demand. It still had little access to Indians and to Indian society outside the confines of a few narrow arenas: jails, barracks, hospitals, and dispensaries. It was frustrated by the elusiveness of the Indian body, by the limits of its own therapeutic capabilities, and by its still-restricted acquaintance with the prevalent diseases of India. It remained essentially state medicine, and if that meant on the one hand that it was invested with a great deal of official authority, it meant on the other that it was also tied to the financial and political constraints of a colonial regime.

2 Colonial Enclaves: The Army and the Jails

Chapter 1 looked at the ways in which Western medicine began to see itself in relation to India's physical and cultural environment and to indigenous society and medical practices. It is now appropriate to turn to two specific colonial arenas, the army and the jails, which exemplified many of these wider ideas but where Western medicine came to occupy a position of particular authority. At a time when the state acknowledged few obligations for the health of the population as a whole, it accepted a special responsibility for the health of the soldiers and prisoners under its control. It was largely within the confines of these privileged sites of observation and experimentation that Western medicine developed its wider understanding of disease in India and the obligations of state medicine in a colonial setting.

But even here, within these favored sites and seemingly secure enclaves, Western medicine did not enjoy an automatic authority. The state did not always welcome the advice and initiatives of its medical officers, and within the barracks and the jails many factors combined to thwart and subvert the "colonizing" ambitions of their medical staff. Nor did developments within the army and the prisons necessarily provide appropriate or acceptable precedents for the extension and elaboration of state medicine into a viable system of public health. To what extent, then, were the barracks and jails medical and sanitary enclaves? How far were they models for the wider colonization of Indian society by Western medicine?

MILITARY MEDICINE

The association between the military and medicine was an intimate one in India—as it was in many other parts of the colonial world. The

61

foremost responsibility of the Indian Medical Service, the origins of which date back to the expansionist decades of the mid eighteenth century, was to provide medical assistance for the armies of the English East India Company. With the abolition of the Company and the takeover of its military forces by the British government following the Mutiny and Rebellion of 1857–58, the IMS was entrusted with the health of the Indian Army. Soldiers of the British Army stationed in India were placed in the charge of the Army Medical Department (from 1898 the Royal Army Medical Corps), which had about four hundred officers in India by the end of the nineteenth century. From less than a hundred doctors and surgeons in the 1780s, the Indian Medical Service had grown by the early 1900s to a corps of six hundred men. They were employed in a wide range of civilian as well as military duties: they ran civil hospitals, mental asylums, and prisons; they supervised dispensaries, staffed medical schools and research institutes, directed the sanitary services, and acted as advisers to the provincial and central governments. They also (except in special cases like the prison service) enjoyed a right to private practice which might significantly augment their official salaries.[1]

Although responsibility for the health of the Indian Army was still described in 1910 as the "first and only indispensable duty" of the IMS, roughly three-fifths of its current strength was deployed in non-military duties. In wartime, however, the military responsibilities of the IMS took precedent over civilian duties, and a large number of officers reverted to service with the Indian Army.[2] The military status of the IMS was further kept alive, if only symbolically, by officers' holding joint army and medical rank. Attempts to divide the IMS into two completely separate civilian and military branches were unsuccessful before World War I, showing how extensively medicine remained the prerogative of the state even in an era of incipient public health. But it was not just that the institutional connections between the military and state medicine were close and enduring. For most of the nineteenth century, the outlook and activities of the medical profession were closely tied to military needs—an association strengthened by the slow development of an independent medical profession in colonial India and hence its comparative inability to act as a critic of state medicine and an alternative source of professional employment, skills, and ideology.

The practical and political consequences of this intimate connection between medicine and the military were enormous and have barely begun to be recognized by India's medical historians, except to some degree by Radhika Ramasubban. She has argued in general terms, rather than through detailed investigation, that the military basis and orientation of Western medicine in colonial India was a primary characteristic of India's "colonial mode of health care," indicative of how the resources of the colonial state were directed almost exclusively to meeting the health needs of the army and the European community while neglecting the great majority of the Indian population. The considerable advances made in public health in nineteenth-century Britain were thus denied to the people of India. Western medicine in India assumed an "enclavist" or "segregated" character. Only after 1918 (and perhaps not until after India's independence in 1947) were significant efforts made to break out of this enclavism and carry Western medicine to the masses.[3]

There is much evidence to support Ramasubban's general line of argument, but it cannot be accepted without some substantial qualifications. Quite apart from the question of how far colonial medicine did reach beyond the confines of the army and European community by 1914, an issue to which we will return in subsequent chapters, there are a number of presumptions about the nature of the relationship between the army and medicine which need to be investigated. First, it would be a mistake to regard the army in India as a single homogeneous constituency. There were enormous differences within the military itself, particularly between the health and medical status of European and Indian soldiers, though these differences had been partly eroded by 1914. Second, the relationship between medicine and the army, though close, was problematic. It was only gradually and with some difficulty that medical and sanitary officers began to command the kind of authority over the army to which many of them believed themselves entitled. The medical profession had a long, hard struggle to demonstrate to the military authorities its competence as a therapeutic and prophylactic agency. Third, it is a matter for investigation whether the medical and sanitary improvements effected in the military cantonments by 1914 were—or were seen to be—relevant to the health needs of the wider civilian population.[4]

But before examining these issues further, we need to consider briefly the size and nature of medicine's military constituency. The army in colonial India was by no means insignificant in either numerical or political terms. There were approximately a quarter of a million soldiers in British India by the 1830s. Of these, approximately forty thousand were Europeans, a third serving directly under the Company. The rest were in regiments of the British Army, first stationed in India in the 1750s to assist Company troops and support imperial interests. Even before the Mutiny of 1857–58 cast doubt upon the reliability of the Company's Indian troops (or "sepoys"), it was often stated that the "ground-work" of British power in India was the presence there of a "substantial body of British soldiers."[5] The scale of the 1857 uprising and the urgent threat it posed to British lives and administrative control further enhanced the perceived need for a strong European military presence. In 1858–59, the Company's European regiments were disbanded, but a force of between 55,000 and 70,000 soldiers of the British Army remained in the country for the rest of the century. This was the largest European force stationed anywhere in the tropical world, and it amounted to roughly a quarter of the entire British Army. Thus, soldiers' health in India was a matter of great imperial, as well as local government, concern.

Before the Mutiny in 1857, the East India Company's Indian regiments had a strength of more than 300,000 men, but their numbers were drastically cut back in the subsequent reorganization of the army to ensure that Britain's military supremacy would not again be imperiled. An increasing proportion of recruits were drawn from the "martial races," particularly from Punjab, the Gurkhas of Nepal, and other "loyal" communities. The Indian Army stood at around 120,000 to 150,000 until World War I prompted a great expansion to meet Britain's wider military needs.

Despite the army's importance to the British conquest of South Asia and its role in the suppression of internal revolts, for most of the nineteenth century the army's main task was to serve as a garrison force, distributed among more than fifty military stations throughout British India, the princely states, and neighboring territories. Although army doctors had particular responsibility for soldiers' health and medical attention during military operations, it was the health of soldiers, especially white soldiers, in the barracks that caused the authorities the greatest concern and posed the greatest difficulties. High levels of sickness and mortality were a heavy drain on imperial finances: they were a cause of military inefficiency and a reckless waste of Britain's scarce military manpower. By one estimate, 100,000 British-born soldiers perished in India between 1815 and 1855—not including the casualties resulting from actual combat. At an estimated cost to the government of £100 each for their recruitment and training, this represented a cumulative (and, it was argued, largely needless) loss of £10 million.[6] Periods of warfare inevitably resulted in high death rates among soldiers, but, as in many other wars fought by European armies abroad during the nineteenth century, this increased mortality owed more to the effects of disease than enemy arms. Of 9,467 losses sustained by British forces during the 1857–58 uprising, only 586 soldiers were killed in action or died of their wounds: the rest perished from disease. "[I]t was disease, and not the enemy that killed them."[7]

The high levels of sickness and mortality, particularly among European troops in India, placed a heavy burden of responsibility upon the military medical services. As the data reproduced later in this chapter indicate, the rate of hospital admissions among white soldiers was extraordinarily high. To cite one specific case, from July 1828 to July 1833 the First Madras European Regiment, with an average strength of 533 men, was stationed on the east coast at Machilipatnam—admittedly a sickly station—and then at Kampti in central India. During this five-year period, there were on average 1,332 hospital admissions annually, the equivalent of 2.5 admissions per soldier each year, and each stay in hospital averaged 12.5 days. In effect, soldiers spent one month out of every twelve in hospital![8] In this, as in other European regiments, the rate of invaliding was also high. In addition to the 140 soldiers who died in hospital (and the 12 who were killed or "died suddenly"), a further 81 were invalided or discharged from the regiment, presumably mainly on health grounds. One of the many tasks of army doctors was to report cases of "malingering" and "shirking" and to decide which soldiers were eligible for sick leave or for invaliding out of the army. This gave medical officers an important, if not always popular, disciplinary role.[9]

From about the 1830s, the high levels of morbidity and mortality among European soldiers in India formed the subject of extensive study by army medical officers. They were prompted by professional responsibility and concern for the health of the soldiers in their charge but were also alert to the opportunities military life in India afforded for the study of tropical diseases and, as Surgeon William

Geddes, the medical officer attached to the First Madras European regiment, put it, for an "accuracy of observation and record" in the study of disease "not generally found in civil society."[10]

The growing use and availability of medical data for the army demonstrated how the statistical techniques gaining favor in Europe and North America at the time, and adapted for the British army and navy by Alexander Tulloch and by William Farr for the vital statistics of England and Wales in the 1830s and 1840s, were rapidly taken up in India.[11] Already by the 1830s, health was being seen as a quantifiable commodity, amenable to comparative analysis as well as clinical investigation. The use of statistical tables by Company surgeons like Geddes represented more than a desire for the accurate observation and recording of disease in the army: it also held out the possibility of showing quantitatively how standards of health among a discrete population, such as soldiers, might improve over time in response to medical and sanitary measures. The possibility of progress was always inherent in this new statistical sense. The availability of statistics for the army also reflected the greater attention given to military than to civilian health. No comparable data existed for India's civilian population until the 1870s, and even then figures were often crude and unreliable, registering only mortality and not morbidity (or, more exactly, in the army and prisons, the number of hospital admissions). Until the last third of the nineteenth century, the army and the jails provided virtually the only significant sites for the collection of vital data.

At first, however, these statistical investigations received little encouragement from the military authorities and resulted almost entirely from individual initiatives. They accordingly drew upon the limited local experience of surgeons at different stations and could not in themselves provide a cogent picture of conditions over time or across the breadth even of a single presidency. They were mere snapshots in a growing album of European ill health and affliction. Many of these observations and reports found their way into the fledgling medical journals of the time, sometimes accompanied by regrets that the military authorities did not pay greater heed to their import.

In 1839 Samuel Rogers, editor of the new *Madras Quarterly Medical Journal*, published an article by an assistant surgeon, James Kellie, on the means by which troops could minimize the risk of contracting malarial fevers while marching through the Gumsur hills.

Coming at a time of growing alarm at the high level of sickness and mortality among troops, particularly on marches, Rogers urged the army authorities to take Kellie's advice seriously, but he was not optimistic that they would: "we suspect the opinion of medical men is not much consulted in this country, prior to the undertaking of campaigns, or the marches of troops." Since "sickness will defeat the finest army," Rogers believed that the prevention of disease was a subject that "ought to be the study of all officers, military as well as medical."[12] Clearly, in the 1830s, it was not.

THE CRISIS OF MILITARY HEALTH

It was not until the 1850s and 1860s that the army's grim record of sickness and mortality came in for more sustained and systematic scrutiny and that political and administrative pressures began to mount in favor of preventive rather than merely curative medicine. Several factors influenced this shift. One was that by mid-century Britain was entering its own era of sanitary reform. The British Army was going through a process of improvement and reorganization, spurred on by official inquiries into such once-neglected matters as barrack accommodations and sanitation.[13] The Crimean War and Florence Nightingale's revelations about medical mismanagement and appalling hospital conditions at Scutari provided a further impetus for reform. Following closely in the wake of the Crimean War, the Rebellion of 1857–58 turned the spotlight onto the condition of British soldiers in India; and Nightingale, who campaigned with dogged determination for a sanitary commission to do for the troops in India what had recently been done for the army in Britain, was at last rewarded in May 1859 by the appointment of a Royal Commission into the Sanitary State of the Army in India.[14] The reform of army health in India thus acquired a political importance and urgency it had never previously enjoyed. Although India's medical establishment remained largely unchanged, the shift from Company raj to Crown rule seemed to promise a change of outlook and a greater sense of British responsibility for Indian welfare.

Statistics compiled in the 1850s and 1860s showed for the first time the full extent of the problem of army health in India. Not only were levels of sickness and mortality generally high in the army, but there was also a striking and (from the imperial perspective) deeply disturbing imbalance between the health of British and Indian soldiers. In

Table 1. Hospital Admissions and Mortality in the Bengal Army,
1818–54

	Admissions as % of total strength	Deaths as % of total strength	Deaths as % of numbers treated
European soldiers	199.70	5.58	2.79
European officers	132.25	2.11	1.60
Indian sepoys	100.84	1.19	1.11

Source: Ewart 1859, 3.

1859 Joseph Ewart of the Bengal Medical Service drew attention to
the remarkable differences in sickness and mortality among the three
main elements of the army of Bengal, as show in table 1.

It was clear from these statistics, and many others like them, that
European officers enjoyed far better health than the European rank-
and-file, but the most striking contrast lay between the Indian sepoys
and British soldiers. The latter were almost twice as likely as Indians
to be admitted to hospital, and more than four-and-a-half times as
likely to die from disease. Even among those hospitalized, European
deaths were more than double those among an equivalent number of
Indian soldiers. Ewart's findings, which were on the whole confirmed
by the Royal Commission when it published its report in 1863, presented a miserable picture of European sickness and mortality over
the previous forty or fifty years (see table 2).

These figures highlighted differences among provinces as well as
among the constituent racial and social elements of the army. The
higher mortality of European soldiers in Bengal (which had much the
largest army) and Madras was particularly marked, but (partly reflecting their heavy losses from disease during the Anglo-Burmese wars of
1824–26 and 1852) Indians had fared especially badly in the army of
the southern presidency compared to Bengal. Although some comparisons were made by the Royal Commission with the health of
soldiers in England and elsewhere, the most pertinent comparison
seemed to be within India itself, between European and Indian soldiers. And in his statistical "digest," Ewart went on to illustrate in relation to specific diseases and for each of the three presidencies the
great disparities between European and Indian health.

Table 2. Mortality among European and Indian Troops, 1803–54

Province	Period	Strength	Deaths	Deaths as % of strength
European soldiers				
Bengal	1812–1854	543,768	37,764	6.94
Bombay	1803–1854	306,978	16,954	5.52
Madras	1829–38, 1842–52	213,587	8,301	3.80
Indian soldiers				
Bengal	1826–53	2,767,347	38,451	1.39
Bombay	1803–54	1,451,166	22,960	1.58
Madras	1827–35, 1842–52	1,242,694	21,759	1.75

Source: Ewart 1859, 19, 36.

The leading recorded causes of sickness and mortality in the army were fevers (which alone accounted for half of all hospital admissions), along with cholera, dysentery, diarrhea, and hepatitis. For Ewart, perhaps even more than for many of his contemporaries, malaria was the "direst foe," the "great enemy of human life," which cut great swathes of sickness through the ranks of British and Indian soldiers and which also made it impossible to contemplate the kind of European colonization in India that was being successfully pursued in Canada.[15] The statistics for this and other diseases showed the apparently discriminatory nature of disease, which felled Europeans by the thousands but seemed to pass more lightly over indigenous troops. Thus, mortality from dysentery and diarrhea was more than eleven times greater among European soldiers in Bengal than among Indians; in Bombay it was nearly nine times greater and in Madras, just over six and a half times.[16] The contrast was even greater with regard to "hepatitis" (a term, as previously noted, contemporaries applied to liver complaints generally). Europeans in Bengal were sixty times more likely to be hospitalized for hepatitis than were Indians and died in almost the same proportion. In Bombay the ratios were 44:1 and 21:1 respectively, and in Madras, a staggering 74:1 and 30:1.[17]

Cholera, one of the most dreaded diseases in India at the time, was a leading cause of military as well as civilian deaths. Between 1818 and 1854, some 8,500 British soldiers were reported to have died from the disease. Over the previous forty years, cholera had been fatal in a third of all reported cases, and in approximately the same proportion among Indian as among European troops. But, relative to their strength, the proportion of cholera deaths was far higher among white than among Indian soldiers. According to Ewart's data, 4,806 European soldiers died of cholera in Bengal between 1818 and 1854 (equivalent to 0.97 percent of the average European strength), while among Indian soldiers in Bengal there had been 4,292 recorded deaths between 1826 and 1852, equal to only 0.16 percent of their strength, a sixth of the European figure. Since cholera was endemic in Bengal, figures for that province were particularly high. In Madras, which was less severely affected, the difference between European and Indian mortality rates was considerably smaller.[18]

Current experience gave fresh urgency to past woes. In 1861, even as the Royal Commission toiled over its report, the British Army was struck by one of the most severe outbreaks of cholera it had yet experienced in India. Among some 20,000 British soldiers and their families stationed in northern India at the time, 1,929 were attacked by cholera and of these 1,231 (64 percent) died. At the cantonment of Mian Mir outside Lahore, 880 out of 2,452 soldiers and their families contracted cholera; 535 (61 percent) died in less than a month. The shock of this stunning mortality among European soldiers (said by the investigating committee to have had few parallels "in modern times and among civilized men") was heightened by the relatively low death rate among Indian troops, even those stationed in the same cantonments. The high death rate among hospital patients (and among the unfortunate soldiers deputed to act as hospital orderlies) pointed to an ignorance of basic hygiene and a fatal assumption that cholera was not a contagious disease.[19] If in England fear of cholera was one of the main imperatives behind the reform of urban public health, in India it served a parallel (if characteristically more restricted) function in the overhaul of army health and sanitation.

Although Ewart and the Royal Commission Report were in broad agreement over their findings, especially the high level of sickness and mortality among European soldiers, they differed in one significant respect. By citing the Bengal figure of 69.4 European deaths per 1,000 over the previous forty years as representative of mortality among white soldiers in India as a whole, the commission (which met in London and never visited India) gave the impression that conditions had been (and remained) uniformly bad. By contrast, Ewart, whose opinions were more representative of the medical profession in India, was at pains to show that mortality and admission rates varied widely among the different presidencies and, above all, had improved markedly in recent decades. Thus, in Bengal the death rate among white soldiers had fallen from 7.59 percent in 1812–31 to 6.41 in the period 1832 to 1851–52, while in Madras it had dropped by 1.30 and in Bombay by 1.49 percent over the corresponding period.[20] Ewart argued that, while there had been little change in the actual level of sickness among European troops, there had been a significant improvement in the rates of recovery among those admitted to hospital. This improvement could not be attributed to sanitary reform, of which there had as yet been very little. The real reason, Ewart believed, lay with changes in therapeutic practice, the gradual abandonment of the old "spoilative" system of treating fevers and other complaints, "the steady displacement of the lancet and mercurialization by the liberal employment of cinchona, the disulphate and bisulphate of quinine, conjoined with promptitude in the administration of tonics, and generous diet during convalescence."[21]

Ironically, historians have tended to ignore the views of writers like Ewart and to accept uncritically the uniformly gloomy view presented by the Royal Commission and by Florence Nightingale, who was personally responsible for much of the text and tone of the commission's report. In consequence, credit for improvements in the army's sickness and mortality rates after the 1850s has gone to the Royal Commission and not to the medical establishment in India, seen, by contrast, as obstructive, obscurantist, and woefully out-of-touch.[22] Certainly, many medical and military officers in India did not take kindly to what they saw as outside meddling in their domestic affairs. The commission was strongly criticized in India at the time by doctors indignant at its apparent failure to acknowledge their own (albeit limited) achievements in military health and hygiene since the 1830s.[23]

The significance of the statistical and sanitary inquiries of the 1850s and 1860s was not that they suddenly threw light into the dark recesses of empire, transforming, as if overnight, the state of army health and military medicine in India. Rather, they gave medical officers and advisers, such as Ewart in Bengal or J. R. Martin (now in London), the opportunity and the confidence to press their professional claims on a previously indifferent administration and, at a time of some therapeutic uncertainty, to stress the urgent necessity and practical value of sanitary reform and preventive medicine. So far, Ewart complained, the government in India had "committed the great mistake of confining the labour of their medical officers to the cure of disease—not to its prevention." In cholera, as with other diseases that blighted the health of the army, he looked forward to the recognition of "the importance, the superlative superiority, of prophylactic over curative science." And he quoted Martin to the effect that "the importance of an efficient medical establishment is so great that we cannot put a money value on it."[24] In the changed political circumstances of the 1860s, this was a message the government was more willing to hear and to heed.

THE REFORM OF ARMY HEALTH

The dire record of military ill health and mortality revealed by the Royal Commission in 1863 was an acutely disturbing one from the imperial standpoint. It suggested the extreme perils of stationing large numbers of European troops in India and the difficulties of safeguarding their health in a tropical environment. Ewart, following the environmentalist tradition of earlier Company surgeons, saw in the army statistics evidence that residence in India was "exceedingly prejudicial to the health and lives of our brave countrymen in arms." In hepatitis and its far lower incidence among Indian than among European troops, he found "a forcible illustration" of "the comparative unadaptability of the European constitution to a tropical climate."[25] The soldiers' dire record of sickness and mortality might possibly have been taken as evidence that because Europeans were (as Ewart reminded his readers) "exotics" in India, they had either to accept this heavy burden of mortality as the climate's inevitable toll or to quit the country entirely. But, in fact, the military statistics were not interpreted as evidence of the unavoidably high cost or impracticality of British dominion over India. The political and economic imperatives behind British rule were too powerful for an established empire in India to be allowed to expire. Colonialism dictated that a solution must be found, and, indeed, the statistics could even be seen to provide proof that sickness and death were not the unavoidable lot of white men in India.

In pointing to a mortality rate for European officers that was 31 per 1,000 *below* that of white soldiers, the Royal Commission concluded that "the lives of nearly half the soldiers, in less unfavourable conditions, might for the future be saved."[26] Ewart likewise commented that:

> The remarkable comparative immunity from disease and death enjoyed by the officers, and the still greater immunity which prevails amongst covenanted civilians [European civil servants], as contrasted with the high ratios of sickness and mortality amongst the constituent members of the ranks, place beyond question or doubt, not only the possibility, but the facile practicability, of greatly improving the health of the latter, and of expanding the present abnormally contracted or narrowed span of their lives.[27]

The difference between the health of European officers and the ranks was believed to reflect their contrasting life-styles and material circumstances. While soldiers and their families were crowded into ill-ventilated and insanitary barracks, which readily became hotbeds of disease, their officers enjoyed more spacious and salubrious quarters, a better diet, more exercise, and more frequent periods of leave. As Ewart commented in discussing the difference in cholera morbidity and death rates between soldiers and officers:

> The preventive qualities of the well-ventilated, airy, capacious and comparatively cool, bungalow, and the superior hygienic, sanitary and dietetic arrangements of the officer, are here contrasted as favourably with the too often ill-positioned, imperfectly ventilated, and contaminated barrack-rooms and general sanitary conditions of the constituents of the ranks, as the palatial residences of Belgravia are with the wretched hovels and polluted cells of St. Giles', Whitechapel, or Bermondsey.[28]

There was a belated recognition, hastened by sanitary reform in England and by Florence Nightingale's work at Scutari, that much of the sickness and mortality experienced in Indian barracks and cantonments was itself a product of the disease-generating conditions in which rank-and-file soldiers lived or the hospitals in which they were confined when sick or wounded. This accorded with the miasmatic theories of the time, in which human "filth" and "effluvia" took their place, as contributory causes of disease, alongside swamps, marshes, rotting animal carcasses, and decaying vegetable matter. Military barracks and hospitals, like jails, meant poor ventilation and concentrated human populations, ideal sites for the generation of miasmas that caused or communicated disease. As J. R. Martin told the Royal Commission, fever, cholera, dysentery, and diarrhea, all diseases common to the army, were "accompanied by profuse discharges, with which the air, water, bedding, linen, closets, walls of hospitals and barracks become more or less infected." Since the unfortunate inmates of such buildings were constantly exposed to such *materies morbi*, Martin said, it was not surprising that they sickened and died in such formidable numbers.[29]

At a time when medicine could claim few therapeutic triumphs of its own, sanitation seemed to hold the key to improved military health and hygiene. The improvements made on the recommendations of the Royal Commission (or already in progress at the time its report was published)—improvements in the siting and construction of barracks, in drainage, conservancy, and water supply—embodied in the small compass of the colonial cantonment many of the doctrines of sanitary science being enunciated in Europe, and they appeared to yield rapid results.[30] As table 3 shows, the health of the army, and especially of its European component, improved dramatically in the decades after 1860, though the greatest advances came only later, shortly before World War I.

Apart from the quinquennium 1915–19, which showed a sharp upturn in sickness and mortality (mainly as a result of the influenza pandemic of 1918–19), the downward trend in both mortality and hospital admissions from the 1860s onward was remarkably consistent. But it is also striking that the health of Indian soldiers, beginning from an apparently superior position in the mid nineteenth century, did not improve at the same rate as the Europeans', with the result that by 1910–14 the rates of sickness and mortality in the two sections of the army had drawn almost level. Although both were adversely affected by epidemic disease in the following quinquennium, sickness and death rates rose higher among Indian than among British troops. However, within the army as a whole, mortality fell to a fifth of what it had been in the 1860s and 1870s.

Table 3. Death Rates and Hospital Admissions among British and Indian Troops in India, 1860–1919 (per 1,000)

	British		Indian	
Period	*Deaths*	*Admissions*	*Deaths*	*Admissions*
1860–64	31.85	—	—	—
1865–69	27.89	—	—	—
1870–74	19.39	—	—	—
1875–79	20.37	1,475.4	19.93	1,322.3
1880–84	16.30	1,500.3	19.00	1,073.8
1885–89	15.11	1,446.3	12.90	930.6
1890–94	15.09	1,468.3	13.48	874.3
1895–99	17.14	1,383.7	11.34	777.2
1900–04	13.03	1,045.9	10.87	711.8
1905–09	8.93	802.5	6.78	633.6
1910–14	4.35	567.2	4.39	544.6
1915–19	8.23	881.7	14.02	788.7

Sources: Balfour and Scott 1924, 128; *India SCAR 1920*, 2, 28.

Although there was a comparable decline in sickness and mortality among British troops generally in this period, reflecting improving health and living conditions in British society in the late nineteenth century, in India this development occurred against a backdrop of soaring Indian mortality between 1880 and 1920. Epidemics of malaria, cholera, plague, and influenza raised annual death rates to 40 or even 50 per 1,000, reaching a peak of 48.6 per 1,000 in 1911–21, before falling back to 36.3 per 1,000 in 1921–31.[31] That such substantial improvements in military health were achieved at a time of high civilian mortality suggests that the causes of sickness and mortality within the army were either intrinsically different from those affecting the Indian population at large or (perhaps additionally) that the army enjoyed a privileged medical status which enabled it to remain effectively isolated from the diseases that ravaged the population outside. These factors will be considered later in this chapter.

In the case of cholera, the disease which more than any other sent shivers of horror through the army ranks and which, as in Europe, was the touchstone by which sanitary progress was commonly judged, mortality and morbidity rates fell impressively and consistently in the

Table 4. Hospital Admissions among British Troops in Bengal, 1859–94 (per 1,000)

	1859–63	*1864–69*	*1870–76*	*1877–94*
Cholera	19.7	9.8	4.3	3.8
Smallpox	2.5	1.9	0.7	0.8
Enteric fever	0.2	0.9	3.7	16.4
Intermittent fever	455.6	393.3	397.3	468.1
Remittent fever	85.4	39.5	29.1	13.8
Simple continued fever	215.0	106.5	147.7	77.0
Apoplexy/heat stroke	4.5	5.3	3.4	4.0
Alcoholism	6.0	4.4	3.3	7.5
Respiratory diseases	76.7	59.0	60.5	47.7
Phthisis	6.8	8.3	8.9	4.7
Dysentery	74.0	39.5	30.0	29.1
Diarrhea	135.4	93.7	59.8	48.2
Hepatitis	63.6	56.3	50.6	25.2
Spleen diseases	—	6.6	7.4	4.5
Scurvy	—	1.1	0.5	1.0
Venereal disease	335.1	213.3	196.5	357.1
All causes	2,039.6	1,565.5	1,478.9	1,562.7

Source: India SCAR 1895, 19.

post-Mutiny decades (see tables 4 and 5). These gains were partly offset by the apparently meteoric rise of enteric fever (typhoid), which began to appear in the army statistics only in the 1860s (earlier cases were probably subsumed in the "continued fever" category), and by the persistence of malaria (classed in the tables mainly as "intermittent" and "remittent" fever) as the greatest single cause of army ill health.

Specific sanitary reform measures, like the provision of piped water or the building of more spacious barrack accommodations, were certainly not incompatible with a belief that disease was caused or aggravated by wider environmental forces. There were few diseases that were not thought to bear the imprint of temperature, humidity, and other climatic or physical influences. But powerful though these factors were reckoned to be, there was a strong and growing conviction that their effects could be moderated, even if they could not be altogether eliminated. The medico-topographical surveys discussed in

Table 5. Mortality among British Troops in Bengal, 1859–94 (per 1,000)

	1859–63	1864–69	1870–76	1877–94
Cholera	11.6	6.5	2.9	2.7
Smallpox	0.4	0.3	0.1	0.1
Enteric fever	0.1	0.5	1.7	4.7
Intermittent fever	0.7	0.7	0.1	0.2
Remittent fever	1.7	1.3	1.0	0.8
Simple continued fever	2.1	1.4	0.5	0.1
Apoplexy/heat stroke	2.2	2.5	1.4	1.2
Alcoholism	0.6	0.4	0.2	0.2
Respiratory diseases	1.0	0.9	1.1	1.2
Phthisis	1.9	1.6	1.3	0.8
Dysentery	5.1	2.1	1.3	0.9
Diarrhea	1.4	0.5	0.1	0.2
Hepatitis	3.6	3.4	2.2	1.3
All causes	36.9	26.6	18.7	18.1

Source: India SCAR 1895, 19.

the previous chapter owed much of their inspiration to military need. Medical topography and military topography, J. R. Martin emphasized, were intimately connected, a point exemplified by the extensive discussion he gave to soldiers' health in his account of the medical topography of Calcutta.[32] Such studies did more than simply describe the local topography and its outstanding physical features. By locating disease within a landscape, they suggested practical measures to avoid the worst effects of disease.

Certainly, some authorities took the view that vast tracts of India were almost uniformly inimical to European health and hence unsuited for permanent military stations. Edmund Parkes in the 1860s dismissed the entire Indo-Gangetic plain, from Calcutta to Delhi and down to Sind, as "more or less malarious"; but others, like T. E. Dempster, took the more discriminating view that in India "healthy and unhealthy localities are everywhere found in close proximity."[33] It was one of the tasks of medical topography, using the health of the civilian population as well as the army's own records as a guide, to locate the safe and avoid the sickly places; and such findings exercised considerable influence on the subsequent siting of military stations. Some, like Berhampore in Bengal, were permanently abandoned because they had proved so persistently unhealthy. Barracks were moved away from swampy and "malarial" ground or were constructed so as to moderate the effects of searing sun or torrential monsoons. Vegetation was cleared to remove its supposedly miasmatic effects: Ewart was among those who urged the "removal and destruction" of all trees and shrubs around military barracks, down "to the last leaf or blade of grass." When it came to combating "malaria," nineteenth-century surgeons were not, by today's lights, very environmentally friendly.[34]

An alternative response, strongly recommended by the commission which investigated the 1861 cholera outbreak in northern India and adopted as standard army and jail procedure for the next thirty-five years, was to evacuate soldiers and prisoners as soon as epidemic cholera or smallpox broke out and to move them into tents in some other (it was hoped, disease-free) locality. It was in this way that the prisoners of Agra jail found themselves camping in the spacious and elegant gardens of the Taj Mahal and Akbar's mausoleum during a cholera outbreak of 1856. John Murray was the doctor in charge at Agra at the time. Thirteen years later, in 1869, citing recent evidence of declining jail and troop mortality, he affirmed that "removal is . . . one of the most efficacious means available for saving life during cholera epidemics."[35] While such elaborate avoidance strategies offered no practical solution to the problems of disease and ill health in civilian society, they probably made some contribution to the decline of cholera and other diseases among the military. Certainly, at the time these measures were confidently believed to be effective.

From his days as presidency surgeon in Calcutta in the 1830s through his presence on the Royal Commission of 1859–63, James Ranald Martin was in the forefront of those current or former Company physicians who advocated even more drastic environmental changes to save European troops from the ravages of India's climate and diseases. "Of all the causes which tend to the premature destruction of the British soldier in our intertropical possessions," he declared in 1856, "none are so powerful as the neglect in selecting proper localities for camps and cantonments." Indeed, "the other ills, although great," sank "into comparative insignificance."[36] Martin was a strong advocate of the establishment of hill stations for the preservation and recovery of European soldiers' health, and by the mid 1850s several military sanatoriums—like Landour and Kussowlie—had been established in the Himalayan foothills or in isolated uplands elsewhere, such as Wellington in the Nilgiris. This specialized form of segregation did more than meet a strictly medical need: it also reflected the continuing belief that Europeans were "exotics," incapable of becoming fully acclimatized to India yet able to find greater physical and mental ease in the hills, an environment more similar to Britain's. But the virtues of hill resorts were also urged on purely medical grounds. Edmund Parkes spoke approvingly in the 1860s of their medical benefits, declaring

> Not only does such a location improve greatly the vigour of the men, who on the hill stations preserve the healthy, ruddy hue of the European, but it prevents many diseases. If properly selected, the vast class of malarious diseases disappears; liver diseases are less common, and bowel complaints, in some stations at any rate, are neither so frequent nor so violent. Digestion and blood-nutrition are greatly improved. Moreover, a proper degree of exercise can be taken, and the best personal hygiene rules easily observed.[37]

Given the enthusiasm of medical experts like Martin and Parkes and the wholehearted endorsement of the Royal Commission in 1863, it was not surprising that the army authorities (who enjoyed summer sojourns of their own in the Olympian heights of Simla, Darjeeling, and Ootacamund) heeded their advice. By the 1870s a sixth of all British troops in India were stationed in the hills, and by the mid 1890s, nearly a quarter (16,500 men).[38] But such changes of environment could never offer more than a partial solution even to the immediate problems of European health and mortality. From a military and political point of view, it was inconvenient, even in an age of telegraphs and trains, to have small and scattered detachments of British soldiers perched on remote hills, away from the main centers of population and the principal scenes of political unrest or communal disturbance. It was acknowledged, too, that not all conditions were improved by a move to cooler climes. Parkes noted the frequency of "hill diarrhoea" among troops and the inconvenient discovery that malaria might be met with even seven thousand feet above sea level.[39] It was found, too, that soldiers (or their innumerable camp followers) brought with them to the hills many of the same causes of ill health—from alcoholism and syphilis to cholera and typhoid—which had previously plagued them in the plains.[40] The limitations of this evasion strategy were a reminder that the essential problems of military, as well as civilian, health had to be tackled in the plains, in and around the teeming cities of India, and could not be neatly resolved by shunting off white soldiers to the hills.

THE HEALTH OF EUROPEAN SOLDIERS

Alcohol

To illustrate the emerging authority of military medicine in colonial India, to pursue further the reasons for the marked differences apparent between European and Indian soldiers in the mid nineteenth century, and to explore the perceived relationship between army and civilian health, we will examine more closely three case studies: alcohol, venereal disease, and enteric fever (typhoid).

While environmentalism remained the dominant paradigm in nineteenth-century medical thought in India, this governing idea was elaborated and amended in various ways. As we saw in chapter 1, one of the main qualifications was the stress placed on moral, social, and cultural traits. This was true not only of the medical discourse on Indian society: it also informed debate about the high levels of sickness and mortality among the European soldiery. Climate and topography might explain why soldiers fell prey to certain diseases or why certain ailments appeared to be severe in the tropics, but social behavior seemed to provide a more fitting, or a complementary, explanation for many other conditions. The readiness of medical and military officers to attribute soldiers' ill health to their habits and conduct gave an important class dimension to debates about disease in the European army. In other contexts, cultural beliefs and social practices were cited to explain Indian susceptibility to disease. But in this instance attitudes were partially reversed, the abstinence of high-caste Hindu soldiers being favorably contrasted with the drunkenness and "indulgence" ascribed to British soldiers.[41]

Drink—like sex—was a troublesome issue for the practitioners of military medicine. Professionally, army doctors had many reasons to regard heavy drinking—"that terrible habit"[42]—as greatly detrimental to soldiers' health and discipline. But it was a measure of their uncertain authority, particularly before the 1850s, that, even within the army that employed them, their advice on this matter was often unheeded or outweighed by more pressing considerations. In the late eighteenth and early nineteenth centuries, an abundance of strong and readily available alcohol was assumed to be necessary to keep British soldiers in India contented and to enable them to endure the tedium and discomfort of barrack life. In time of war, hard liquor was expected to sustain the soldiers' powers of endurance and fuel their reckless courage. It was their reward in victory, their comfort in defeat and adversity. Many military and medical officers further believed that heavy drinking was "natural" to the laboring classes from which the bulk of British soldiers were drawn. Intemperance was seen to be an intrinsic, if deplorable, part of working-class culture, and therefore little could be done to change it.[43] It was also argued that it was better to supply soldiers with as much drink as they wanted in the barracks than to allow them to wander off into the neighboring bazaars where the "country liquor" was even more injurious to health and where military discipline was difficult to enforce.[44]

But alcohol was also a major disciplinary and medical issue. In the view of many military officers and medical men, it was a leading cause of crime and insubordination within the army as well a major source of "inefficiency" resulting from drinking bouts and alcohol-related illnesses. In 1819 the commander-in-chief of the Bengal Army drew attention to "the destruction of health, the defiance of control, the commission of crimes and the brutalizing depravity which are the consequences of the fatal habit of inebriety." The brutalizing effects both of drink and the harsh punishments meted out for drunken insubordination and crime were a common theme, too, of the medical literature. But the commander-in-chief went some way toward expressing the army's acceptance of this savage state of affairs, because European soldiers spent most of their time in India confined to barracks, "exhausted by the enervating effects of the climate[,] without pursuits of industry [and] interest or of amusement to occupy their time and engage their minds."[45]

In consequence, despite protests from medical officers like Martin, who blamed the government for encouraging the "moral and physical poison" of drink with one hand, while exercising the disciplinary lash of corporal punishment with the other,[46] heavy drinking long remained an institutionalized part of army life in India. Two drams of "ardent spirits" were issued daily to each soldier, in addition to virtually as much beer, wine, and brandy as he chose to consume in the army canteen. The First European Regiment of the Madras Army, a body of about five hundred men, was probably not atypical when in 1830 it drank its way through ten thousand gallons of arrack in a single year—in addition to prodigious amounts of brandy, gin, wine, and beer.[47] Not until 1854 was the daily spirit ration curtailed and some attempt made to encourage soldiers to drink beer rather than hard liquor. No improvement was immediately apparent. The British Army in India, Dr. Sutherland told the Royal Commission on the Sanitary State of the Army, "presents the largest amount of drunkenness of, perhaps, any body of men in existence, as it certainly does of disease produced directly or indirectly by intemperance."[48] The number of deaths from delirium tremens was said to be sixteen times greater among white soldiers in India than among civilians in Britain, and the extraordinarily high incidence of hepatic disorders was similarly taken to be due mainly to excessive and continual drinking of hard spirits.[49]

How much this equating of drink with disease was warranted and how much it reflected a moral rather than a medical judgment is hard to ascertain. It is likely that some apparently drink-related illnesses arose from other causes. Liver complaints might have been the result of amoebic dysentery and viral hepatitis (hepatitis and liver abscesses were listed separately only in the army returns from 1888 onward). A connection between amoebic dysentery and abscess of the liver was not fully recognized before the mid 1890s and was only conclusively established by Leonard Rogers in 1902. In 1898, Patrick Manson, "the father of modern tropical medicine," still clung to the position that the reason why European soldiers were so much more subject than Indians to liver abscesses was "over-indulgence in stimulating food and alcoholic drinks."[50]

Inasmuch as the problem of hepatitis and alcohol-related disease was seen to be specific to the European army and its "indulgent" lifestyle, it was thought to be amenable to local solutions, within the army "enclave," and not to require changes in colonial society in general. Insofar as it was a degenerative condition associated with long-serving soldiers, the incidence of liver disease was reduced by the introduction of shorter terms of service in the British Army in the 1870s. Until the 1840s soldiers had enlisted in the British Army for life—or until discharged for health reasons. In 1847 the Limited Enlistment Act allowed for voluntary discharge after ten years in the infantry but with the possibility of reenlistment for eleven more years. The army reforms of 1870 brought this down still further to six years active service, followed by an equivalent period in the reserves. The young soldiers in their teens and twenties who came to predominate in the army in India by the late nineteenth century were thus less likely to be hospitalized with alcohol-related complaints than old sots of sergeants in their forties or fifties.

A gradual reduction in the amount of alcohol, especially hard liquor, consumed in cantonments, the availability of alternative forms of recreation through regimental libraries, sports, and gardens, and even the slow growth of a temperance movement in the army, might also have contributed to a fall in the incidence of alcoholism and liver disease. Nonetheless, the striking disparity between white and Indian soldiers remained. In 1895 mortality from abscess of the liver was calculated to be seventy times greater among European than Indian troops, and as late as 1910 it was still the largest single cause of death in the British Army in India after enteric fever.[51]

Venereal Disease

The history of venereal disease in the army in India also reflected the institution's social composition and internal management, but it says much, too, about the limited effectiveness—and contradictory opinions—of army doctors. Syphilis and gonorrhea added little directly to the sum of European military mortality in India, but for much of the nineteenth century, VD was the largest single cause of hospital admissions among European soldiers, exceeding even the high number of fever cases. It was also a common cause of invaliding. Three things "break up the constitution of a man. . . in India," Dr. Colvin Smith told the Royal Commission in 1861: "a malarious climate, . . . intemperance and syphilis."[52]

During the second half of the century, the number of patients hospitalized for venereal disease, already high, increased still further with the influx of British soldiers during the Mutiny campaigns. From 177 admissions per 1,000 men in 1855, the rate in Bengal rose to 359 in 1859 but sank back again to 167 in 1867. The introduction of the short-service system in 1870 resulted in an increased proportion of young, unmarried soldiers in the British Army in India: by 1880 41 percent of soldiers were under 25, with a further 34 percent between the ages of 25 and 29. In consequence, the incidence of VD began to climb steeply again, more than doubling from 205 per 1,000 in 1875 to 522 in 1895. This was the equivalent of more than half the army hospitalized with VD each year and represented the loss of more than a million military man-days. Among Indian soldiers, by contrast, the reported incidence of venereal disease was much smaller, though also tending to increase. From 27 in 1877, the incidence per 1,000 reached 41 in 1890, but declined again to 31 in 1895.[53]

Colonial medicine identified VD almost exclusively as a military problem, a complaint "pernicious to the constitutions and discipline" specifically of European troops.[54] Syphilis was numerically much the most significant of the venereal diseases involved. Although Europeans had introduced the disease into India in the sixteenth and seventeenth centuries, and though soldiers and sailors remained a major source of infection, it was thought of as a disease that threatened the army from without, especially from contact with low-caste Indian prostitutes. The extent of VD among India's civilian population was unknown and almost entirely uninvestigated before the 1920s. The disease assumed significance for state medicine only when white soldiers were thought to be at risk, though as early as 1808 one British doctor rated it next to smallpox among the "most destructive and most perilous disease[s] in India" and claimed that one in every ten adult Indian males was infected with it.[55]

The problem of venereal disease in the European army revolved around two issues. The first was the social composition and sexual conduct of the army. Few white soldiers in India after the 1850s were married, and with the advent of the short-service system their numbers declined still further. Officially, 12 percent of British soldiers abroad were allowed to have wives "on the strength," but the actual proportion was far smaller. In 1890 only 2,544, or 3.7 percent, of the 66,194 British soldiers in India were married. In the infantry, which made up the bulk of the army, the proportion was as low as 2.8 percent.[56] The army authorities accepted that, given the paucity of women of their own race and class and the want of other recreational activities, British soldiers inevitably consorted with Indian prostitutes and so risked repeated exposure to venereal disease. But, as with heavy drinking, the authorities tended to regard such sexual behavior as a part of the "animal" passions of the lower classes and thus not possible to prohibit effectively. Prostitution was certainly regarded as preferable to masturbation, which was thought to be physically weakening and mentally damaging. It was sometimes argued that unmarried men made better soldiers or that a private's wage was insufficient to support a European wife and children in India. For a variety of reasons, then, the army preferred tacitly to condone prostitution than to bear the financial and administrative responsibility of a greater number of wives and children.[57] In the early years of the nineteenth century, concubinage with Indian women was suggested as a possible option and a likely check to the spread of venereal disease, but in the changed moral and racial climate of the mid nineteenth century, this was no longer considered desirable.[58]

The second issue raised by the prevalence of venereal disease in the army was the possibility of effective medical surveillance and control. Lock hospitals for the detention and treatment of prostitutes infected with venereal disease had been in use by the army since the beginning of the nineteenth century, but their morality and their practical value in controlling venereal disease were always matters of controversy, with opinion veering first one way, then the other.[59] Certainly, there was no unanimity of medical opinion, even as to whether mercury was effective in curing the disease or, as with the use of mercurials in the treatment of other illnesses, merely wrecked the patient's constitution.[60]

In 1868 the government in India followed recent metropolitan precedents and formally sanctioned, through its own Contagious Diseases Act, the medical inspection of army prostitutes and the use of lock hospitals for their treatment and detention. But the system was difficult to operate effectively, and doubts were raised as much about its practical utility as its moral acceptability. Prostitutes evaded medical examination and lock hospitals whenever they could, and soldiers' sexual appetites could not be confined to the small number of licensed and inspected prostitutes attached to the army. Surgeon-Major D. Blair Brown, writing in the late 1880s when controversy over the Contagious Diseases Act was at its height, advanced several objections to the inspection of prostitutes. The examinations, he believed, were too cursory to allow for accurate diagnosis, and hence the protection claimed was "but a poor and insignificant one, greatly overbalanced by the absurd ideas prevalent regarding medical men's powers of detection, and the so-called cleanliness of women." He even suspected that medical examinations so carelessly performed actually communicated the "syphilitic poison" from one woman to another. Brown was frankly skeptical about doctors' ability to cure the disease: hospitalizing soldiers and then releasing them as soon as the primary lesions disappeared was, in his view, only a form of "temporary treatment," and not a real cure.[61]

In his 1881 annual report, the Government of India's Sanitary Commissioner, J. M. Cuningham, remarked that "year by year it becomes more and more evident that, however successful such a system promised to be when it was originally adopted, its practical working has proved a complete failure."[62] Not every doctor agreed—or accepted moral arguments against medical inspections and lock hospitals. The *Indian Medical Gazette*, the unofficial voice of the IMS, was inclined to believe that the system could be effective, if properly implemented. Commenting on Cuningham's report and noting the continuing rise of venereal disease among British soldiers, an editorial in the *Gazette* remarked in 1883 that, since the "conditions of propagation of this class of disorders" were "more special, definite, and accurately known" than those for any other contagious diseases, VD ought to be particularly amenable to preventive measures, especially in a community "so isolated, so subject to observation and control as the European army in India." In demonstrating that VD had *not* been brought under effective control in the fifteen years since the act had first come into force, Cuningham's admission amounted, the journal claimed, to a "record of sanitary incompetence."[63] And while the medical profession debated the reasons for the apparent failure of lock hospitals to check venereal disease in the army, outside critics focused on the offensive and coercive manner in which the inspections were said to be carried out and the immorality of state-sponsored "harlotry." As one official aptly remarked in the 1880s, the operation of the Contagious Diseases Act touched "closely on the habits of the people."[64] This was an area in which state medicine, driven by the need to protect its military enclaves, found itself both powerless to devise effective measures of control and in danger of provoking a public outcry by its clumsy attempts at medical policing.

The abolition of Britain's own Contagious Diseases Act in 1886 increased the pressure for India to follow suit. Agitation by Christian missionaries in India and their allies in England persuaded the House of Commons to pass a resolution in June 1888 condemning the compulsory examination of women and calling for an end to lock hospitals and the licensing of army prostitutes.[65] Against its own inclinations, the Government of India was obliged to comply with the wishes of Parliament and the secretary of state, but it viewed the repeal of the Contagious Diseases Act with grave misgivings. Ironically, in this instance, the government and the military authorities showed greater confidence in the power of medicine than did many doctors themselves. The secretary of the Government of India's Military Department noted despairingly, shortly after the act's repeal, that the problem of venereal disease in the army was now "almost beyond human control" and "almost without a remedy."[66]

In fact, the prospects for the army were not quite as dismal as his lament suggested. Although cases of venereal disease continued to rise over the next few years, they peaked in 1895 (at 522 cases per 1,000 men) and then declined sharply. By 1900 they had fallen to 298, and by 1913 to 53, barely a tenth of the rate twenty years earlier. This striking reversal appears to have been achieved through tighter cantonment regulations (which quietly restored some of the controls over prostitution formally surrendered through the abolition of the Contagious Diseases Act), along with moral pressure and educational propaganda by doctors, chaplains, and army officers.[67] From 1910, trials with the new drug Salvarsan, a compound of arsenic, proved successful in treating soldiers' syphilis.[68] An effective medical solution had at last been found to a long-standing moral and military problem.

Enteric Fever

The medical and administrative difficulties of preserving the health of European soldiers in India were further exemplified by enteric fever (typhoid). A disease unrecognized in India before the 1850s (though its symptoms had previously been noted by Annesley, Twining, and others), enteric fever entered the army's statistical returns only in the early 1870s. But thereafter, it grew with great rapidity to become within two decades a leading cause of illness and mortality among British troops. Recorded deaths from enteric fever rose from 1.6 per 1,000 men in 1877 to a peak of 6.1 in 1889; cases increased from 5.6 per 1,000 in 1881 to 36.9 in 1898, but fell back to 16.1 in 1905 and 4.6 in 1910.[69]

Like cholera or hepatitis, enteric fever seemed to present yet another example of the perversely discriminatory nature of disease in

India and, even more than cholera, the remoteness of the army's medical problems and priorities from those of the Indian population. Until the 1890s almost all the cases recorded were among Europeans: Indians were thought to be virtually immune to the disease. As was later realized, this was because many Indians encountered typhoid in childhood, acquiring subsequent immunity to the disease (though they could still be carriers). In addition, the characteristic rash of rose-pink spots that accompanied enteric fever was reputedly less visible on dark Indian skin than on pale European skin. The ban on conducting postmortems on Indian soldiers made it impossible to identify the internal marks of the disease (the ulceration of the small intestines and Peyer's patches): thus, the greater accessibility of prison corpses made India's jails a richer field for medical research.[70] By 1914, however, the position had been reversed, with an increasing number of cases and fatalities reported among Indian soldiers (as a result of better diagnosis and improved laboratory techniques) at a time when the disease had already greatly diminished as a threat to the lives of European soldiers.

Quite apart from the difficulties surrounding the identification of enteric fever, the introduction of the short-service system in the 1870s is likely to have increased the relative incidence of the disease among European troops by creating a changing pool of young susceptible males, many of whom contracted enteric fever from food, water, and flies within days or weeks of arriving in India. Thus, it was young soldiers who were most at risk from enteric fever, as they were from VD. It was calculated in 1890 that there were 10.2 deaths from enteric fever among every 1,000 British soldiers during their first two years of service in India. This fell to 3.0 deaths per 1,000 after three to five years, and 2.2 per 1,000 after six to ten years in India.[71]

At first, the mysterious etiology of enteric fever and the apparent immunity of Indians to the disease prompted fresh speculation about the influence of climate and environment on India's diseases and fostered doubts about its contagiousness. The army's success in combating cholera since the 1860s through improved sanitation and filtered water supplies (even while controversy raged over its origins and transmission) made it harder for many doctors to accept that enteric fever, too, might be connected with defective sanitation and hygiene.[72] But, especially after enteric fever had been traced by Karl Joseph Eberth in 1880 to a specific bacillus, it was increasingly accepted as a "filth disease," brought into the army barracks through contaminated food, drink, and sewage. Like malaria, plague, and many other diseases at the time, enteric fever fed the growing antipathy between Europeans and Indians and provoked demands for greater physical as well as social distance between the races.[73] European vulnerability was no longer attributed to any constitutional susceptibility or even, in the main, to the adverse effects of climate, but instead to perennial reservoirs of disease among the "native" population. Under the combined and heady influence of the germ theory and late nineteenth-century doctrines of race and empire, enteric fever came (at least in military circles) to epitomize disease as an insidious enemy, infiltrating the sanitized world of the cantonment from the neighboring bazaars, through Indian camp servants, prostitutes, and suppliers of milk and fruit, menacing innocent young British soldiers whenever they ventured beyond the sheltering safety of the cantonment environment.

Between the 1890s and 1914, enteric fever and veneral disease, though clearly very different in their clinical character, were frequently compared and seen to share a common origin in the "native" (or *sadr*) bazaars that huddled close to every cantonment. As a medical officer at Lucknow lamented in 1894, after the introduction of a new water supply had failed to protect soldiers from enteric fever,

> Within the regimental lines there is no insanitary influence
> which should cause the disease. Without the regimental lines
> things are different. The cantonment sudder bazar has grown to
> the proportions of a small city, and is crowded with natives of
> all classes and their dirty surroundings. There are various attrac-
> tions to the soldier in the shape of billiard rooms, treating
> shops, prostitutes' quarters, which afford the soldier ample
> opportunity of exposing himself to infection of all kinds. . . .
> The appalling number of admissions for venereal disease shows
> where he spends his leisure hours. It does not appear to me un-
> reasonable to suppose that where he contracts venereal disease
> he also contracts enteric fever.[74]

Why, asked the Government of India's sanitary commissioner in 1890, was enteric fever common among European soldiers but rare among Indians? "Natives," he answered, live "generation after generation" in an environment "saturated in specific filth" and so gained immunity to the disease. But when young soldiers "from comparatively pure England" went to India, they fell ready prey to the disease. Cantonments might have become "oases of purity," but they were still set "amidst a desert of filth."[75]

Because enteric fever was seen to strike specifically at Europeans, especially young white soldiers, there were powerful racial and political pressures for making its control a high medical and administrative priority. The perceived nature of the disease and the medical techniques that were becoming available by 1900 encouraged a preventive strategy which sought to isolate or protect British soldiers from likely sources of the disease. Apart from discouraging soldiers from frequenting the bazaars, a vigorous campaign was conducted to educate soldiers about the hazards of bazaar food and drink. Fly screens were put on the doors and windows of messes and food halls. A careful watch was kept on milk supplied to cantonments (in the knowledge that Indians diluted it with water to increase its volume). Known typhoid cases were isolated or moved to two special convalescent stations (one at Naini Tal in north India, the other at Wellington in the Nilgiris) to prevent them from communicating the disease to others.[76]

But the greatest reliance was placed on the antityphoid vaccine developed by Almroth Wright of the Royal Army Medical College at Netley and first tried out on four thousand British soldiers in India in 1898–99.[77] By 1913, 93 percent of British soldiers in India had been inoculated against enteric fever and enjoyed a high degree of protection against the disease. But the campaign did not stop with the soldiers themselves. The Indian cooks, mess servants, and others who prepared or handled food were also inoculated—or dismissed, if they were identified as carriers. As the extent of enteric fever among Indian soldiers began to be recognized, prophylactic measures were extended to them as well. But by 1914, only about a tenth of the Indian soldiers had been inoculated. As far as the British Army was concerned, however, the result of these intensive measures was that enteric fever, once so menacing, was in the space of less than two decades reduced to "almost negligible proportions."[78] But if this was a further demonstration of the extreme value of medical science to the army in India by World War I, it was also a reminder of how specific both the problems and the solutions of military medicine might be and how far removed from wider considerations of Indian public health.

INDIAN SOLDIERS

In keeping with the army and medical service's own priorities, this discussion of military medicine so far has focused on the European army in India, but what of the Indian Army? The statistical evidence produced in the 1850s and 1860s suggested that the health of Indian soldiers was greatly superior to that of their European counterparts, a finding which encouraged a generally complacent view of Indian health and mortality. Martin referred in 1856 to the "remarkable condition of health" apparently enjoyed by Indian soldiers, especially when compared with the dire record of European health.[79] Lower levels of sickness and mortality among Indians were attributed to their constitutional adaptation to the climate or to social and cultural characteristics—such as abstinence from alcohol—which contrasted with the Europeans' "indulgence" in food and drink. Given the large part played by sexually transmitted and alcohol-related diseases in the European army, Indian soldiers were indeed probably better off.

Indians might have enjoyed better health for other reasons, too. In South Asia's pathogen-rich environment, Indians were likely to have experienced childhood exposure, and hence acquired subsequent immunity, to a number of diseases—such as enteric fever—which wreaked such havoc among Europeans in India. But as the century progressed, as the empire expanded into new disease environments, as army recruitment policies changed to draw heavily upon selected "martial races," so Indian soldiers, too, began to face many of the kinds of "relocation costs"—to use Philip Curtin's phrase—previously incurred by Europeans. In one of the best-documented instances of this, Gurkhas, stationed far from their homes in Nepal, were found to suffer from enteric fever and venereal diseases like their European comrades-in-arms, and for much the same sociological and epidemiological reasons.[80]

But it is important to be wary of the statistical record, especially as far as Indian soldiers are concerned. The stark comparisons made between the health of European and Indian soldiers in the 1850s and 1860s were in many ways misleading, reflecting preconceptions of greater European vulnerability and a relative ignorance of the actual state of Indian health even within the privileged confines of the army. Indian soldiers formed a far less medicalized and hospitalized community than their European counterparts. In the 1830s there were three surgeon-doctors for each regiment of white soldiers, but only one for each Indian regiment.[81] Many cantonments had a "native hospital," but it was smaller and flimsier than its European counterpart, and it accommodated fewer patients. In the 1830s at Mirat (Meerut), one of the principal cantonments of northern India, the military hospital for a European force of 400 men had four wards, including one reserved for soldiers' wives and another for contagious diseases, with 12 to 14 beds in each, and a medical staff of eight, including a European surgeon and his assistant. The hospital for the station's 1,500 Indian soldiers, located in the same compound, was barely a fifth of the size. It had only one 14-bed ward, with four "native doctors" and a dresser. Between January 1833 and June 1837, 1,557 European soldiers were admitted to the hospital in Mirat (of whom 43 died) compared with 851 Indians (26 died).[82]

The hospital in which the Indian soldier was treated before World War I was not even a "dieted institution." The equipment was likely to consist, "at the best, of beds, mattresses, and pillows, a small stock of blankets, a pair of medical panniers, and a somewhat scanty supply of medical and surgical necessities." Hospital clothing was not provided, nor were there any fans or punkahs. The patient brought his own bedding and clothing. He was expected to subsist on his rations, "supplemented by such medical comforts as were specially ordered for him." These conditions substantially changed only after 1914.[83]

Given the violent purges, venesections, and mercurials favored by Western medical practitioners in early nineteenth-century India, which appear to have had such a deleterious effect on the health of European soldiers (but which were more rarely employed on Indian patients), Indian soldiers were probably fortunate to have escaped more active medical attention before the 1850s. Indian soldiers might have profited from neglect in a second respect, too. Instead of being housed in barracks, like European soldiers, they were allocated vacant ground on which to erect their own huts; they were also given an allowance (*batta*) to purchase and prepare their own food. Thus, they were spared the ill-ventilated, overcrowded, and insanitary barracks and the common messes in which epidemics of cholera spread so rapidly among European troops and caused such heavy mortality.[84]

But it is likely, too, that because less importance was attached to

Indian soldiers' health, a great deal of morbidity (recorded in the form of hospital admissions) simply passed unreported. One possible illustration is the much lower rate of venereal disease recorded among Indian than British troops. This may, indeed, reflect social and cultural differences, particularly the fact that many Indian soldiers lived in the army lines with their wives and families, while among Europeans, as we have seen, this was rare. But it is easy to exaggerate the difference. The point was made in the 1880s that "in India it is notorious that native soldiers are rarely examined for venereal diseases, though they trade with the same women as the Europeans."[85] Since it was European health that was the focus of military and medical concern, the incidence of Indian infection (though likely to have been lower than the Europeans') could well have been considerably underreported. European soldiers were relatively expensive to recruit, train, and maintain: Indians were cheaper, a more readily available—and hence more expendable—commodity. Sepoys suffering from chronic diseases were more easily discharged from the army than white soldiers and their deaths omitted from the list of fatalities.

As the century advanced, the material disadvantages of Indian soldiers became more evident. Frail huts of bamboo and matting afforded scant protection against monsoon rains and the cold weather months: not surprisingly, Indians suffered far more than Europeans from rheumatism, pneumonia, bronchitis, pleurisy, and other respiratory infections. The far greater sickness and mortality among Indian than European soldiers in the influenza epidemics of 1890 and 1918–19 (in which pneumonia was a common complication) was one indication of their greater susceptibility to viral and respiratory infections.[86] The inadequate diets of Indian soldiers might also have contributed to their poor health. Paid a fixed allowance for their food, they tended to be insufficiently compensated when grain prices rose sharply in times of shortage and incipient famine. Like the civilian population, they felt the pinch of hunger and even occasionally participated in food riots.[87] Attempting to feed their families as well as themselves left them malnourished, weakened, and further exposed to disease. The health of Indian soldiers thus reflected the fortunes of the agrarian economy and the prevalence of epidemic disease much more than did the Europeans'. Debilitating conditions that were rare among British soldiers—beriberi, guinea worm, and hookworm—

further indicated the way in which disease tended to reflect material as well as cultural circumstances.[88]

The relative neglect of Indian soldiers and the privileging of European health represents, in part, the replication within the army of a ruling bias and a racial prioritizing that was evident in colonial society as a whole. In this respect the army was typical, not exceptional. And, as in that wider society, colonial indifference toward, or neglect of, Indian health was strengthened and rationalized by indigenous resistance, or at least by the expectation of Indian resistance. The Indian Army revealed a deeply paradoxical situation. In some ways it epitomized the strength of the colonial regime's authority over its indigenous subjects and the highly effective incorporation of Indian military manpower into a vast system of imperial control. Indian soldiers played a critical part in the establishment and the maintenance of colonial rule in South Asia and in the wider world. Equally, it was the imposition of a European system of military discipline and order (with the accompanying drill, uniforms, regular pay, and white officer corps) which first distinguished the English (and, briefly, French) sepoy regiments from the kinds of armies previously known in South Asia.

And yet the army also epitomized many of the intrinsic weaknesses of colonial rule. The soldiers resisted some of the more extreme or culturally threatening forms of regimentation and bodily colonization. The mutiny which broke out at Vellore in south India in 1806 was partly inspired by officers' attempts to make sepoys look more like European soldiers by removing their caste marks and replacing their turbans with hats and leather cockades. The Mutiny of 1857, with its "greased cartridges," was a further and still more persuasive demonstration that Indian soldiers would not simply accept whatever their white officers ordered them to do.[89]

These eruptions of military discontent—and the degree of civilian support they seemed capable of commanding—encouraged the conviction that the preservation of British power in India was best served by respecting Indians' religious beliefs and social practices as far as these were compatible with military discipline and order. This cautious and conservative approach was duly reflected in medical and sanitary practice. Measures that might be deemed appropriate, even imperative, among European soldiers were often thought unsuitable among Indian soldiers for fear of offending caste and religion, stirring up discontent, or goading them to mutiny.[90]

Thus, the general unwillingness of Indian soldiers to seek Western medical attention was compounded—at least until the last third of the nineteenth century—by the relative indifference of the medical and military authorities and by a pragmatic policy of nonintervention or noncoercion toward them. According to the report of the Royal Commission on the Sanitary State of the Army in 1863, the Indian soldier had "an instinctive horror of barracks" and retired "from duty to the lines, where he finds his hut, into which not even the doctor dares to penetrate. The sepoy there is free; his hut is his home."[91] John Murray, describing conditions in the Mirat cantonment twenty years earlier, also noted that "natives generally have an aversion to entering hospital. Those not obliged to attend regular regimental duty seldom apply for advice, till their diseases are far advanced."[92] The virtual ban on conducting postmortems on Indian soldiers was a further sign of caution, as was a reluctance to subject them to anything which might smack of medical experimentation. By contrast, European soldiers, alive or dead, were one of the mainstays of medical research in India.

But there were exceptions to this noninterventionist policy. Vaccination against smallpox became compulsory for Indian Army recruits by the 1860s and was even extensively practiced among their families by the 1890s. Perhaps it was accepted less as a medical measure than as a "mark" (*tika*) of service under the British.[93] In fact, open resistance to medical and sanitary measures by Indian soldiers was rare. Evasion and rumor were more common. When they were ill, Indian soldiers turned to the practitioners of various forms of indigenous medicine in the neighboring towns and bazaars or followed their own folk and religious remedies.[94]

But, as the century progressed and memories of 1857 receded, Indian soldiers became more fully integrated into the colonial system of military medicine and, if only as a spin-off from measures designed primarily to protect European health, they became increasingly subject to the new skills and techniques of Western medicine. To vaccination against smallpox were added, by the early 1900s, inoculation against typhoid and plague and prophylactic doses of quinine. Many of these procedures to which Indians were now subjected would have been thought, a few decades earlier, likely to incur dangerous opposition. Moreover, the army authorities were becoming more interventionist in other ways affecting the welfare of Indian soldiers. By 1900 Indian soldiers were being moved out of their huts into barracks built for that purpose, and despite some opposition, they were being fed in army messes rather than left to fend for themselves in regimental lines.[95] In time, as the medicalization of the Indian Army progressed, returning soldiers might even have been an important agency for the dissemination of Western medical ideas and practices, especially in the towns and villages of the Punjab, the province from which a large proportion of the late nineteenth-century army was recruited.[96]

The growing power of military medicine over the lives of Indian and British soldiers was aptly reflected in the following official account published shortly after World War I:

> The object aimed at is to maintain in the soldier a high standard of physical health and fitness, and to increase his powers of resisting disease. For this reason, the medical services are required to concern themselves with every department of the soldier's life, with the climatic and hygienic conditions of the cantonments in which the troops are stationed, with the hygienic suitability of the barracks in which the soldier lives, with the clothes he is required to wear, the equipment that he is required to carry, the quality and composition of the ration which he is given to eat, and with the character and degree of the physical training which he is required to undergo.[97]

OUT OF THE ENCLAVE?

Where, then, does this history of expanding medical responsibility and authority within the army leave relations between the military and civilian society in India? The discussion so far has tended to reinforce a broadly enclavist argument by stressing the way in which many of the army's medical problems and their solutions were seen to be sui generis and to require greater or more effective segregation between the sanitized oasis of the cantonment and the disease environment outside. The apparent success of this enclavism is illustrated by declining mortality rates within the army at a time when epidemics of malaria, cholera, plague, influenza, and other diseases were causing heavy, and rising, mortality in civilian society.

But it would be easy to exaggerate the perceived or practical isolation of military medicine. It was very evident to the sanitary reformers of the 1850s and 1860s that the health of the army could not be guaranteed merely by improving conditions within the barracks. The point was made by Dr. Sutherland in the résumé he prepared for the Royal Commission on the Sanitary State of the Army in India:

At almost every station the sanitary condition of the native population is intimately connected with the sanitary condition of the troops. The two are bound up together so closely that the sanitary improvement of the army must involve one of two courses, either the removal of the troops away from the civil population, or the sanitary improvement of stations, as one part of the sanitary improvement of native cities and towns, and of the country.[98]

That army and civilian health were "intimately connected" was a view shared by the Royal Commission as a whole and featured prominently in its report. It was also a position formally accepted by the Government of India. When the secretary of state for India wrote in 1863 urging the appointment of provincial sanitary commissioners to carry out the recommendations of the Royal Commission, the Government of India dutifully replied that while the "diminution of mortality in the army and the improvement generally of its sanitary state was the primary object which the Government had in view," it also understood that "the full improvement in the health of the European troops . . . would not be brought about by measures solely directed to the amelioration of the sanitary condition of the soldier as such" and that "the interests of the community at large were as much concerned as those of the army."[99]

It was, however, one thing formally to acknowledge an "intimate" connection and quite another to make the financial commitments and forge the institutional structures necessary to extend to civilians the benefits of the medical and sanitary reforms being effected within the army. And it was here that the Government of India and the administrations of the constituent provinces proved, over the next thirty years, to be generally negligent. Even when measures of "public health" were introduced—such as the Contagious Diseases Act of 1868 or the Vaccination Acts a decade later—they barely concealed a continuing preoccupation with the health of Europeans, especially soldiers.

Another way in which what happened in the barracks was related to civilian life outside was through the moral argument, more fervently voiced by Florence Nightingale in London than by the medical profession in India, that sanitation *was* civilization. In her view, it was a terrible blight on Britain's record as a civilized nation that its soldiers lived in India in conditions of disease, intemperance, and squalor. But she equally believed that Britain had a civilizing and sanitizing mission that extended beyond its own soldiers to India's "native" population. In May 1863, as the labors of the Sanitary Commission drew wearily to a close, Nightingale reflected: "This is the dawn of a new day for India in sanitary things, not only as regards our Army, but as regards the native population." In an address in October that year, she described India as "the focus of epidemics" and the home of cholera. It was a land of "domestic filth," a place where plague and pestilence were "the ordinary state of things." The vital question, then, was "no less an one than this: How to create a public health department for India; how to bring a higher civilization into India." A year later, in September 1864, she wrote to Sir John Lawrence, the new viceroy of India and a trusted ally in the fight against disease, "you are conquering India anew by civilization, taking possession of the Empire for the first time by knowledge instead of by the sword."[100] Nightingale's practical impact upon sanitary policy and medical ideas in India was not as great as her admirers have liked to believe. But in linking health and sanitation with civilization, with the wider purpose and moral legitimacy of British rule in India, she was giving voice to sentiments that were shared by many medical and sanitary officers in India.

MEDICINE'S PRISON DOMAIN

Apart from the army, the prison was one of the few areas where the colonial state had direct access to the body of its Indian subjects. Indeed, prison life involved a degree of state regulation in such matters as accommodations and diet not to be found in the Indian Army until the very end of the nineteenth century. And yet in the prisons, as in the army, medicine only gradually acquired a position of authority.

The history of medical involvement in colonial penology dates effectively from the 1830s. In 1838 a committee, appointed by the Government of India to report on jail discipline, proposed the reform of Indian prisons along broadly Benthamite lines. But, significantly, the fourteen members of the committee did not include a single doctor, and medical authorities were not consulted in its inquiry. Although the health of prisoners was one of the issues discussed, questions of sickness, diet, and medical care were subordinated to the need for stricter discipline and more effective control of prison inmates.[101] A report on the "medical management of the native jails," prepared in 1835 by James Hutchinson, secretary of the Bengal Medical Board, had previously revealed the alarming extent of sickness and mortality and argued that it was morally indefensible for a "humane" and "civilized" government to allow, as was often the case, a short sentence of imprisonment to become—through the neglect of prisoners' health—in effect a sentence of death.[102] But Hutchinson's report (and a second edition published in 1845 in the wake of the Prison Discipline Committee) went largely unheeded, and the unfavorable comparison he made between Indian mortality in the army and the jails was casually brushed aside.[103]

One reason for this was that the judiciary, then largely responsible for prison administration in India, was not professionally interested in prisoners' health. Judges and magistrates believed that prisons should be made more deterrent and not provide conditions in any way superior to those endured by the poorest classes outside. Improving prisoners' diet, accommodations, and general conditions of health was seen to run counter to this deterrent strategy.[104]

An additional factor was the lowly status of civil surgeons and their limited influence over how prisons were run. Thirty years later, R. T. Lyons, an assistant surgeon with the Bengal Army, blamed the sickness and mortality which prevailed in Indian prisons before the 1860s on the magistrates and judges who, he said, ignored medical advice and drew their own unscientific conclusions about prison conditions. According to Lyons:

> The teachings of medical science were disdained by the judicial administrators; and the opinions of medical officers . . . were held in scorn. The status formerly allotted to the civil surgeon was inferior, as it would appear that he was regarded less as a public officer than as a member of the household of the judge's wife. This low estimate of his position weakened his influence in the official atmosphere. From neglect of the precepts of the medical sciences, and from erroneous considerations, arose the system of prison economy which fills a sad page in the history of the administration of former days.[105]

In the mid 1850s, however, the situation began to change. Under the influence of prison reform in Britain, and as part of wider changes in the administrative and judicial structure of colonial rule in India, new central jails were constructed (with London's Pentonville prison as their model) to replace the old, disease-ridden, and crumbling local lockups. Separate jail departments were established in the provinces, and in the absence of a professional prison service, IMS doctors were appointed as jail superintendents or became provincial inspectors-general. The latters' responsibilities, as stated in the Bombay prison legislation of 1856, encompassed the "internal economy, discipline, and management of jails." The larger prisons also had their own medical officers, whose wide-ranging duties (as in the army) included disciplinary, as well as specifically medical, functions.[106]

Previously shunned, from the 1860s onward members of the IMS were appointed to serve on several committees of inquiry into prison conditions and had an influential voice in their deliberations and recommendations, particularly on matters of diet, accommodation, and disciplinary punishments. Just as high mortality in the European army provoked official concern in the 1850s and 1860s and gave medical men new responsibilities and opportunities to carry out sanitary reforms, so at approximately the same time prison health was also coming under official scrutiny and gave fresh scope for medical zeal and sanitary action. In 1864 high death rates in the prisons forced the Government of India to appoint an inquiry committee, which, unlike the Prison Discipline committee eighteen years earlier, included medical personnel. It was followed in 1877 by an Indian Jails Conference, in which medical authorities again played a prominent part, and in 1889 by a two-man committee of inquiry into jail administration consisting of Dr. W. Walker, surgeon-general and sanitary commissioner with the Government of India, and Surgeon-Major A. S. Lethbridge, inspector-general of prisons for Bengal. Although the colonial administration undoubtedly regarded the health of prisoners as a matter of far less urgency and importance than that of European soldiers, many medical officers held a strong conviction that high levels of sickness and mortality were no more acceptable in the jails than in the army—and no less amenable to medical and sanitary measures.

The health of prisoners, announced F. J. Mouat in 1856, shortly after his appointment as inspector of jails for Bengal, was "a matter of very grave and serious importance." In words which echoed Hutchinson's remarks twenty years earlier and amounted to a personal manifesto for prison reform, Mouat declared that "no practice regarding convicts is justifiable, which would render an imprisonment of three or five years equivalent to a sentence of death, upon a large proportion of those convicted of crimes not deserving of so severe a punishment." There was at present a "large amount of preventible mortality" in the jails of Bengal: hence, his "great anxiety on the subject."[107]

Mouat came to the prison service after an already distinguished medical career: he had recently been professor of medicine at Calcutta's Medical College and was the author of an *Atlas of Anatomical Plates of the Human Body* (with descriptions in Hindustani), as well as a highly critical report on mortality among indentured laborers traveling to the West Indies.[108] He was not, therefore, a man likely to keep his opinions quietly to himself. During his long term of office (he retired in 1869), Mouat insisted upon the special qualifications and responsibilities of the medical profession for the superintendence, management, and discipline of India's prison population. He protested when (as on a visit to Alipur Jail in Calcutta in 1855) he found that slack attendance to duty by medical officers had serious consequences for prisoners' health. He campaigned energetically for better diets (an issue we return to later in this chapter) and in the end had some success in forcing the government to listen to him, and he asserted the right of medical officers to decide the appropriate form prisoners' work tasks and disciplinary punishments should take. "Refractory prisoners, those confined for murder and the graver crimes, and all of whom examples require to be made," he stated in the 1850s, "should be put upon the severest labour their health will bear." But he added: "The only limit to each task should be the physical endurance and health of the prisoners" and "to regulate these, the advice of the medical officer in charge of the jail is always available."[109] In Mouat's view, then, medical officers were to be the prime movers alike in penal policy and in penal practice: health was the principal criterion by which prison discipline and efficiency should be judged.

This was not a view the government, or even other medical officers, necessarily shared. A half-century after Mouat, the Indian Jails Committee of 1919–20 found some IMS officers as enthusiastic as he had been about the unique qualifications of doctors to be prison superintendents. Major H. P. Cameron, the Madras inspector-general of prisons, said in his evidence that the IMS officer (he was one himself) was "peculiarly suited" to run a jail: "He is a trained scientist with expert knowledge in military law, organization, administration, sanitation, psychiatry and tropical medicine." He dismissed suggestions that there was no work for a medical man in jail as "arrant nonsense. Not only is there plenty of clinical work, but a jail provides ideal scope for research work and the practice of preventive medicine."[110] Other witnesses, however, presented a rather different picture. Lieutenant-Colonel Fearnside, formerly superintendent of Coimbatore Jail, said that an IMS officer who was "found to be of no use in the Medical Department" was shunted off to the Jails Department instead.[111]

Clearly, not every IMS officer was an enthusiast for the kinds of research opportunities a jail provided or felt particularly qualified to manage prison inmates. Some felt tainted by the criminal associations of the prison. Prison work burdened busy doctors with extra duties— without the financial compensation of private practice. Some civil surgeons neglected their jails or made merely perfunctory visits. Lieutenant-Colonel John Mulvaney, previously superintendent of Alipur Jail, dubbed the Jails Department "the Cinderella of the Indian medical service" and claimed that "in most cases" the duties of civil surgeons in district jails were "whittled down to the automatic signing of documents, an occasional tour of the jail, and a hurried examination of the more serious cases in hospital, the whole occupying, on an average, perhaps 15 minutes." He also asserted that nine-tenths of the work was done through an interpreter, further emphasizing the superintendent's remoteness from the day-to-day management of the jail. Indeed, Mulvaney, whose experience had left him bitterly disillusioned, claimed that the internal management of the jail was largely in the hands of the convicts themselves (especially the convict warders) and that "in very many instances" the regulations laid down in the Indian jail code were simply "a dead letter." "The moral condition of the convicts was deplorable" and discipline could be maintained only by "repressive severity."[112]

HEALTH IN THE JAILS

Nonetheless, the prison was an important site of medical observation and control, if only because the rest of Indian society was otherwise relatively inaccessible to colonial power and knowledge.[113] At a time when most of India lay beyond any kind of medical and statistical purview, prisoners could be classified and counted, and by the 1830s and 1840s data were being compiled for the prisons, as for the army, showing the number of hospital admissions, the principal causes of sickness and death, and the rates of morbidity and mortality among prisoners in particular jails.

Remarkably, the exceptional nature of prison conditions was often overlooked in this early period, and prisons were taken as a guide to the prevalent diseases and general state of health of the civilian population. In his discussion of epidemic cholera in Bengal in 1820, James Jameson remarked that prison statistics provided "a pretty good criterion by which to judge of the health of their respective districts," a view shared by F. P. Strong in the 24 Parganas district of Bengal in the 1830s.[114] By mid-century, however, evidence was accumulating, as in the army, to show the full extent of prison mortality, especially during epidemics of cholera and malaria and in times of dearth. It was noted, for instance, in 1866, a famine year, that the level of mortality inside the prisons of the Madras Presidency was four times greater than that recorded for the outside population: 100, as against 25, deaths per 1,000.[115]

The relatively small size of the prison population in nineteenth-century India made the collection and analysis of statistical data a manageable task. In 1838 the prison population of British India was stated to be 56,632 out of a total of 91.5 million people.[116] But since there was some confusion about how the statistics should be compiled—particularly whether undertrial prisoners should be included—this figure is doubtless unreliable. By 1880, when we are on firmer statistical ground, the prison population had risen to 106,763, almost double the 1838 figure, but still a tiny fraction of India's total population. In Bengal and Madras, prisoners constituted less than 0.1 percent of the population. In 1914 there were 114,113 prisoners in India (including the penal settlement at Port Blair in the Andaman islands), and with mounting political unrest, numbers began to rise substantially thereafter.[117] Women and Europeans formed only a small part of the prison population.

Apart from changes in the law, in the organization of the police, and in sentencing policy of the courts, two factors governed the size of the prison population during the nineteenth century. One was the prodigious mortality. In the first sixty years of the century, annual death rates not infrequently reached 25 percent: a quarter of all the prisoners in a jail might perish in a single year. As in the army, cholera, malaria, dysentery, and diarrhea were the main causes of

Table 6. Sickness in Bengal Jails, 1863–92

Period	Average daily numbers	Average daily sick	Daily sick per 1,000
1863–67	19,997	766	46.7
1868–72	18,338	651	35.4
1873–77	20,670	777	37.5
1878–82	17,464	883	50.6
1883–87	14,239	683	45.7
1888–92	15,254	641	42.1
1863–92	17,329	733	42.3

Source: *IMG* 1893, 28, 293.

death. In Mangalore Jail in 1838, 151 out of 263 prisoners (57 percent) died in a single year, more than half of them from cholera; at Mirat Jail during the cholera epidemic of 1861 (which so badly affected British soldiers and their families), mortality among prisoners soared to 62 percent. In the prisons of Bengal 40,550 deaths from disease (more than a fifth of them from cholera) were recorded in the quarter-century between 1843 and 1867, though this was equivalent to no more than 8.2 percent of the total number of prisoners during that period.[118] Even after the 1860s, as tables 6 and 7 show for Bengal, levels of sickness and mortality remained extremely high, with cholera retaining a place among the leading causes of mortality.

Another factor which affected both the size of prison populations and the prisoners' health was the occurrence of food shortages and famines. High grain prices, loss of agrarian employment, and fear of imminent starvation caused a sharp rise in rural crime levels, and these in turn swelled prison populations, sometimes by as much as a third their normal size.[119] Because of the debilitated state of under-trial prisoners and convicts, cholera and dysentery spread quickly among them or were rapidly communicated from the new arrivals to other prisoners. In Bengal there were clear peaks of jail mortality in 1866 (when, following famine in Orissa, prison numbers rose to 20,633, and there were 684 cholera deaths among 2,223 fatalities from all causes) and again in 1876, when the same deadly combination of famine and cholera resulted in 1,242 deaths, 975 of them from cholera.[120]

Table 7. Mortality in Bengal Jails, 1863–92

	Cholera deaths	Other causes	Total deaths	Cholera deaths per 1,000	Other deaths per 1,000	All deaths per 1,000
1863–67	315	1,060	1,370	17.1	58.1	75.2
1868–72	125	756	880	6.6	41.2	47.8
1873–77	157	909	1,067	6.5	43.8	51.2
1878–82	165	1,106	1,271	9.2	63.2	72.4
1883–87	68	598	666	4.6	41.6	46.2
1888–92	83	521	604	5.6	34.2	39.6
1863–92	152	824	976	8.8	47.8	56.3

Source: IMG 1893, 28, 293.

"There can be no question that the excessive death-rate in Indian jails is a great reproach," remarked J. M. Cuningham, the Government of India's sanitary commissioner in 1880, but he had few ideas to offer as to how an average annual death rate of more than 50 per 1,000 could be brought down to more acceptable levels.[121] The kinds of improvements made in the barracks were slow to affect sickness and mortality in the jails. It was more difficult to isolate the prison from the epidemics and famines that raged outside; sanitary conditions were even more primitive in the prisons than in the army barracks; and the state was more reluctant to invest in prisoners' health than in that of European, or even Indian, soldiers. Although, as in the army, cholera gradually declined, malaria and dysentery remained major causes of sickness and death until World War I. Tuberculosis, a disease which reflected the persistent problem of prison overcrowding, was increasingly prevalent. There was criticism, too, that prison hospitals were failing to keep pace with standards of hygiene and medical care outside. In 1919 Mulvaney described Bengal's jails as "more deadly to live in than the notoriously insanitary towns of the province," and he gave a graphic account of conditions in a jail hospital:

> Here, perhaps, we see a patient in the throes of tenesmus, squatting on the floor and trying, supported by his nurse, to ease himself of his bloody flux, for bed-pans are infrequent. There again, may be, is a patient awaiting the busy *mehtar* to cleanse him of the excrement in which he has lain, possibly half the night. And here again is the wasted form of a chronic dysenteric, his back riddled with bed-sores from the iron laths of his comfortless bed, filthy to a degree, his lips covered with sores, his face by flies, and his body smeared with excrement. . . . Why seek for higher causes of jail mortality?[122]

Prison mortality *was* falling—in 1910 it stood at 21.6 per 1,000 prisoners for the whole of India—but that was still five times higher than in the Indian Army. In 1913 prison mortality in mainland India reached its lowest recorded level of 15.5 per 1,000, but that was still a level unknown in the army since the early 1880s (see table 8).[123]

Given the grim plethora of sickness and disease in the jails and the close involvement of medical officers in their administration, it is not surprising that the prisons became important sites of medical observation and experimentation. This phenomenon was not unique to colo-

Table 8. Hospital Admissions and Deaths in Indian Jails, 1910*
(per 1,000)

	Admissions	Deaths
Cholera	0.4	0.21
Smallpox	0.2	0.03
Enteric fever	0.8	0.22
Malaria	231.5	1.37
Pyrexia of uncertain origin	8.8	0.05
Tubercule of the lung	9.4	3.98
Pneumonia	11.9	3.08
Respiratory diseases	30.3	0.89
Influenza	1.8	—
Dysentery	62.3	3.90
Diarrhea	35.6	0.73
Anemic debility	9.7	0.47
Abscess, ulcer, boil	58.8	—
All causes (including others not listed)	663.8	21.62

*Including Burma and the Andamans.
Source: *India SCAR 1910*, 87.

nial India, but because of the continuing paucity of statistical and clinical information about disease among the Indian population in general and the cultural and political obstacles to physical access to the body of the colonized elsewhere in Indian society, the prison occupied a position of exceptional prominence and importance.[124] Thus, early accounts of cholera and dysentery, like later studies of enteric fever, cerebrospinal fever, tuberculosis, kala-azar, and ankylostomiasis (hookworm infestation) drew heavily upon the observation of prison populations. The investigation of many of these conditions was of particular significance because they were common among plantation workers, and so their identification and treatment had important economic consequences, especially for the European tea planters of northeastern India.[125]

Within the confines of the prison, observations could be made, and experiments conducted, that were judged to be impractical or impolitic elsewhere. For instance, given the extreme difficulty colonial physicians encountered in obtaining corpses for dissection and the intensity of Indian opposition to this practice, the jail was one of the few possible sources for cadavers. A researcher who had access to the corpses of Indian prisoners considered himself particularly fortunate.[126] By the 1860s it was standard practice to conduct a postmortem on every prisoner who died, particularly if there were suspicious circumstances or the cause of death could not otherwise be ascertained. Such a procedure was rare in the Indian Army. The dissection of prisoners was an additional punishment, a medical addendum to the sentence decreed by the courts. Bizarrely, there was even some suggestion that postmortems might have a deterrent effect. The *Bengal Jail Manual* directed that the bodies of prisoners could not be removed from prison until an inquest had been held—so as to "prevent the escape of prisoners from jail by feigning dead."[127]

The prison also made possible trials and experiments with various prophylactic drugs and inoculations. "In no cases are preventive and prophylactic measures so efficacious as among bodies of men so completely under control, as are prisoners in jails," Mouat declared in 1856.[128] Indeed, it was to a great extent possible in prison to ignore or override the cultural and social obstacles that were seen to be the bane of Western medicine elsewhere in India. At a time when vaccination against smallpox still encountered strong resistance and evasion in India, it was compulsory for prisoners. One of the tasks of a prison's medical officer was to inspect new prisoners and determine whether they had previously been vaccinated (or were otherwise protected against smallpox). According to a circular order of the Bengal Government in 1855, all unprotected convicts were to be vaccinated on entering the jail "as a matter of jail discipline."[129] Even a man in the Punjab sent to prison in 1911 for refusing to have his daughter vaccinated found himself compulsorily vaccinated.[130]

Early trials in inoculating against plague, cholera, and typhoid were also carried out on selected (and reputedly voluntary) groups of prisoners during the 1890s and early 1900s. At Gaya Jail in Bihar in 1894, the Russian bacteriologist Waldemar M. Haffkine inoculated 215 out of 433 prisoners against cholera; three years later, in January 1897, roughly half of the inmates of Bombay's House of Correction were inoculated with his experimental antiplague serum. In both cases, the results derived from prisoners (along with plantation workers and soldiers) provided evidence for the safety and effectiveness of these prophylactic measures and their suitability for public use. But the conduct of such experiments, especially in the heightened political atmosphere of the late 1890s, provoked adverse comment and gave rise to suggestions that prisoners' participation had been less than voluntary.[131]

The use of quinine as a prophylactic against malaria (by far the largest single cause of admissions to jail hospitals) was also experimented with because of the facilities jails offered for the administration of strictly regulated doses and careful observation of their effects. At a time when quinine encountered strong public resistance—because of its bitter taste, "heating" effect, and apparently doubtful efficacy—the captive clientele of the prison provided a unique opportunity to show its effectiveness. The drug was first given to prisoners in the late nineteenth century, but its systematic use dates from 1907 when G. F. W. Braide, inspector-general of prisons in the Punjab, directed jail superintendents in the province to give prisoners regular weekly doses of sulphate of quinine during months when malaria was common. Ramadan fell that year during the malarial season, but instructions were issued that Muslim prisoners were not to be omitted but should receive their dose after sundown: "in no case" would the distribution of quinine "be suspended or vigilance over it be relaxed during the period of the fast." Braide attached great importance to adequate and consistent dosage (inconsistent usage was one reason why quinine often appeared ineffective) and urged prison officers to use their authority to ensure that every prisoner "actually receive[d] the exact quantity of the drug fixed by the rules in force at the appointed times."

The following year, 1908, proved to be one of the worst malaria years on record. In the four months from August to November, an estimated 90 percent of the population of Punjab was hit by malaria; 50 percent fell seriously ill. Over four hundred thousand deaths were reported, and the loss of productive labor was so great as to cause the government concern. But Braide's quinine policy seemed to be vindicated because sickness and mortality rates among prisoners were significantly below those of the general population. That 90 percent of the public fell ill, but only 10 percent of prisoners, was cited as proof of the value of quinine prophylaxis, and the public was duly urged to follow the example of the jails.[132]

DISCIPLINE AND DIET

By contrast with the Indian Army, the prisons were an institutional arena in which the state early in the nineteenth century found itself responsible for feeding as well as housing Indians. This raised a series of critical issues: about the relationship between discipline and diet, about the extent to which caste and religion should be recognized within the prison, and about the importance of food as a factor in labor productivity and the physical condition of the Indian population.

Diet was a focus for prisoners' resistance to disciplinary control. In one of the most sustained episodes of this kind, prisoners in the jails of the Bengal Presidency in the early 1840s openly resisted the introduction of a common messing system. Previously, prisoners had been allowed to buy and prepare their own food and were given a money dole by the prison authorities for the purpose. This enabled them not only to follow religious and caste observances relating to the preparation and consumption of food but also to relieve the tedium of prison life by haggling with the traders who came to the jail or by bartering for other commodities. The withdrawal of this right was part of a deliberate policy to tighten the screw of jail discipline and to curb the few freedoms prisoners still enjoyed. In order to make prison life more punitive and deterrent, the government decided that prisoners would only receive food prepared for them by prison cooks and eat it alongside other prisoners, regardless of their caste. This unwelcome innovation sparked protests, hunger strikes, assaults, and eventually rioting, which was suppressed with armed might and bloodshed.[133]

But although resistance had been quelled, these disturbances and others which followed[134] were taken to show the expediency of respecting caste as far as this was compatible with prison economy and discipline. The East India Company's Court of Directors in London remarked that any benefits that might be gained by the messing system were unlikely to be "commensurate with the difficulties and risks attending its introduction." While the directors appreciated "the danger and inexpediency of giving way to insubordination," they felt sure that the Bengal government would not persist in "any measures calculated to excite alarm and discontent as interfering with the religious opinions and feelings of the natives."[135] It was some evidence of administrative willingness to accommodate such "opinions and feelings" that when Mouat visited Bihar jail in 1856 he found 53 cooks preparing food for 504 prisoners. "It is true that the prejudices of caste in Bihar are very strong," he commented, "yet it seems preposterous that men of the same caste cannot take food from the hands of each other, and that every petty sub-division of the same fraternity, should have rules and practices of its own."[136]

For medical officers like Mouat, jail diets were an important scientific as well as disciplinary issue, thus reflecting both aspects of the doctor's dual role within the prison system. Given that remarkably little was known about Indian diets before the late nineteenth century (particularly about the quantities of food consumed), the prison provided a critical site for observation and experimentation of much wider utility. These investigations began as early as the 1840s. In 1846 Dr. A. H. Leith conducted an inquiry into the health of Indian prisoners at Bombay's House of Correction, where levels of sickness and mortality had been persistently high. He found the prison's location and the amount of work exacted from the prisoners unobjectionable, and so focused on the jail's diet, which consisted of rice and dal, plus a little salt and ghee. When, at Leith's suggestion, an improved diet was introduced with an antiscorbutic pickle and wheat flour instead of rice, scurvy disappeared, sickness rates fell, and the weight and general health of prisoners improved.[137]

Critical comments made by Mouat in 1856 following his first tour of inspection on the deficiencies of jail diets in Bengal led to revived interest in the subject. His recommendations for an improved diet met with no immediate response in Calcutta, but in 1861 (after his report had attracted comment in London) the Government of India asked each province to report on the jail diets currently in use and to compare them with those of the laboring population outside (from whom the prison population was largely drawn). The resulting surveys offer some fascinating insights into patterns of food consumption at the time, and it is indicative of the skewed nature of medical and social science in colonial India that this pioneering survey of the food habits of the general population should have arisen out of a (rather reluctant) concern for prison health.[138]

Several further dietary investigations followed, and there was much heated debate and acrimony between medical and prison officers about the quantity of food and the varieties of diet most appropriate for Indian prisoners. Some doctors argued from an economistic and disciplinarian position that the food given to prisoners should not be better than that consumed by the poorest classes outside. Too generous a diet (as they saw it) would make prisoners a privileged class, living in greater comfort and security than men of their class ever enjoyed outside. This would make prison conditions an invitation to crime rather than a deterrent and, in a country where the poor were legion, would involve the state in enormous and unwarranted expense. Diet had to be subservient to the needs of discipline and deterrence.[139]

But others, like Mouat in Bengal and W. R. Cornish, the Madras sanitary commissioner, argued that the health of prisoners should, within reasonable limits, be the prime consideration. The state had an obligation to keep prisoners not merely alive but in a sound physical condition, and this should not be sacrificed by denying them items like fresh vegetables, meat, and ghee essential (from a medical and dietetic viewpoint) for their health. A more varied, nutritious, and substantial diet would support a healthier prison population and thus reduce the cost of medical attention. It would also make prisoners a more reliable and productive labor force, something Mouat, who wanted to turn prisons into industrial workshops, as much to lessen the financial burden on the state as to reform prisoners' lives, was especially keen on.[140]

In fact, prison policy between the 1860s and the 1920s dithered uncertainly between these two positions, with prisoners serving as involuntary guinea pigs for the latest experiments in disciplinary dietetics.[141] But, despite these uncertainties, dietary investigations had an importance beyond the prisons themselves. They provided a standard by which food or money doles were given to those who sought state relief during the frequent famines of the late nineteenth century, providing evidence of how much—more often, how little— food was required to sustain life and labor.[142] Colonial knowledge, born of the prison, thus supplied a standard of wider social and economic utility.

Prison data were also used to make "scientific" pronouncements not only about dietary and physiological differences between Indians and Europeans but also between the inhabitants of different parts of India. In 1912 Professor D. McCay of Calcutta's Medical College contrasted jail diets in Bengal with those in the United Provinces (formerly the North-Western Provinces), then used the results to explain the apparent physical frailty of rice-eating Bengalis compared with the robust and martial manliness of the Sikhs and Rajputs of northwestern India, with their diet of dairy products, wheat, and meat. According to McCay, dietary differences explained why prisoners in UP (and hence the agrarian classes from which they came) were on a "distinctly higher plane of physical development" than those of Bengal.

> The general muscularity of the body is decidedly better and their capabilities of labour are greater. They are smarter on their feet, more brisk and more alive to the incidents of everyday life, and they do not present such slackness and tonelessness as one is accustomed to observe in the people of Lower Bengal.[143]

Despite the narrowness of his evidence, McCay was clearly not thinking of the health and welfare of prison populations alone but also of how dietary "faults" could be corrected to the common advantage of prisoners, peasant cultivators, and the state. In this instance, jail dietaries were taken as indicators of the importance of food (rather than purely cultural, hereditary, or environmental factors) "in the formation and development of those attributes and qualities of mind and body that are alike the pride of the soldier and the envy of inferior races."[144] It seemed no more inappropriate to McCay than to many earlier colonial physicians to read civilian health from convict physiology.

CONCLUSION

The army and the jails of colonial India were exceptional sites of medical observation and control. At a time when the health of the mass of the population was still largely unknown and unexplored, they offered unique opportunities for medical investigation and experimentation. Over the course of the nineteenth century, these enclaves were progressively colonized by Western medical and sanitary practices, and the authority and responsibility of the state's medical service correspondingly increased. In the army, this increased medical activity was impelled by the political and strategic importance of protecting the lives of the European soldiers on whom British power was seen so critically to depend. Although the health of the army could not be detached entirely from the issue of civilian health, the problem was treated to a large extent in isolation from Indian society, just as, within the army, the health of European soldiers received much greater attention than that of Indians. Many of the health problems of the army were seen either to be specific to the force and its European component alone, or best dealt with by transforming cantonments into sanitary "oases" and cutting them off, as much as possible, from the teeming pathogens outside the barrack gates. This exercise in sanitary segregation was fairly successful, as the striking improvements in army sickness and mortality rates showed, especially after the 1890s. Improvements in the health of Indian soldiers were partly a by-product of this European advance; the health of Indian prisoners lagged far behind.

But although both the army and the prisons can be seen as medical and sanitary enclaves, they were not irrelevant to, or unrepresentative of, the broader character and ambitions of Western medicine and colonial rule in India. What happened in the army or the jail was often symptomatic of outside trends. The favoring of Europeans over Indians—in health as in so much else—was a common, almost universal, colonial phenomenon before 1914. Similarly, the increasing incorporation of Indians into the Western system of medicine and public health, despite Indian resistance (or rumors of resistance) closely paralleled wider trends. Pioneering arenas for a variety of statistical and clinical (and, in the case of the prisons, dietary) investigations, the army and even more the jails served as observatories and laboratories for medical ideas and techniques which were ultimately seen to be relevant to the wider population and especially to productive labor. The army and the jails in their different ways constituted exemplary sites, perceived models of how Western medical and sanitary practices might—in theory, at least—be deployed in the wider society.

But what kind of a model or institutional base did military and prison medicine provide? In the Indian Medical Service, the army and jails possessed an agency through which medical expertise could be extended into other spheres, but it was a tiny elite, almost entirely European in composition before 1914 and tied professionally and politically to the state's own needs and priorities. It was no substitute for a more independent, publicly minded medical profession. One impediment in translating military and prison medicine into public health was the inbuilt disposition to see health and sanitation as disciplinary matters, to be imposed by force, if necessary, on an ignorant, superstitious, or simply lethargic population, as part of a top-down, state-driven regime rather than as part of a voluntary, community-based movement of self-help and self-improvement. In such circumstances, the needs of the state, not the wishes of the people, were bound to be paramount. Equally, if caste and religion—the great qualifiers when dealing with Indian society—were understood to be major obstacles to medicalization and sanitation in the prisons and the Indian Army, what prospect was there for the successful introduction of medicine and sanitary reform in society at large? A closer look at the relationship of state medicine with three of the main epidemic diseases of the nineteenth century—smallpox, cholera, and plague—provides some answers.

3 Smallpox: The Body of the Goddess

British physicians in nineteenth-century India ranked smallpox among the most prevalent and destructive of all epidemic diseases. The "scourge of India," smallpox reputedly claimed more victims than "all other diseases combined," its "tenacity and malignity" making it "one of the most violent and severe diseases to which the human race is liable."[1] Smallpox accounted for several million deaths in the late nineteenth century alone, amounting on average to more than one hundred thousand fatal cases a year.

But it was not just the prodigious mortality caused by smallpox that made it appear an exceptionally menacing disease: there was also the horrific nature of the disease itself. An acute contagious viral infection, smallpox (*Variola major*) produced an intense, burning fever, followed by multiple cutaneous eruptions and pustules which clustered thickest on the face and limbs, but in the most extreme, confluent, form covered almost every inch of the body's surface. A third or more of those seized by smallpox died, usually within two weeks of the first symptoms of the disease. But even those who escaped death were likely to be disfigured or incapacitated for the rest of their lives—their faces transformed into pockmarked lunar landscapes, the sight in one or both eyes dimmed or destroyed through ulceration of the cornea. Some authorities attributed three-quarters of all blindness in India to the effects of smallpox.[2]

In the absence of adequate statistical data before the 1870s, it is impossible to gauge the full extent of the devastation caused by this disease. In Calcutta, a city of more than a third of a million people, mortality from smallpox was put at 11,000 between 1837 and 1851

(6,100 deaths occurring during the epidemic of 1849–50 alone), with a further 9,549 deaths between 1851 and 1869.[3] By the later decades of the century, when more reliable and comprehensive mortality statistics were being compiled, the full extent of the ravages of smallpox became evident, though as vaccination became more widespread and effective, mortality from the disease began to decline appreciably (see table 9).

A similar downward trend is indicated in table 10, but here it can be seen that there were marked differences in mortality between one quinquennium and another, reflecting the incidence of major epidemics, and between one administrative area and another (particularly between "well-vaccinated" provinces, like the North-Western Provinces, Bombay, and Madras, and Bengal, with its record of "continual failure"[4]).

Some of the most telling evidence for the prevalence of smallpox in nineteenth-century India is, however, circumstantial rather than statistical. Pringle in 1869 estimated that in the populous Doab, between the Ganges and Yamuna rivers of northern India, as many as ninety-five percent of the population were exposed to smallpox at some stage of life. Examination of prisoners, schoolchildren, and laborers in the 1870s in northern and eastern India largely confirmed this impression. Since smallpox erupted epidemically roughly every five to seven years in most parts of India, its principal victims were children born since the previous epidemic. So common was the disease in northern India, Pringle maintained, that "it has become quite a saying among the agricultural and even wealthier classes never to count children as permanent members of the family until they have been attacked with and recovered from smallpox."[5] In a similar vein, Sir Sayyid Ahmad Khan, introducing a bill for compulsory vaccination in the Viceroy's Legislative Council in 1879, said that smallpox was

> the inevitable bridge which every child has to cross before entering into life; and recovery from the disease is considered second birth. . . . Other diseases are looked upon as accidental; but small-pox is regarded, as indeed it is, [as] almost universal. It touches the keenest of human susceptibilities; for there are thousands in this country who, though spared by it from death, still have traces of its violence in the deep marks on the face or the loss of an eye.[6]

Table 9. Smallpox Mortality and Vaccination in British India, 1871–1900

	Average annual number of smallpox deaths	Smallpox deaths per 1,000 population	Average annual number of successful vaccinations
1871–80	168,964	0.93	3,951,709
1881–90	121,680	0.63	5,024,352
1891–1900	81,233	0.38	6,778,624

Source: Imperial Gazetteer 1907, 525.

Table 10. Average Annual Smallpox Deaths, 1875–1904 (per million)

	Bengal	North-Western Provinces	Punjab	Bombay	Central Provinces	Madras	British India
1875–79	196	1,704	1,430	590	1,848	1,428	976
1880–84	280	1,782	550	376	490	1,000	804
1885–89	98	482	632	218	856	860	410
1890–94	208	440	334	152	158	960	430
1895–99	204	580	774	172	420	438	432
1900–04	438	152	532	262	440	600	392

Source: Leonard 1926, 4.

A disease so widely prevalent, so destructive of human life, and so fearful in its physical manifestations could not but impress itself forcefully upon the minds of Indians and Europeans and have a profound impact upon their conceptualization of disease. One route to comprehending and gaining some form of control over smallpox lay through religion. Understood as a divine presence rather than as a disease, smallpox occupied a prominent place in Hindu beliefs and rituals: the goddess Sitala and other deities identified with smallpox were worshipped and propitiated in virtually every part of the country. A second route, not incompatible with the first and acknowledging Sitala's rights over the body, was through variolation, inoculation with live smallpox matter to produce a controlled and moderated form of the disease and so protect the individual against subsequent attack. A third path, vaccination, introduced into India by the British in the early nineteenth century, went further in the preemption of natural smallpox through prophylactic intervention, by using cowpox vaccine rather than live smallpox matter. But vaccination did more than substitute one regulatory technique for another. For whereas variolation was commonly seen as a religious act as well as an effective means of prevention, vaccination was secular in character and alien in origin, representing a significant extension of state power over the individual and community.

Although Western medicine could no more cure smallpox than could its Indian counterparts, the advent of vaccination encouraged British physicians to see smallpox as a preventable disease—at a time when the control of most other major diseases lay beyond their therapeutic grasp. Because of its relative simplicity and cheapness and because it at first appeared to be such an unequivocal demonstration of the effectiveness of Western medicine, vaccination was taken up by the colonial state and became emblematic of its self-declared humanity and benevolence toward the people of India. And yet, despite what the British saw as vaccination's indisputable benefits and despite the importance initially attached to it, vaccination was slow to gain public acceptance or to be practiced on a sufficient scale to have a marked effect on smallpox mortality. It took almost the whole of the nineteenth century for vaccination to become established as an acceptable form of mass prophylaxis in India, and a further seventy-five years beyond that before the dreaded disease was finally eradicated.

At one level, vaccination can be seen as a remarkable demonstration of the interventionist ambitions and capabilities of Western medicine in India. By the closing decades of British rule, vaccination and revaccination were being performed on an enormous scale. In the province of Madras alone between 1936 and 1945 there were, on average, 4.3 million vaccinations a year, equivalent to almost 10 percent of the population. In 1947, the year of Britain's departure, 21.3 million vaccinations and revaccinations were performed throughout the whole country.[7] Medical activity on such a scale suggests a high level of administrative commitment as well as a fair degree of public acceptance. But, as this chapter will show, vaccination was held back not just by the strength of indigenous opposition and rival systems of belief and prophylaxis but also by technical difficulties and the reluctance of the colonial state to take on the political and financial burden of mass vaccination.

GODDESS OF SMALLPOX

Across northern India, from Sind and Gujarat in the west, through northern and central India to Bengal, Assam, and Orissa in the east, smallpox was identified with a goddess known generally as Sitala but also simply but expressively called Mata, "Mother." In some areas "sitala" was the name given both to the disease and to the deity who presided over it. In Bengal she was sometimes called Basanta or Basanta-chandi (spring goddess) and the disease *basanta rog* (spring disease), after the season in which smallpox was most prevalent and in which the goddess was most widely celebrated.[8] Sitala did not appear in the original Hindu pantheon, and her probable origins were as a folk deity who only gradually and partially found recognition in Brahminical Hinduism.

William Crooke in the 1890s included her among Hinduism's lesser and more rustic divinities as a "godling of disease." In so doing, Crooke echoed the earlier colonial and missionary representations of Sitala and other disease deities as "devils" and "demons," but this characterization hardly did justice to the importance of Sitala in modern Hinduism or to the diverse forms her worship has taken.[9] As Crooke pointed out, in the countryside of northern India Sitala was sometimes thought of as one of seven disease goddesses or sisters, but she enjoyed a prominence and a potency unmatched by other disease deities. In Bengal there were few temples devoted to Sitala, often only a small shrine, a symbolic pot, or piece of decorated stone. There were, however, major sites of Sitala worship in northern India. One was at Gurgaon, just south of Delhi, where pilgrims gathered in large numbers each March, at the start of the smallpox season, to seek the goddess's protection for their children or in fulfillment of earlier vows. There were similar Sitala fairs and shrines in western India. Perhaps because smallpox was above all a disease of children, or because they were thought better able than men to intercede with a female deity, women played a leading part in the worship of Sitala, in pilgrimages, in making vows, reciting prayers and songs, or in offering sweets and "cooling" drinks and fruits to the goddess.[10]

Inasmuch as there was any special priesthood associated with Sitala, her servants were neither women nor Brahmins, India's principal priestly caste, but members of lower but "clean" Sudra castes. The Malis, a caste of gardeners and cultivators in northern India, and their namesakes the Malis (or Malakaras) of Bengal, who were petty shopkeepers, garland-makers, and, like the north Indian Malis, variolators, enjoyed close identification with the goddess. According to James Wise, a British surgeon long resident in Dhaka, Malakaras supervised arrangements for the annual festival of Sitala, held on the first day of the month of Caitra (March 15), when the goddess was venerated with offerings of curd, coconuts, and plantains.[11] This date is also mentioned by Lawrence A. Babb in his account of Hinduism in Chhattisgarh in today's Madhya Pradesh. Significantly, it marks the start of the hot season there and the time of year when smallpox was most likely to occur. But other days in the Hindu calendar were also sacred to Sitala, such as the seventh day of the month of Sravan (July–August).[12] Although firmly rooted in the Hindu tradition, in some parts of India (such as Bengal and Punjab), Sitala was also worshipped (or at least propitiated in times of epidemic danger) by Muslims, converts from Hinduism who in this, as in many of their other religious beliefs, still adhered to a common folk culture. It was one of the fervent aims of the Faraizis, a Muslim reform movement active in eastern Bengal in the nineteenth century, to purge their community of this continuing faith in Sitala.[13]

Although Sitala was often referred to as "the goddess of smallpox" or simply "the smallpox goddess," smallpox was understood to be a manifestation of her personality and presence rather than her essential character. The disease was her "sport" or "play" and had to be tolerated accordingly or given the respect and honor due to the visiting goddess. Smallpox was conceptualized not as a disease but rather as a form of divine possession, and the burning fever and pustules that marked her entry into the body demanded ritual rather than therapeutic responses. To some Hindus, recourse to any form of prophylaxis or treatment was impious, likely to provoke the goddess and further imperil the child in whose body she currently resided.

Sitala means "the Cool One," and this has been interpreted as a euphemistic way of avoiding reference to one of the most obvious and alarming aspect of the disease—its intense fever. But as Susan Wadley has argued, it is better understood as the intrinsic desire of the goddess to be cool, a desire from which she is constantly thwarted by human neglect or misconduct and, in consequence, by her own fiery rage. Although in some areas, festivals in Sitala's honor were accompanied by the sacrifice of goats, chickens, and other animals, more commonly worship was made by offering such "cooling" substances as curd, plantains, cold rice, and sweets. During festivities for the heat-abhorring goddess, the preparation of cooked food was prohibited, domestic fires were extinguished, and sex, a "heating" activity, was banned.[14]

Similarly, when an attack of smallpox occurred, cooling drinks were offered to the patient as the abode of the goddess, and his or her feverish body was washed with cold water or soothed with the wetted leaves of the *neem* (or margosa), Sitala's favorite tree. When no ritual specialists attended the patient, women of the household fanned and cooled the body, or sang songs in praise of the *devi* (goddess):

O Mother, giver of salvation to the world, thou art kind to the poor.
My kine have strayed into the forest of Sitala.
O Mother, giver of salvation to the world, thou art kind to the poor.
What can avail if God gives [a child] to any one? One gets it only when Sitala gives; the giver of salvation to the world.
When Sitala is wroth with one, one finds no pleasure in milk, in the milk-pot, in the son in the cradle, in the house or the courtyard. O Mother, giver of salvation to the world.
Thou art land and water, and thou art the most powerful of all.
Thou art queen of three regions. O Mother, giver of salvation to the world.[15]

But often Malis, or members of other castes favored by Sitala, were called to attend the goddess. According to Wise, in eastern Bengal as soon as smallpox made its appearance in a Hindu household, a Mali was summoned:

> His first act is to forbid the introduction of meat, and all food requiring oil or spices for its preparation. He then ties a lock of hair, a cowrie shell, a piece of turmeric, and an article of gold on the right wrist of the patient. The sick person is then laid on the "Manjh-patta", the young and unexpanded leaf of the plantain tree, and milk is prescribed as the sole article of food. He is fanned with a branch of the sacred Nim, and anyone entering the chamber is sprinkled with water. Should the fever become aggravated and delirium ensue, or if a child cries much and sleeps little, the Mali performs the Mata pujah. This consists in bathing the image of the goddess causing the disease, and giving a draught of water to drink.[16]

To relieve the irritation of the skin, the Mali sprinkled the body with a cooling talc of ground lentils, turmeric, flour, and powdered shell. As the disease reached its climax on the evening of the seventh day, he placed a water pot in the sickroom, accompanied by offerings of rice, coconut, sugar, flowers, and *neem* leaves, and recited prayers to Sitala for hours at a time. Once the pustules had ripened, the Mali gave the patient physical relief by piercing them with a sharp thorn. Finally, as the patient recovered and the scabs peeled off, the Mali performed a final Sitala *puja* and then retired with a share of the offerings and a fee for his services.[17]

Thus perceived, Sitala was both the source of smallpox and the means of gaining protection from it, or rather (given the virtual universality of the disease) of ensuring that the child experienced it in a mild and "proper" form, without the dangerous complications that might result from incurring her wrath. The body was Sitala's temple, the shrine at which devotees worshipped and praised an all-powerful but difficult deity. The physical heat experienced was understood as ritual heat, an expression of the ambivalent strength of *sakti*, Hinduism's female principle, a potentially fierce and destructive force which, if ritually appeased and accommodated, could be transformed into protection, good fortune, and fertility.

The visitation of the goddess might connote possession in a second sense, too. The wishes of the smallpox sufferer were respected because they were taken to represent the voice of the goddess herself. Victims were believed to have oracular powers, and their requests or commands were honored accordingly. The delirium and hallucinations caused by the disease might have contributed to this belief. But possession in the spiritual sense was not necessarily confined to those actually seized by smallpox. During epidemics, women sometimes declared themselves possessed by Sitala and, going into a trance, revealed the goddess's wishes or the reason for her anger. In nineteenth-century Bengal, some mediums attributed the wrath of the goddess to the activities of vaccinators, thereby perhaps articulating a collective unease at the arrival of this alien practice, but there were also contrary cases of possessed women welcoming vaccination in Sitala's name.[18]

VARIOLATION

Neither the texts of Ayurvedic medicine nor its practitioners, the *vaidyas*, could offer much help and comfort to those who were threatened by smallpox. Two of the oldest and most revered texts, the *Caraka Samhita* and *Susruta Samhita*, compiled before the fifth century A.D., made only passing reference to an eruptive disease called *masurika* (from the resemblance of the pustule to a lentil, *masura*) and implied that it was only a minor ailment. It has, therefore, been suggested that smallpox either was not present in India when these works were compiled or had yet to assume its more malignant form. Only with later works, like the *Madhavanidana*, dating from the eighth or ninth century, are more detailed descriptions of smallpox to be found, indicating the severity that had by then come to characterize the disease.[19]

Like other diseases in the Ayurvedic corpus, *masurika* or smallpox was understood in terms of a humoral construction of the body. Disease was conceptualized as the result of a derangement or imbalance among the three humors (*tridosha*)—wind, bile, and phlegm—which jointly governed the physiological processes of the body. In a healthy individual, all three humors existed in harmony; sickness arose from an excess or disorder of one humor.[20] The causes of these imbalances and excesses were many and various. An unnamed medical treatise (probably the *Astangahrdaya Samhita*) cited by Radha Kanta Deb, a leading Calcutta Hindu, in 1831 ascribed smallpox to the eating of pungent, acidic, or saline substances and unwholesome mixtures such as fish with milk. It could also be caused by taking food before the previous meal had been properly digested, by drinking impure water, by exposure to foul air, or by unpropitious planets.[21] The most the experienced *vaidya* could do was to use his diagnostic skills to identify the specific form of the disease, principally through the character of the pustules, and to prescribe cooling drafts and embrocations, administer purgatives to flush the body of its poisons, and prohibit foods likely to produce or prolong the derangement of the humors. But the general impression given in the nineteenth century is that the disease was considered, even by physicians themselves, to be beyond their powers to prevent or to relieve. Thus, the only appropriate course was to seek the intercession of Sitala, a deity who had crept into Ayurvedic texts only in relatively recent times. "As soon as the nature of the disease is determined," reported James Wise, "the Kabiraj [doctor] retires, and a Malakar [attendant of Sitala] is summoned." Or, as Ramchandra Mallick told the Smallpox Commission in Calcutta in 1850, Hindus believed the disease to be "above all medical cure . . . a patient is entirely at the mercy of Situla."[22]

But one way of anticipating the almost certain visitation of smallpox and of gaining protection against its worst ravages was through variolation. This was among the commonest and most effective forms of indigenous medical practice in India until it was displaced by Jennerian vaccination in the second half of the nineteenth century, though, as many contemporary accounts attest, it was seen more as a religious ceremony and a ritual invocation of Sitala than as a medical procedure as such.

There are many accounts of variolation in eastern and northern India in the eighteenth and nineteenth centuries, most of them written by European doctors and surgeons. These accounts differ somewhat in the procedures they describe (reflecting local variations, changes over time, or perhaps simply the reporter's uncertain knowledge), but they also vary in their evaluation of variolation. Before about 1800 the accounts are largely favorable. Thereafter, with the introduction of the rival practice of vaccination, they tend to be more skeptical or even frankly contemptuous. It seems likely, too, that as variolation fell into official disfavor and measures were introduced for its suppression, the nature of the practice changed, becoming more secretive and devoid of the prohibitions and prescriptions that had contributed to its earlier effectiveness.

The most frequently cited account of smallpox inoculation in Bengal was that given by J. Z. Holwell in 1767 to the College of Physicians in London. It was based upon observations made during his long residence in India and, by presenting variolation in India in an attractive light, Holwell hoped to reassure people in Britain of its safety and reliability at a time when inoculation was still a novelty there and doubts persisted about its effects. It was thus a more sympathetic account than those left by many doctors in the second half of the nineteenth century when variolation was under attack.

Holwell understood the inoculators in Bengal to be "a particular tribe of Bramins. . . delegated annually for this service" from Vrindaban, Allahabad, and Varanasi. They arrived in the districts where they were to work in small parties of three or four "some weeks before the usual return of the disease," which in Bengal was usually February or early March. They "inoculate indifferently," Holwell explained, "on any part" of the body, but preferred the outside of the arm, midway between the wrist and the elbow on males and between the elbow and shoulder on females. The inoculator rubbed the chosen place for eight to ten minutes with a piece of cloth, then

> with a small instrument he wounds, by many slight touches, about the compass of a silver groat, just making the smallest appearance of blood, then opening a linen double rag (which he always keeps in a cloth round his waist) takes from thence a small pledget of cotton charged with variolous matter, which he moistens with two or three drops of the Ganges water, and applies it to the wound, fixing it on with a slight bandage, and ordering it to remain on for six hours without being moved.[23]

According to Holwell, the variolous matter used was taken from the pustules produced by the previous year's inoculations, "for they never inoculate with fresh matter, nor with matter from the disease caught in the natural way, however distinct and mild the species." This use of old and carefully selected smallpox matter was undoubtedly important, for in artificially introducing the disease in a more attenuated form than if it had been acquired naturally, the inoculators were likely to reproduce the disease not in its full severity but still in sufficient strength to have a prophylactic effect.

Holwell also drew attention to the carefully controlled environment in which these skilled and experienced inoculators performed their craft. Pregnant women, unprotected adults, and others who might be vulnerable to attack from smallpox were removed from the place of inoculation. A series of dietary restrictions was also imposed, and though these can have had little practical effect upon the operation's success, they emphasized the importance and danger attached to variolation and the need to observe due care to prevent the disease from becoming contagious. The consumption of fish, milk, and ghee was prohibited for a month before variolation and for another month after it. The inoculator ordered the patient to be fed a regimen consisting of "all the refrigerating things the climate and season produces"—plantains, sugarcane, watermelons, rice, white poppy-seed gruel, and cold water. Holwell found these dietary directions "rational enough," agreeing, for example, that fish was "a viscid and inflammatory diet, tending to foul and obstruct the cutaneous glands and excretory ducts, and to create in the stomach and first passages a tough, slimy phlegm, highly injurious to the human constitution."

Early on the day after the inoculation, large quantities of cold water were poured over the patient's head, and this practice was repeated night and morning until a fever developed at the close of the sixth day. It was then discontinued for three days while the eruptions began, and then the cold-water treatment was resumed until the scabs fell off. At this stage the pustules were opened with a sharp-pointed thorn and the pus drained off, a procedure repeated several times until the fluid ceased to flow. This practice not only relieved the patient's physical discomfort but also gave the inoculators the variolous matter they needed for the following year's inoculations.[24]

Given the nature of his audience, Holwell was understandably more interested in describing the medical rather than the religious aspects of inoculation in India, but he did note that from the first rubbing of the arm to the final tying of the bandage the variolator recited continuously from the "Aughtorrah Bhade" (*Atharva Veda*), praising the "goddess of spots." On recovery, a thanksgiving *puja* was held in the goddess's honor, and only then did the inoculator receive his payment ("which from the poor is a pund [sic] of cowries, equal to about a penny sterling"). Holwell's identification of the inoculators as Brahmins and his references to the Vedas were perhaps intended to reassure the West of the prestige and antiquity of variolation in India.[25] The smallpox produced by variolation was, he further explained, of a mild nature. The number of pustules was small (between fifty and two hundred), and there was little risk either of the disease spreading by contagion to the unprotected or of its causing the death of the inoculees. Despite the "multitudes" inoculated every year in Bengal, Holwell declared, the practice "adds no malignity to the disease taken in the natural way, nor spreads the infection, as is commonly imagined in Europe."[26]

Holwell's account is largely confirmed by that given nearly fifty years later in 1831 by Radha Kanta Deb. While Holwell does not give the inoculators a title, Deb calls them *tikadars*, meaning those who make a *tika*, or mark. Since he, too, was writing for a medical audience, this time European doctors and surgeons in Bengal, Deb also stressed the medical aspects of variolation rather than its religious side:

> On some lucky day of the month of Phalgoon (February, March) and Chaitra (March, April), the Tikadars inoculate the healthy boys and girls, by thrusting or punching their arms with a pointed iron instrument, and infusing the pus previously collected in a cotton, from the good sort of ripened natural smallpox; and cause them to bathe and eat chilly and juicy food, repeatedly, until they excite a fever, which comes on violently in 6 or 7 days, accompanied by smallpox. The fever goes off in 3 days, when all the pocks are visible, which are sprinkled over with a little water on the 5th day, to make them rise up, and then stained with bruised raw turmeric on the 7th, in order to make them ripen well the sooner. They are afterwards broken with the thorn of a shrub, called "Bainch" (Flacourtia sapadia), on the 9th or 10th day. This treatment terminates, and the patient perfectly recovers in three weeks; during which time, all the patients of a family are kept in a separate room, with great care, without allowing the approach of any unclean person; and also their parents and domestics live abstemiously, and worship the goddess "Situla", which presides over the smallpox, and other eruptive distempers. The Tikadars are remunerated according to the circumstances of the parents or patients; but they commonly charge the poor people one or two Rupees per each head.[27]

Like Holwell, Radha Kanta Deb gave no indication how widely variolation was practiced in India. Its extent became apparent only later in the century when the British set about trying to suppress the practice. Information for the years 1848–67 showed that almost 82 percent of prisoners in Bengal's jails had been inoculated, while a series of "vaccine censuses" in the 1870s revealed that variolation was "the universal practice" over much of Bengal, Assam, Bihar, and Orissa, with more than 60 percent of the population having undergone inoculation. A survey of 17,697 people in the Bengal Presidency in 1872–73 (mainly prisoners, schoolchildren, dispensary patients, and laborers) indicated that 66 percent had been inoculated, 5 percent vaccinated, 18 percent had had smallpox, and 11 percent remained unprotected.[28] Beyond eastern India, variolation was also common in the eastern districts of the North-Western Provinces (in Varanasi division especially), in the hills of Kumaon and Punjab through to Rawalpindi in the northwest, further south in Rajasthan, Sind, Kutch, and Gujarat, and in scattered parts of Maharashtra (particularly the Konkan coast) and central India. For reasons that are not clear, it was virtually unknown in northern India west of Varanasi, in Avadh and the Delhi area, in Nepal, Hyderabad, and Mysore. It seems to have been rare (except in some northern districts of the Madras Presidency where it was practiced by Oriya Brahmins) over almost the whole of Dravidian India, the region where, perhaps only coincidentally, Mariamma replaced Sitala as the goddess of smallpox.[29]

Although inoculation was most widely practiced among Hindus— and was opposed by some Muslim communities—it was by no means restricted to them. In Rajasthan, according to one recent report, variolation was "confined exclusively to the Muslim community." This was certainly not the case in India as a whole, but in the northwest generally, variolation was closely associated with Muslims and was even said to have been introduced by them.[30] Certain social groups were less likely to be protected by variolation than others. Untouchables were rarely, if ever, inoculated, because contact with them would be ritually polluting to caste-Hindu inoculators; nor perhaps would they have been able to pay the fees required. This meant that as many as twenty percent of the population might have escaped (or been denied) variolation, thus maintaining a large pool of susceptible adults and children. Many tribal populations apparently had no acquaintance with variolation. Women were not excluded (though they are not mentioned as variolators), but it was a measure of the inferior value placed on their lives that they commanded a fee only half that asked for male inoculees (upcountry, usually two annas rather than four). The vaccine census for 1872–73 suggests (admittedly on the basis of a small sample) that schoolgirls in Bengal were less likely to have been inoculated than schoolboys.[31]

The variolators, or *tikadars*, were also a far more diverse group than Holwell's reference to "a particular tribe of Bramins" would suggest. Radha Kanta Deb reported that in Bengal they included men from several castes—"viz. low Brahmun . . . , Acharjya or Daivagna, (astrologer or calculator of nativities), Coombhakar, or Coomar (potter), Sankhakar or Sankharee (shell-cutter or conchmaker) &c." He also refuted the claim (at least as far as Calcutta was concerned) that they came from such distant places as Varanasi. Those he knew of either lived in Calcutta or came from the neighboring districts of Burdwan, Hughli, and Nadia. "The Vaidya, or Physicians of this country," he added, "never follow this profession, as they abhor the touching of blood, purulent matter, &c."[32]

A report of 1850 identified the forty-two *tikadars* then resident in Calcutta as belonging mostly to low-status artisanal or petty trading castes: Malis, Tantis, Kumars, and Napits (barbers). In eastern Bengal, Wise described variolation as "one of the chief occupations" of the Malis (whom we have already met as ritual specialists of Sitala), but he also mentions Napits as inoculators.[33] In Balasore district of Orissa, hereditary inoculators were said to be Mastan or "low" Brahmins. In one part of Bihar, Francis Buchanan found variolation practiced by a class of people called Gotpachcha or Pachaniya, who he said were mostly Malis, though they tried to pass themselves off as Brahmins; in Rangpur in northern Bengal, the inoculators were Rojas, whose other skills included conjuring, exorcism, and curing snakebites. Northern and central Indian variolators included Brahmins, barbers, and members of diverse artisanal and agricultural castes, among them Malis, Muslim weavers, and Sindurias (vermilion sellers). On the west coast, variolation was practiced by agrarian castes like the Kunbis, and even, in Portuguese Goa, by the lower ranks of the Catholic clergy. For virtually all variolators, inoculation was a supplementary source of income, providing seasonal employment during the postharvest months when agricultural work was light. It was seldom an exclusive occupation.[34]

Nonetheless, the scale of the inoculators' annual enterprise was remarkable. Dozens of *tikadars* worked in each district of eastern India during the inoculating season, moving from house to house, village to village, inoculating several members of a household at a time and returning to drain pustules and see each patient through the various stages of fever and recovery. No less striking was the apparent willingness of villagers to pay for this service. Some of the more renowned inoculators earned substantial sums of money, and their skill won them respect as well as material reward. One *tikadar* in Calcutta reputedly earned Rs 12,000 a year, but Rs 80 to 90 a month during the inoculating season was probably more common, at least in northern India.[35]

Clearly, there were great variations in the status of the inoculators and the manner of their practice. Buchanan, himself a physician, stressed the low-caste status of many practitioners in up-country Bengal and Bihar, observing that "they are by no means respected nor considered as on a footing with the practitioner of medicine."[36] But this does not appear to have been the case everywhere, or else the variolators would not have been as well rewarded as some of them undoubtedly were, nor would their dietary bans and ritual prescriptions have been as faithfully observed they appear to have been. *Tikadars*, many of whom were hereditary practitioners of their craft, were often well known to, and respected by, the families and villages they served. According to one account from the North-Western Provinces, "Each village has its own inoculator, who is known and treated as a kind of family physician in smallpox cases."[37] However, the more widely British opposition to variolation became known and enforced, the more secretive the practice became. Many *tikadars* were forced to abandon their hereditary calling or switched to vaccination, and it seems likely that less reputable and less skilled inoculators took over, who "had not the influence necessary to make the people conform to the rules for preventing the spread of the disease."[38]

That inoculation was not generally performed by "high" Brahmins or by *vaidya*s did not mean it was devoid of religious significance and simply a craft like setting bones, curing snakebites, or delivering babies. Sitala's sanction was considered essential to the success of variolation. *Tikadars* freely acknowledged that they were trespassing on her territory when they chanted her praise or asked her blessing while at work. For both practitioners and observers, variolation was "practically a religious ceremony," and without Sitala its success and the safety of the person inoculated could not be guaranteed. O'Malley, describing variolation in Orissa at the turn of the century, explained how the inoculator began with "a solemn offering" to Sitala and performed *puja* to the goddess repeatedly during the operation. Even during the period of convalescence following the operation,

> the patient is humoured, dealt gently with, and never scolded, even if fractious, as it is believed that the deity presiding over small-pox is in the child's system, and any castigation or abuse might offend the goddess and draw down her wrath upon the child, in the form of confluent small-pox and death.[39]

Hence, variolation was generally understood as a way of invoking the protective power of the goddess. Unlike vaccination, it celebrated, rather than violated, Sitala's rights over the body.

VACCINATION

Smallpox occupied a paradoxical place in the history of European medical ideas and practices in nineteenth-century India. Despite the prevalence of the disease and the threat it posed to European as well as Indian lives, it was not seen as a disease peculiar to India, nor did it form part of the nineteenth-century literature on the "diseases of warm climates." It was absent from such influential treatises as James Annesley's *Sketches of the Most Prevalent Diseases of India* or William Twining's *Clinical Illustrations of the More Important Diseases of Bengal*, works which, for all their expansive titles, aptly reflected the narrow purview of medical thought in India at the time. Nor did it appear in Patrick Manson's *Manual* of tropical diseases published in 1898.

Smallpox stood apart from other diseases for a number of reasons. First, it was almost as familiar a disease in late eighteenth- and early nineteenth-century Europe as it was in India. It was so common, endemically and epidemically, that it provoked little specific comment and became a "tropical disease" only after World War I, following its virtual elimination from Europe and North America.[40] Second, the contagious nature of smallpox was well known, even if it could not yet be explained scientifically. It provided a model of disease transmission with which other diseases were more often contrasted than compared. Smallpox presented none of the difficulties posed by malarial "miasma" or by the uncertain "contagion" of cholera. Third, there was little to connect smallpox with an Indian or tropical environment. Charles Morehead, who was something of an exception in discussing the disease at all, noted the far greater seasonal concentration of smallpox mortality in India than in Europe (with as many as half the deaths from the disease falling during the spring months).[41] But otherwise, the disease seemed essentially the same as that known in Europe. Paradoxically, the sameness of the disease in Europe and Asia diverted attention toward its very different cultural context in India. The propitiation of Sitala looked all the more obscure and absurd to medical practitioners who confidently believed that they possessed a scientific understanding of the disease, just as the advent of vaccination gave added emphasis to variolation as the offending cause—rather than warm climates or tropical miasmas—which kept this virulent, but eminently "preventable," disease in circulation.

A leading cause of Indian mortality, smallpox was also greatly feared among Europeans in eighteenth- and early nineteenth-century India. Between the 1780s and early 1800s, the British in Calcutta had some recourse to variolation, more in emulation of its recent adoption in Europe than of long-standing Indian practice. Otherwise, they fled "from those terrors which were always created by the prevalence of smallpox," taking refuge in the countryside until the epidemic season had passed.[42]

With the rapid adoption of vaccination after its introduction into Bombay in June 1802, Europeans felt less vulnerable to smallpox than to many other diseases encountered in India and against which they could acquire no comparable protection, such as cholera and typhoid. In 1806 the British community in Bengal sent Edward Jenner £4,000 in gratitude for its deliverance from smallpox; two further gifts, amounting to £3,383, followed shortly afterward from Madras and Bombay.[43] But the epidemics which swept through the countryside and towns every six or seven years still posed a partial threat to unprotected (or poorly vaccinated) Europeans. In the 1849–50 epidemic in Calcutta, seventy-six Europeans were admitted to the city's General Hospital with smallpox and, of these, twenty died. Most of the victims were from the poorer classes of Europeans, mainly soldiers and sailors. Wealthier white residents in Calcutta were better protected, not only by vaccination but also by the spaciousness of their houses and gardens and their limited contact with Indians. In Bombay, smallpox mortality was thought to be only a sixth among

Europeans what it was among Indians, because of the protection conferred by vaccination.[44]

Diminished susceptibility to the disease did not mean that smallpox ceased to be a matter of European concern. Vaccination was so poorly performed in Bengal, according to one British visitor, as to be "worthless," and until revaccination was introduced in the second half of the century, immunity could be short-lived as well as deficient. Children were thought to be at risk from Indian servants who might transmit the disease from their "obscure homes in the bazar." In the opinion of the Smallpox Commissioners in Calcutta in 1850, the homes of the poor—small, overcrowded, and ill ventilated—were "permanent storehouses of every pestilential disease," smallpox included.[45]

In such circumstances, vaccination policy was partly an in-depth defense of European health. Careful watch was kept on the environs of Simla, as a European hill resort and summer capital of the Government of India, to minimize the potential risk from smallpox, and as late as 1893 one of the arguments for the introduction of compulsory vaccination in Pune (Poona) was "in consideration of the proximity of the city to the large European population of the cantonment and the constant intercommunication which exists between the city and the cantonment."[46] Some degree of contact with Indians being unavoidable, one of the priorities of Western medicine was to erect a *cordon sanitaire* around the white community, with those closest to it— domestic servants, soldiers, plantation laborers—among the first to be targeted for vaccination. Demands that inoculation be prohibited and vaccination made compulsory were thus prompted in part by a desire to save European, rather than Indian, lives.

But vaccination was never intended exclusively for the white population of India. Indeed, the speed with which it was taken up as a cardinal feature of state medicine in India is an important demonstration of the extent to which Western medicine was not governed by a purely enclavist mentality, though it soon became clear that the enthusiasm of the medical profession was not well supported by the financial constraints and political pragmatism of the government itself. Vaccination was introduced at a critical moment in the history of colonialism in India. For a regime but recently established by force of arms and with the struggle against the Marathas still unresolved, vaccination offered a welcome opportunity to give "fresh proof" of the

East India Company's "humane and benevolent" intentions toward its subjects, "an additional mark of the fostering care of the British Government" in India.[47] Although the protection of white soldiers and civilians was certainly an immediate consideration in the minds of the colonial authorities, it was not their only or even paramount concern—as the governor of Bombay made clear in 1803. In declaring his "great joy" at the successful introduction of vaccination a few months earlier, he remarked that "the prestige that we have achieved by this one act has been the source of much good will from the people—it is a great reward."[48]

Some administrators saw the rewards of smallpox vaccination in material as well as political terms. Lord Bentinck, governor of Madras, in approving official expenditure on vaccination in 1805, declared himself "happy in the reflection that no expense was ever made for objects of greater individual happiness or of public advantage." In a country where the state derived so large a share of its income from the cultivation of the land, "every life saved," he reasoned, "is additional revenue and an increase to the population and to the prosperity of the Company's territories in an incalculable ratio."[49]

At first, Europeans confidently anticipated that the population of India would take up with as much "gratitude" as their own a discovery which conferred "such inestimable benefits to mankind." There was an ill-judged expectation, too, that Hindus, with their famed reverence for the cow, would seize "with the greatest ardour" this latest bovine gift to humanity.[50] But hopes of a ready and appreciative acceptance of vaccination were soon dashed. "The circumstances of the disease [cowpox] coming originally from the cow," John Shoolbred, superintendent-general of vaccination in Bengal, was forced to acknowledge in 1804, were a "very strong objection to its adoption." Within ten years of the vaccine's introduction, medical officers were lamenting "the prejudices and indolence of the natives" and "the doctrines of fatalism, which inculcate resignation to the ravages of the small pox."[51] As a result, it seemed, the number of vaccinations remained stubbornly low. In the years 1803–06, there were between 11,000 and 18,000 vaccinations in the whole of eastern and northern India. Between 1818 and 1829, the number of operations in the vast and populous Bengal Presidency averaged only 30,000 a year, and though it reached nearly 62,000 in 1828–29, it sank back again to barely 15,000 in 1832, and as late as 1843 had scarcely regained the level of fifteen years earlier.[52]

Such an apparently negative result (which in fact, as will shortly be seen, partly reflected government parsimony) confirmed many British medical officers in their prejudices about Indians. As early as 1804, less than two years after the introduction of vaccination to Bengal, Shoolbred castigated Hindus for being "naturally averse to all innovation" and denounced the province's laboring classes as "stupid and insensible" for failing to recognize instantly vaccination's "inestimable value to mankind."[53] In 1831 Dr. W. Cameron, deploring the lack of progress in vaccination since Shoolbred's report, blamed the "astonishing indifference" of the bulk of the inhabitants of Bengal to "the very great blessing Government offers to them, through vaccination."[54] Duncan Stewart, a later superintendent-general of vaccination in the 1840s, likewise railed against Hindu ingratitude and ignorance. He blamed "the trammels of a degrading religion, by which their thoughts are chained, their reasoning faculties hoodwinked and their mutual affections thwarted." Even offers of "the most simple, obvious, and unquestionable temporal advantage" to the recipient were, he claimed, unacceptable to Hindus if they entailed "the slightest deviation from ancient usage."[55] Nor were such vehement sentiments confined either to Bengal or to the early part of the century. In 1878, for instance, the sanitary commissioner for the North-Western Provinces attributed the limited impact which vaccination had had in the region to circumstances peculiar to the people of India, principally their "natural apathy, . . . their disinclination to accept a new thing, and their unreasonable religious beliefs or caste prejudices."[56]

A corollary to this angry reaction was to see inoculation and inoculators as the main obstacles to vaccination's rightful success and the principal reason why smallpox remained so virulent in India. According to Cameron in 1831, the suppression of inoculation was "indispensable to the interests of humanity," and he supported this claim by alleging that the ten to fifteen *tikadar*s currently active in Calcutta were "the great means by which variola is kept in existence" there. Fearing the loss of their "influence and emolument," the *tikadar*s, Cameron further claimed, deliberately and selfishly spread "falsehoods and ridiculous stories" about vaccination so as to prejudice the people against it.[57] A Smallpox Commission, set up in March 1850 in the wake of recent epidemics and numbering three Bengalis among its seven members (including Pandit Madhusudan Gupta, lecturer in anatomy at Calcutta's Medical College), largely concurred with Cameron's hostile opinions. Indeed, the commissioners went even further, stating:

> We think that he might truly have added that, in a country where practices such as *Suttee* and *Infanticide* were, until lately, deemed justifiable on the score of religious usage, neither will there be wanting bigots to mislead the ignorant Hindoos, and to prejudice their credulous and simple minds, against whatever may be falsely represented to them as an innovation, or an interference with their religious privileges . . . the time has come and can no longer be deferred when this murderous trade should be suppressed.[58]

In calling for variolation to be prohibited, the commissioners described it as the duty of the government "to save from wilful self-destruction the ignorant and thoughtless millions, whom Providence has committed to its charge and protection."[59] For the present the government declined to accept such a weighty responsibility, but it was widely held—at least in medical circles—that variolation was dangerous on three counts. First, it was said that it obstructed the progress of the safer and superior practice of vaccination; second, that it often caused a severe or fatal attack of the disease in those inoculated; and, third, that by propagating natural smallpox, variolation gave rise to epidemics of the disease. Shoolbred, for instance, contended (on the basis more of hearsay than of hard evidence) that *tikadars* in Bengal privately confessed to causing one death for every two hundred inoculations they performed. He contrasted this with a figure of one death for every three hundred operations when variolation had been practiced in Europe and, believing that it was "certainly less favourable here than in Europe," concluded that it caused the death of one in every sixty or seventy people inoculated in India.[60]

It is worth recalling, however, how safe the Indian practice of variolation had appeared to Holwell only a few decades earlier and the stress he placed on the *tikadars'* precautionary measures. Francis Buchanan, Shoolbred's contemporary, had also presented variolation in a far more favorable light, estimating at only one percent the number of deaths caused.[61] Nor did all later commentators regard variolation quite as negatively as Shoolbred. In the late 1860s T. E. Charles, the current superintendent-general of vaccination, concluded from a careful review of the evidence that the likely mortality among inoculees was probably no more than about one percent and that variolation was rarely a cause of epidemics *when* the traditional restrictions were followed. Like James Wise, the civil surgeon at Dhaka, he argued that it was premature to try to prohibit variolation while vaccination was still widely shunned by the people of eastern India and thus not yet able to provide an "efficient substitute." Banning variolation, Charles believed, would "constitute a great hardship" to the people and deny them a readily available and trusted form of prophylaxis. Although making clear his own faith in the superiority of vaccination, Charles went so far as to suggest that the *tikadar*s be licensed and brought under state regulation, but, given the growing strength of feeling against the inoculators, this was not a policy the government was prepared to pursue.[62]

Despite Charles and Wise, the general imputation from the early nineteenth century onward was that variolation was indeed a "murderous trade," that it was sustained only through the narrow self-interest of the *tikadar*s, and that vaccination could never entirely succeed until it had been suppressed. That vaccination also encountered considerable opposition and apathy in Britain was seldom mentioned: that part of Britain's experience of vaccination was generally not for export.[63] Instead, Indians' religion, their social practices, and customs were made to bear the burden of responsibility. In fact, although cultural resistance was undoubtedly an important factor in vaccination's slow progress in India, it was by no means the only inhibiting factor.

VACCINATION ON TRIAL

Despite the claims made for the simplicity and effectiveness of vaccination, many technical and practical difficulties stood in the way of its successful use in India. Commentators today who contrast variolation with vaccination are apt to forget how crude and unreliable the latter often was during the nineteenth century.

There was, first of all, a problem of supply. Cowpox was rare in India; some sources suggest it was entirely absent. In consequence, until the 1890s much of the vaccine used was imported from Britain. The first vaccine reached India in June 1802 through a relay of children vaccinated from arm to arm from Baghdad to Bombay.[64] Subsequently, vaccine crusts or sealed tubes of lymph were sent by sea or brought overland from Britain, but by the time the lymph came to be used, it was many months old and often inert or otherwise unfit for use. This was one reason for the initially high level of unsuccessful operations in India.[65]

Once the vaccine was established locally, attempts were made (as in Britain) to maintain the supply through arm-to-arm vaccinations. But the vaccine was often "lost" in the process of human transmission, or parents refused to allow their children to be used to supply lymph for the vaccination of others. During the hottest months of the year, vaccination was either ineffective or tended to produce "foul sloughing sores." As a result, vaccination was largely confined to the cooler, drier months between September and March—vaccination, like variolation, had its season—and added to the difficulties of maintaining an adequate supply of lymph from one year to the next.[66] Although arm-to-arm vaccination had the advantage of being relatively cheap—in Bengal in the 1870s each successful vaccination cost less than two annas—there were suggestions, as in Europe, that it was responsible for transmitting diseases such as syphilis and leprosy. One hostile Tamil newspaper asked in 1891 how doctors had ever imagined that transferring "pus" from one body to another would not produce such "baneful effects."[67]

As long as vaccination relied on imported lymph and the arm-to-arm method of propagation, the scale of operations in India was necessarily very limited. In Bombay, a province where vaccination was pursued more enthusiastically than in Bengal, and where inoculation was a less formidable rival, only 446,000 vaccinations were performed between 1846 and 1850, with a further 849,000 following between 1851 and 1855. At this mid-century stage, vaccination was reaching only about 1.5 percent of the population.[68]

Thereafter, however, significant technical advances were made. In the cool of the Kumaon hills in the North-Western Provinces, vaccine crusts and lymph were collected for use in the neighboring plains: some twenty thousand crusts were dispatched in this manner in 1867–68 alone.[69] In the 1850s Bombay's Vaccination Department began experimenting with the production of calf lymph as a way of overcoming the practical limitations imposed by purely human sources of supply, but it was twenty years before the calf-to-arm technique was sufficiently reliable for more general use. Even then it was hampered by the difficulty, especially in rural areas, of moving calves from place to place with the vaccinators. This form of vaccination was also three times more expensive, and partly for this reason arm-to-arm vaccination persisted in parts of Bengal until World War I. By that time, however, calf lymph, preserved with lanolin or glycerine, was being produced in sufficient quantities to end dependence on imported supplies. A Vaccine Institute, established at Belgaum in the Bombay Presidency in 1907, was manufacturing two hundred thousand doses of calf vaccine a year by 1911, and the King Institute of Preventive Medicine at Guindy, Madras, had a similar output of vaccine. Electric refrigeration also made it easier to store vaccine until required.[70] By 1914 vaccination was a far more efficient and reliable operation than it had been thirty or forty years earlier.

Only after these technical advances had been made could the scale of vaccination be substantially increased. From 350,000 operations annually in British India in 1850, the figure rose to 4.5 million in 1877, 5 million in 1883, 6 million in 1888, reaching 7 million five years later and 8 million by the end of the century.[71] In the period 1867–76 it was estimated that less than a third of the children in the North-Western Provinces were vaccinated: by 1908 nearly 50 percent of infants under a year old in the United Provinces (as it had been renamed) had been vaccinated. In Bombay the advance was even more dramatic, with some 80 percent of children being vaccinated by the end of the century, but that still left at least 20 percent unprotected.[72] In Bengal vaccination lagged far behind most other provinces. In 1873 it was reckoned that for a population of 68 million people, at least 2 million vaccinations a year were needed, but they currently amounted to barely a third of that number. By 1900, when the figure of 2 million primary vaccinations a year had been reached, more than 20 percent of the targeted age group, those under a year old, were still being missed.[73] It was this failure to vaccinate one in five children which prevented further substantial progress in reducing smallpox mortality in India until after independence.

The persistence of the arm-to-arm method highlights one reason for vaccination's long-lasting unpopularity. Unlike variolation by *tikadars*, in which old crusts were generally used (sanctified with a sprinkling of Ganges water), vaccination transferred body fluids directly from one individual to another. For most Hindus this was offensively polluting, especially since low-caste or Untouchable children were often the only vaccinifers available; high-caste parents went to great lengths to ensure that their children were not used in this way.[74] The extraction of lymph from a child's arm could, besides, be a painfully distressing experience. According to Surgeon-Captain H. J. Dyson, Bengal's sanitary commissioner, in 1893:

> The child, attended by its weeping mother, is taken round the town or village, and sometimes from one village to another, and after all the lymph has been extracted from the vesicles on its arms, it is a common practice for the vaccinators to squeeze the inflammed base of the vaccine pustules further in order to obtain serum for more vaccinations. The agony of this practice is obviously intense, and sometimes causes long periods of suffering from severe and deep ulcers. It also sometimes happens that the infants thus used die from tetanus, exhaustion, and continued fever. It is therefore not surprising that the present attitude of the people of Bengal is still more or less hostile towards vaccination, and that parents covertly hide away their children from the vaccinators.[75]

Dyson recommended that calf lymph should replace arm-to-arm vaccination as quickly as possible—despite the greater expense involved.

Substituting calf lymph, however, created problems of its own. Many Hindus believed that taking lymph from calves involved cruelty to the animals and so was objectionable on religious grounds. Opposition was particularly intense in those towns of western India where animal vaccination was first introduced in the 1870s and 1880s. A few municipalities bluntly refused to allocate funds for the purpose, and some contractors succumbed to pressure not to supply heifers for vaccination purposes. Attempts to bypass objections to the use of cows, as sacred animals, by conducting trials with donkeys, goats, and sundry other animals, were not well received.[76] In time, however, opposition died away, partly because many Indians clearly preferred calf vaccine to the pain and inconvenience of the old arm-to-arm method.

Vaccination was disliked for other reasons, too. Unlike the *tikadars*, the vaccinators (except perhaps when they were former variolators) were strangers to the community: there was no reason to trust them, every reason to fear them. One explanation given for the unpopularity of vaccination in Punjab in the 1870s was the "brutality and dishonesty of native vaccinators." Only if the operator's palm was "greased with silver" would the child be spared "needless torture."[77] Whereas inoculation had been performed on children between about three and ten years old, vaccinators sought out infants under a year old, far too young, their mothers believed, to be exposed to such an ordeal and to risk the "evil eye."[78] Paradoxically, the mildness of the reaction normally produced by vaccination—one of its virtues in British eyes—was taken by some Indians as evidence of its ineffectiveness compared to inoculation. Skepticism was increased by the high failure rate from vaccination compared to the lifelong immunity conferred by variolation. There was, then, a not unfounded "want of faith in the protective power of vaccination."[79] A further objection—more relevant to revaccination than to primary vaccination—was that it exposed women of postpubertal age to a male vaccinator's touch. It was not until the 1880s that a few female vaccinators were appointed, and then only in small numbers and in urban areas. Even as late as 1935, there were only eighty-two for the whole of British India.[80]

But perhaps the greatest objection to vaccination was its raw secularity. There was no ritual and dietary preparation; no Sitala prayers or Ganges water; no appeal to the goddess of smallpox to guide the child safely through such a dangerous defile. Since there was "no preparation of the body or poojah," no "blessing could . . . attend it." Vaccination was seen as an "irreligious" act, an encroachment on the prerogative of the goddess without any attempt to "conciliate her with worship."[81] It treated smallpox purely as a disease, stripped of any religious significance—if indeed it was seen to have any connection with disease at all and not to be merely the "mark" the colonial state made on its subjects. The Khutris, a leading trading caste in Punjab, were said in the 1870s to oppose vaccination precisely because it represented a "mark of subjection to the British Government."[82]

Other castes and communities wondered why the British were so keen to put their *tika* upon the people. Rumor claimed that it was a deliberate attempt to violate caste and religion and force conversion to Christianity. Those vaccinated would be sacrificed to ensure the successful completion of a bridge or railway embankment, or it was said that vaccination was the prelude to a new impost or forced labor overseas.[83] One of the most persistent beliefs was that the British were searching for a child with white blood or milk in his veins. This was Kalki, the last avatar of Vishnu, who would "expel the English and become Emperor of India." Or it was the Mahdi, the Muslims' long-awaited Prophet, who would drive the infidels out of India unless first found and destroyed. Or, yet again, it was Sitala herself whom the British were seeking out with their cruel knives and needles. Thus was the body of the goddess threatened by the actions of the godless.[84] Vaccination was construed as a site of conflict between malevolent British intent and something Indian, something sacred, that was under threat of violation and destruction.

But it would be wrong to represent vaccination and variolation solely in antagonistic terms or to allow no room for accommodation between Sitala and secular medicine. Parents and vaccinators alike were involved in a process of tacit compromise. Accepting that vaccination was either desirable or unavoidable, many middle-class households treated it exactly as they had variolation, choosing an auspicious day for the operation, observing the old rituals and dietary taboos, employing a priest or paying the vaccinator to invoke the goddess of smallpox, and thanking Sitala Devi rather than Jenner Sahib for the child's safe passage.[85]

In many ways rivals for control over the body, variolation and vaccination were in some respects kindred forms of prophylaxis. The basic technique was not visibly very different: smallpox scabs or vaccine crusts, incisions made on the arm with a knife or a needle. Both vaccination and variolation had their due season, their itinerant practitioners. Even that richly polysemic word *tika* came to embrace both forms of prophylactic practice: in some parts of northern India it was the vaccinator who became the *tikawala sahib*.[86] And yet this very capacity for accommodation also emphasizes the extent to which what was being resisted was not so much vaccination as such as the abrupt, even brutal, manner of its delivery. Conversely, opposition to vaccination tended to be particularly stubborn in regions like Avadh or in the tribal tracts of central India where there had been no previous acquaintance with variolation to prepare the way for vaccination and where any form of human intervention was seen as contrary to divine will.[87]

AGENCY

Confident that vaccination would gain rapid acceptance in India, the British at first gave little thought to the need for a permanent vaccination agency. It was assumed that, once the practice had become popular, Indians would take it up for themselves at minimal cost to the state. The colonial administration would thus have the prestige of introducing vaccination without being excessively burdened with its cost. It was not long, however, before this early optimism evaporated and the state's financial commitment to vaccination was viewed with growing concern. As early as 1808 the Government of India advised caution over expenditure on vaccination, and further orders in 1811 called for reductions in vaccination staff as soon as the practice became widely accepted. In 1829 the Government of Bengal went further and decided that the expense of running thirty vaccination stations was not justified by the results, and all but six of them were closed. This was one reason why the progress of vaccination in the province was so slow.[88]

Bombay, by contrast, pioneered a more ambitious vaccination program. At the direction of the governor, Mountstuart Elphinstone, a plan was devised in 1827 to carry vaccination directly to the rural population rather than, as in Bengal, waiting for them to present themselves at a vaccination center. The Bombay Presidency was divided into four vaccination circles, each with its own team of itinerant vaccinators. These were to visit each village in their area at least once a year and provide free vaccination for as many children as possible. The vaccinators were Indians, but, following a common pattern of colonial administration, they were placed under European superintendents, who were to examine their work and periodically check their returns. According to S. P. James, the Bombay system had two "great merits:" first, "it brought vaccination to the doors of the people—too lazy, too poor, or too ignorant to seek it," and second, "it ensured the examination by the European medical officer of every case operated upon."[89] Following its apparent success in Bombay, the scheme was taken up elsewhere, for instance in Punjab in 1864 and Madras in 1865.

Bengal, however, declined to follow suit. In 1839 it launched its own system, providing vaccination through public dispensaries under the charge of civil surgeons, and clung to this for the rest of the colonial period. One reason for the difference was that, unlike the *raiyat- wari* provinces of Bombay and Madras, where the government had close administrative contact with revenue-paying peasant proprietors, Bengal and Bihar local authority had been partly delegated by the Permanent Settlement of 1793 to big landlords, or zamindars, thus leaving the state with little immediate contact with the rural population. This important social and administrative difference, as well as the strength of variolation in eastern India, helps to explain why vaccination was far less advanced in Bengal by 1914 than in western and southern India.

But the Bombay system had limitations of its own. There were reports of vaccinators submitting false returns, exaggerating the number of vaccinations performed, being too illiterate to fill in their forms correctly, or being bribed not to vaccinate at all. Low-caste vaccinators were thought to command little respect from villagers, and too much was seen to depend upon an unreliable, and often corrupt and coercive, subordinate agency. Morehead, who looked to trained Indian practitioners to spread Western medicine in a way Europeans would never be able to do, was dismayed by the vaccinators in the Bombay Presidency, commenting on the "ignorance, dishonesty, and unskilfulness of much of the native agency employed."[90] "Bad vaccination is ruin to the cause," declared Surgeon-Major F. Pearson in the North-Western Provinces in 1872, and, remarked the Madras sanitary commissioner in a similar vein in 1884, "nothing tends more to injure the cause of vaccination than incompetent and untrustworthy agency."[91] It was common enough for European officials to blame their Indian subordinates for administrative deficiencies, even when the problem was, as here, far more complex. But in this instance, the vaccinators' ignorance and dishonesty was seen as a serious impediment to the further extension of state vaccination and a further reason why compulsory vaccination might be "unwise and inexpedient" in India.[92]

The creation of a special vaccination staff and the establishment of provincial vaccination departments in the 1850s and 1860s were not in themselves sufficient, therefore, to guarantee the success of vaccination. In Bengal, where the challenge from the *tikadars* was greatest, the government adopted a series of expedients to try to supplant them. Soon after vaccination was introduced, attempts were made to induce leading variolators to take up vaccination and to persuade Brahmin pandits to issue public declarations that there was nothing in the *sastras*, the sacred texts, that prohibited vaccination or made variolation a religious obligation for Hindus. This attempt to annex the authority of the pandits had little evident effect (though it was repeated in

1870), and the number of *tikadar*s in Calcutta appears actually to have increased during the first half of the century.[93]

Further attempts at co-opting variolators were made in northern and eastern India in the 1870s. In 1873 Bengal alone counted 472 former *tikadar*s among its vaccinators, and five years later, at the height of the recruitment drive, there were nearly a thousand of them. It was further hoped that by allowing the practitioners to charge for their services (as they had previously for variolation), vaccination would in time become independent of state subsidy.[94] But the scheme met with such scant success that it was abandoned In 1878. Villagers would not pay for a vaccination they did not want, and vaccinators could collect their fees only with difficulty—or by reverting to variolation. Having earned substantial sums in the past, many leading *tikadar*s were unwilling to forgo the profit and prestige of their old calling to become state vaccinators on a paltry Rs 10 to 18 a month. European medical officers also had a strong antipathy to recruiting low-caste variolators, like the Malis and Napits, whom they regarded as dirty, shabby, untrustworthy, and an insult to their professional pride.[95]

In the early decades of the nineteenth century, vaccination stood in the forefront of British attempts to promote Western medicine in India. By the second half of the century, however, despite the considerable expansion of vaccination that was taking place, it was being seen in more routine, even menial, terms. This view was supported by a strong conviction that the vaccinators were an inappropriate instrument for the more general dissemination of Western medical and sanitary ideas. When it was proposed in 1871 by J. M. Cuningham, the Government of India's sanitary commissioner, to merge the provincial vaccination departments with the newly established sanitary departments (partly for reasons of economy, partly because the restricted "vaccination season" left vaccinators idle for several months of the year), there was a strong outcry from Bengal. T. E. Charles, the provincial superintendent of vaccination, explained that many of Bengal's vaccinators were erstwhile inoculators who were illiterate or barely able to read and write. Their mental capacity was "of a low order"; they knew nothing about medicine, had no influence with the people, and could not take on other duties without harming their vaccination work. Combining sanitation work with vaccination would, he concluded, merely create new opportunities for extortion and oppression and further jeopardize public support. An added difficulty, raised by F. Powell, superintendent of vaccination for Bengal's Metropolitan Circle, was that the majority of vaccinators in and around Calcutta were Brahmins whose caste status precluded them from doing manual work or inspecting latrines. He confirmed that the vaccinators "know nothing of sanitation or of the causes of disease." They were illiterate; the only thing they knew how to do was vaccinate.[96] To be sure, not all provinces took such a negative view of their vaccinators' abilities, and some entrusted their vaccination staff with packets of quinine or simple medicines for distribution in rural areas. But in general the feeling remained, in Bengal as elsewhere, that vaccination was a distinctive form of medical activity which did not provide a suitable base or blueprint for the wider development of state medicine and public health in India.

Given the perceived limitations of the vaccinators, an alternative ploy was to look beyond the state's own agency to "natives of rank" who might, by their example and influence, promote vaccination among their families, followers, and friends. This top-down strategy produced some early successes—including the grandson of the king of Delhi and other members of the Mughal royal family, and the wife of the peshwa in Pune in the first decade of vaccination in India[97]— but their example failed to persuade others to follow their lead. It proved comparatively easy to vaccinate members of the lowest castes, partly because they were more readily offered up by the village authorities than were children of higher castes. But high-caste evasion and reluctant low-caste compliance seemed an unsatisfactory basis for an effective vaccination strategy. There appeared, not for the first time in the history of Western medicine in India, to be a danger that vaccination (and the system of medicine it stood for) would be seen to be fit only for the low castes and Untouchables and unacceptable, on grounds of caste and religion, to high-status communities.

Looking to urban and rural elites for support was a vaccination policy much favored in the North-Western Provinces and Avadh where, after the suppression of the Mutiny and Rebellion of 1857–58, British power acknowledged a dependence upon the loyalty and authority of the "chiefs and landlords of the people." Among those whose "wisdom and philanthropy" were successfully invoked in the cause of vaccination in the 1870s and 1880s were the maharajas of

Varanasi, Balrampur, and Tehri.[98] This was in many ways a conservative policy: it endorsed the authority of the zamindars and rajas over their tenants and dependents while acknowledging the remoteness of the colonial state from the mass of the people. It made authority (the authority, in this instance, of the raja over the body of his subject) the key issue rather than understanding or desire (as in the voluntary use of variolation).

In his report on operations in Varanasi division for 1878–79, the vaccination superintendent, J. MacGregor, argued that the social standing of those vaccinated was more significant than the actual numbers involved. "An alteration in social custom," he believed, "to be successful in India, as in other countries, must take firm root in the upper strata before it penetrates downwards to the masses." It was accordingly essential for vaccinators to win the trust and support of the local "leaders" of society. "It has been found from experience," MacGregor continued,

> that when a zamindar's child is vaccinated, the *ryots* submit their children, with only the slender amount of pressure required to remove the *vis inertia* of apathy. When, on the other hand, the zamindar is an absentee or malcontent, the vaccinator is obliged to find his recruits among those out-casts who live in the slums, or in the outskirts, of the village.[99]

While, in the countryside, zamindars and rajas might lend their support to vaccination less from conviction than because their authority was being invoked, in the towns and cities, vaccination might find genuine enthusiasts among Indian newspaper editors, lawyers, teachers, and government servants. In Varanasi, for instance, in addition to the support received from the maharaja, the administration welcomed the energetic work of Pandit Bishan Dutt, a deputy superintendent of vaccination and a Brahmin, who wrote a vernacular treatise in praise of vaccination and used his personal influence with the high castes of the area to win them over. Rai Bakhtawar Singh, a judge of the Small Cause Court at Varanasi, was another enthusiastic and influential supporter.[100]

Community hierarchy and solidarity were also invoked in attempts to spread vaccination among resistant communities, and a great deal of effort went into finding out who commanded influence and the intermediaries through whom they could be successfully approached.

This effort, too, tended to reflect, and in turn reinforce, the British understanding of India as a caste-bound, communally ordered, inegalitarian society. Pragmatically, it strengthened the conviction that, if they were to be successful and not arouse strong public opposition, medical policies in India had to conform to the contours of indigenous society rather than blindly follow British precepts.

The Kansaris of Calcutta, brassmakers and devout Hindus, provide an illustration of this strategy at work. In the 1860s, when the carriage of T. E. Charles, the superintendent-general of vaccination, visited their neighborhood, the alarm was given and every door barricaded against him. Kansaris even consulted lawyers to find out how best to protect themselves from the threat of vaccination. The British response to their defiance was not, however, to resort to coercion but to try to gain influence with the Kansaris' patron, Babu Tarrucknath Pramanick, a man of great wealth and intense religious feeling. Issen Chunder Banerjee, one of the clerks in Charles's office, undertook to win over the Kansaris and spend his Sundays and spare time among them. As a Brahmin (rather than as a government servant) and as a man familiar with Hindu scriptures, he was able to counter the religious arguments against vaccination and gradually to win the trust and respect of the community's leader. In 1873 the grandchildren of Tarrucknath Pramanick were vaccinated, and other members of the community followed soon after.[101]

A similar quest for influence through community leaders characterized the protracted campaign to bring vaccination to the four million Faraizis of eastern Bengal.[102] But some of urban India's most affluent and powerful residents, the Marwaris and Banias, were among the most adamant opponents of vaccination—partly from the strength of their religious convictions (which made them suspicious, for example, of animal vaccination), but also because, as merchants and moneylenders, they remained largely untouched by Westernizing influences. This was a source of resistance the vaccinators found difficult to overcome, whether by persuasion or by recourse to the law.[103]

VACCINATION AND THE LAW

Frustration at the slow progress of vaccination, at continuing high levels of smallpox mortality, and the persistence of variolation produced strong pressure from the medical profession for legislative action and for state intervention in a field previously left largely to laissez-faire. The first move in this direction came as early as 1804, when Lord Wellesley's government formally banned variolation in Calcutta in 1804. But this decree was never enforced, and for several decades no fresh initiative was taken. Fifty years after Wellesley and following the report of Calcutta's Smallpox Commission, another governor-general, Lord Dalhousie, declared that it was as impossible to prohibit variolation as it was to "make the monsoon penal."[104]

The issue was revived in 1872 when the Bombay government submitted to the Government of India a draft compulsory vaccination bill for its approval. J. M. Cuningham, the Government of India's sanitary commissioner, whose antipathy to state intervention (rather than any obvious medical competence) might explain his long tenure of that office, expressed grave doubts about the use of compulsion. "In all sanitary legislation in this country," he argued,

> it is essential that the people should first be alive to the benefits of the proposed law. It would be much better to postpone compulsory vaccination for a time, until the benefits of vaccination are more fully appreciated, than to introduce a measure, however good in itself, if the people are not as yet prepared for it.[105]

His views were readily endorsed by the government itself. Without entering into the technical arguments for vaccination, Sir John Strachey of the Viceroy's Council minuted that it would be "unwise to the last degree to force upon the people a measure of so absolutely novel a character." He thought that the likely result would be "to make vaccination unpopular in the extreme and to defeat the object that is desired." The "prejudices of the people" could only be overcome by demonstrating "with patience and time and, above all, the utmost care," that vaccination was effective and reliable.[106]

But, despite the Government of India's equivocation, the provincial administrations were becoming convinced of the need for legislative action. Metropolitan precedent was one factor in this. Recent enactments in Britain in 1853 and 1867, outlawing variolation and making vaccination compulsory, set an example for India to follow. By Act IV of 1865, the Government of Bengal implemented the recommendations of the Smallpox Commission of 1850 and prohibited the practice of variolation in Calcutta and its suburbs: failure to obey the ban was to be punished with three months' imprisonment or a fine of Rs 200 (or both), and recent inoculees were prohibited from entering the city for forty days on pain of the same penalty.[107] In 1866 the ban was extended to surrounding villages, and by 1890 it had been extended to many other areas of the Bengal Presidency as well. This was a significant factor in turning the tide against variolation in Bengal. Although the actual number of prosecutions under the act was small, variolation was steadily driven underground in areas where it had formerly been openly and widely practiced. By the end of the century, a form of prophylaxis once commonplace in Bengal had become almost extinct.[108]

Another factor driving provincial governments toward legislation was concern about the continuing vulnerability of their principal cities. Bombay, a rapidly growing commercial and industrial center, suffered severely from smallpox epidemics during the 1860s and 1870s, reaching a peak in 1875–77 when the impact of the disease was exacerbated by the effects of famine and the influx of unprotected migrants into the city in search of relief; the result was a steep surge in smallpox mortality (see figure 1). As with the plague epidemic which struck Bombay twenty years later, this epidemic invasion of one of India's leading cities forced the government to act. The Government of Bombay, with the reluctant concurrence of its superior in Calcutta, passed a Vaccination Act, Act I of 1877, which came into force in September 1877 and made vaccination within six months of birth compulsory for all babies born within Bombay municipality and for unprotected children under fourteen years of age arriving from outside the city. Failure to comply was punished with six months in prison, a fine of Rs 1,000, or both. The act also banned variolation and prohibited anyone from entering the city within forty days of being inoculated on pain of three months in jail, Rs 200 fine, or both. Significantly, it was the recent development of an adequate supply of animal lymph which made compulsory vaccination possible in a city of 650,000 people.[109]

The marked increase in infants vaccinated under a year old and the decline in the number of smallpox deaths in Bombay following the introduction of compulsory vaccination strengthened the case for similar measures elsewhere. Although there had been talk of "mutinies" and "massacres" if compulsion were used in Bombay, in practice, the act encountered little active resistance. The voluntary system had proved "ineffectual," the Government of Bombay argued, not so

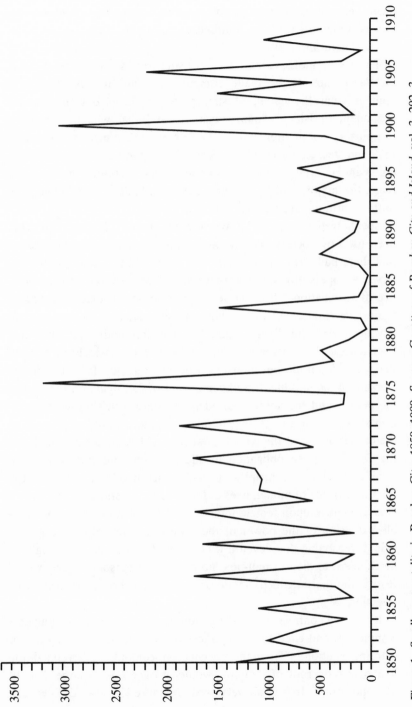

Figure 1. Smallpox mortality in Bombay City, 1850–1909. *Source: Gazetteer of Bombay City and Island*, vol. 3, 202–3.

much because of the strength of religious opposition to vaccination, as was commonly assumed, but because of public "indifference, indolence or ignorance."[110]

There was, moreover, growing pressure from some Indian quarters for vaccination to be made compulsory. Thus it was Sir Sayyid Ahmad Khan, the leading Muslim spokesman of his day and a major proponent of Islamic "modernization" in India, who introduced a compulsory vaccination bill in the Viceroy's Council in September 1879 and steered it through its second reading in February the following year. He argued that without compulsion, vaccination would not reach the majority of India's unprotected infants and left them prey to the continuing scourge of smallpox.

Speaking the language of Western rationality which had so often been used by doctors and officials against Indians, he acknowledged that there had been a time when the people of India "had prejudices, to which superstition and ignorance had given birth, against the practice of vaccination." But, he declared, "the hatred that once existed against vaccination is now a thing of the past, at least in the more advanced parts of British India." Education and experience had "opened the eyes of the people," and it was now widely recognized that vaccination did not interfere with religious beliefs, not even the worship of Sitala. Only "apathy and want of foresight" on the part of the people and the absence of adequate state provision for vaccination stood in the way of its general acceptance. Citing as precedents the earlier action of the colonial state, Sayyid Ahmad Khan said that the British had an obligation to alleviate suffering and protect the weak and helpless, principles, he said, which had led to the abolition of "the sacrifice of human lives at the altar of superstition, and put an effective check upon female infanticide." He pleaded for a comparable extension of the power of the state over the rights of the individual, reasoning that "even if it be granted that a man has a right, if he chooses, to die of small-pox, no respect for personal liberty would justify the harm which he does to his neighbours by conveying infection."[111]

It was, by contrast, the colonial administrators who argued against compulsion and cited the "prejudices of the people" as a reason for extreme caution. "To make vaccination compulsory," replied the lieutenant-governor of Punjab, "would at once raise a large amount of opposition." It was all very well, remarked a second European member of the council, for the "enlightened minority" of Indians to favor compulsion, but the government had to reckon with the views of the great majority of the people, the "unenlightened masses," whose religious feelings might be whipped up by designing agitators. Eventually the bill was passed, but only when its proposer had been able to assure the council that it was merely permissive legislation and would be confined to those municipalities and cantonments that actively wanted vaccination.[112]

Quite apart from the ever-present financial considerations, the colonial regime remained nervous of a backlash against compulsory vaccination and coercive state medicine. Northern India was thought to be particularly volatile. The mere rumor of compulsory vaccination had been enough, it was pointed out, to set off a scare and threaten disturbances in Delhi in 1870–71.[113] The strength of the public reaction against antiplague measures in 1896–1900 (discussed in chapter 5) further suggested the political risks medical interventionism might entail for an alien government. In consequence, the Government of India allowed only a gradual extension of the 1880 Vaccination Act. By 1906 it had been introduced in only 441 towns and cantonments, representing a mere 7 percent of the total population of British India. Very few small towns and villages were included before the 1930s, and even in 1950, three years after Indian independence, vaccination was compulsory in no more than 732 of the country's 842 municipalities and barely half of its 408,000 villages.[114]

The Vaccination Act was also notoriously difficult to enforce. The registration of births, even in leading municipalities like Bombay, remained so incomplete that vaccination staff had no clear idea of the number of infants of the age appropriate for vaccination. In Bombay, as in other large commercial and industrial cities, there was the added complication of high rates of immigration from the countryside, with many babies and children arriving unvaccinated and undetected. Prosecutions were rare, partly because of a lack of interest by the police, magistrates, and municipal authorities. In some urban areas in the 1880s and 1890s, the Vaccination Act was frankly admitted to be a "dead letter."[115] As a result, upward of 20 percent of infants in even the best-vaccinated urban areas escaped vaccination. Although immunization significantly reduced the absolute number of susceptibles in the community and helped to break the chain of epidemiological transmission, a substantial pool of unprotected children and adults remained, among whom smallpox continued to circulate. Across British India as a whole, epidemics were becoming less frequent and less deadly by the early years of the twentieth century, but (as the figures for Bombay city in figure 1 show) they did not cease to claim thousands of lives and, indeed, included a growing proportion of adults who had failed to gain either natural or artificial protection in their infancy.[116]

The assertion that vaccination made smallpox a preventable disease was thus only partly valid given the political and cultural constraints on its deployment in nineteenth- and early twentieth-century India. From time to time it was urged that vaccination, to be effective, must also be accompanied by the isolation of all smallpox cases and their contacts; but this was always rejected as entailing an intolerable degree of interference in the lives of the people and requiring an army of medical subordinates for its implementation.[117] Again, the experience of the early plague years showed the practical obstacles and political snares such sweeping measures were likely to encounter. In consequence, smallpox was never made a notifiable disease in colonial India, and it was not until the international eradication campaign of the 1960s and 1970s that smallpox was tackled in a sufficiently systematic way to contrive its final extinction in India.

CONCLUSION

Smallpox was almost as familiar to eighteenth- and nineteenth-century Europe as it was to South Asia. Because it seemed to pose few of the problems presented by cholera, malaria, and other "diseases of warm climates," medical intervention against it at first appeared relatively straightforward—uncomplicated by mysterious miasmas and other environmental forces over which medicine and sanitation could exercise little control. Its basic mode of transmission was well known (if not well understood), and vaccination offered a potentially effective form of prophylaxis. Despite its potential, vaccination, in many ways the pioneer and exemplar of public health policy in India, ran into repeated difficulties. To some extent these mirrored Europe's own experience: the reluctance of people to seek vaccination (except when pressed to do so by epidemics or the law), the low level of immunity conferred (until the development of improved vaccine preservation techniques and the introduction of revaccination), and the problems of creating a reliable vaccinating agency.

And yet in many other ways the history of vaccination was expressive of a peculiarly colonial predicament in which the administration was culturally and politically distant from the lives of its subjects.

Belief in a smallpox deity provided an alternative, religious, explanation for the incidence of the disease and prescribed ritual observances that were at variance with Western medical secularism. In variolation, too, vaccination found an entrenched and formidable adversary, sustained by its own specialized agency and sanctioned by popular religious belief. It enjoyed the confidence of the people in the areas where it was widely practiced and (until late in the century) was often more readily available and actively sought than state vaccination. Disdainful alike of folk belief and indigenous practice, the colonial medical establishment was loath to compromise either with Sitala or with variolation. But while there could be no question of outlawing disease deities, the British saw the defeat of variolation as essential to the success of their own medical enterprise. Medical monopoly, not cultural pluralism, was their goal. Finding persuasion, co-option, and enlistment of "natives of rank" inadequate for the purpose, the colonial administration turned reluctantly to the law to prohibit variolation and hasten public acceptance of vaccination. An exotic, without root on Indian soil, vaccination long remained closely identified with foreign rule, attracting fears and suspicions that ranged far beyond doubts about its medical efficacy. By the 1880s, however, vaccination had begun to win support among the Indian middle classes, some of whom urged more active intervention than the state was itself prepared to countenance.

Vaccination against smallpox in nineteenth-century India was thus only partly constrained by popular opposition and apathy. The ambivalent or hesitant attitude of the state and the divided nature of medical opinion were also critical factors. Seeing the health of its European subjects and servants as its first priority, the state was reluctant to make the financial and administrative commitment necessary for an effective assault on smallpox. The sheer size and expense of such an undertaking was always a deterrent. Medical opinion, although often trenchant in its opposition to variolation and confident in its claims for the efficacy of vaccination, at times also voiced a reluctance to impose vaccination on an unwilling populace or to ban variolation before its own system of medicine had gained wider acceptance. Vaccination had been warmly welcomed by the colonial administration in the early decades of the nineteenth century as a token of its benevolence and proof of the superiority of Western science over Eastern "prejudice." But from an abiding sense of political insecurity, heightened by the events of 1857–58 and by rumbling discontent over this and other forms of medical intervention, the state shied away from a more energetic vaccination program lest it provoke resistance and revolt. Fear of the political consequences of compulsion was a powerful brake on medical interventionism. It encouraged greater reliance, in this field of colonial activity as in many others, on persuasion, on Indian intermediaries, and a gradualist approach to social change.

4 Cholera: Disease as Disorder

Few diseases in nineteenth-century India appeared to be as violently destructive as epidemic cholera. None provoked more sustained medical controversy, and, until the plague epidemic of the 1890s, none was the cause of greater administrative concern. In an environment in which epidemiology and empire repeatedly intersected, cholera was a highly political disease, one that seemed to threaten the slender basis of British power in India and to stand at the critical point of interaction between colonial state and indigenous society. Elsewhere in the world, the significance of invading cholera lay mainly in its capacity to open up fissures within society, particularly between the rich and the poor, or between the host society and immigrant communities. In India, its country of origin, cholera was important rather in terms of the dividing line it repeatedly drew between European rulers and their Indian subjects and the questions it posed about the terms on which the British held India.[1]

A disease scarcely recognized by the West before the early nineteenth century, cholera rapidly stamped its authority on India and the world. Already in 1819, two years after it first forced itself upon the attention of East India Company physicians, it was being described as one of the "most formidable and fatal diseases" to have "visited India in modern times."[2] Few diseases, noted James Annesley in 1825, "have excited more interest among medical men, or more terror in the mind of the Indian community at large, than the epidemic cholera."[3] The view of cholera as an exceptionally destructive and terrifying disease was soon shared by writers in Europe. A contributor to a London journal in 1831, reflecting on the remorseless advance of cholera from Asia into Europe, remarked that "within the annals of medicine there are few, if indeed any, diseases which are attended with such a frightful array of symptoms, or which destroy their unfortunate victims with such relentless fury, as the pestilential cholera."[4]

Cholera struck suddenly and unpredictably. A person in apparently sound health at one moment might be seized the next by violent vomiting and uncontrollable purging. The massive loss of body fluids that followed produced some of cholera's most alarming symptoms—the agonizing cramps, the cold, clammy surface of the skin, the deathly pallor—which led rapidly to death, often within hours of the first seizure. "This disease is characterized by the suddenness of its attack," explained the secretary to the Madras Medical Board in August 1818:

> It commences with a sense of heat in the epigastrium and slight watery purgings accompanied by a great languor and depression of spirits, with a diminished temperature of the surface of the body. The uneasiness at stomach and watery purging with a most remarkable prostration of strength increase rapidly; spasms are felt in the extremities, the pulse becomes very small and languid, and unless these symptoms are arrested by medicine, the vomiting and purging of a glary nearly colourless matter becomes more urgent—the cramp extends from the feet and legs to the muscles of the abdomen, thorax and arms—affecting those of a robust habit and in whom the attack is severe, with most excruciating pains, and exhausting the vital energies so rapidly that the patient in six or eight hours loses his pulse at the wrist; his body is bedewed with a cold clammy sweat, the eyes, dull and heavy, are covered with a film, occasionally suffused with blood and insensible to the stimulus of light, and in this state of the disease he is often afflicted with deafness, the breathing becomes greatly affected, and is sometimes performed . . . with much labor and a sort of grunting—the tongue is generally white, sometimes but seldom parched.
>
> During this awful and rapid progress of symptoms the countenance . . . becomes collapsed, the eye sinks, the patient has occasionally the appearance of being comatose and is roused for a few moments with difficulty, the extremities become cold and the circulation gradually dies away.
>
> In the progress of the disease the patient complains of great, and in some instances, insatiable thirst, having a strong desire

for cold fluids—the secretion as well as the excretion of bile
would appear to be entirely suppressed—the burning uneasiness
in the stomach extends to the whole alimentary canal, and a
total want of urine is observed in all the worst cases of disease.

In this severe epidemic, death has hitherto been observed to
ensue from 10 to 24 hours from the commencement of the
attack.[5]

Where smallpox was all raging heat and burning possession,
cholera was deadly chill and fearful isolation. If smallpox could be
ennobled by association with a fiery goddess, cholera spoke only of
the vile pollution of diarrhea and vomit. While there was a predicta-
bility about the contagiousness of smallpox, the apparent randomness
with which cholera seized its victims made it a peculiarly baffling disease, an "inscrutable malady," to European and Indian alike.[6] It
seemed to follow no logical "line of progression" in its forays into the
Indian countryside, "but with the greatest irregularity and caprice,
pounced upon a village here or there." It selected one village and in-
explicably spared its neighbors, though alike in every apparent respect; it might suddenly vanish, only mysteriously to reappear a few
months later in precisely the same place.[7] The elusiveness of its
identity made cholera a disease open to a variety of different cultural
and political interpretations, many of which identified disease with
"disorder."

THE TRAIL OF MORTALITY

The exceptional virulence of the disease was registered not only in
personal experience and clinical observation but also in the mounting
testimony of Indian mortality. Cholera, like smallpox, was one of the
mainstays of nineteenth-century medical statistics in India. Because
the collection of vital data did not begin in earnest until the late
1860s, it is impossible to arrive at an accurate figure for the number
of deaths caused by cholera during the nineteenth century, especially
during its earlier decades. But from such imperfect statistics as are
available, it would appear that at least 15 million deaths occurred in
British India alone between 1817, the year in which the century's first
major epidemic erupted in Bengal, and 1865, when mortality data began to be collected systematically for the first time. A further 23 million cholera deaths were recorded between 1865 and 1947, a figure
likely to understate the full extent of the mortality.

The epidemic of 1817–21 has been described as "probably the most terrible of all Indian cholera epidemics,"[8] but, because it struck when medical statistics was still in its infancy, no overall estimate of the death toll was attempted at the time, and such figures as were produced were almost invariably qualified by doubts about their accuracy. The only attempt at a comprehensive figure was made not in India but in France by the physician Alexandre Moreau de Jonnès in 1831. Although based on information from India, his calculations were informed and inflated by the alarm cholera was already causing in Europe. On the basis of mortality figures for certain areas of Bengal and among troops of the East India Company—a dubious guide to civilian mortality—Moreau de Jonnès calculated that cholera affected one-tenth of the population of British India and killed one-sixteenth. For the period 1817–31, he postulated an average annual mortality of 1.25 million, arriving at a figure of 18 million deaths overall.[9] Other commentators made estimates that were even more profligate, suggesting that for the whole of India, the number of cholera deaths might have been as high as 40 or 50 million in only fourteen years.[10] It is little wonder Europe feared the return of epidemic destruction on the scale of the Black Death that had caused such massive mortality in the fourteenth century.

The death toll in 1817–21 was undoubtedly great, but there is no evidence to suggest that it was as uniformly high as Moreau de Jonnès presumed. In some respects the 1817–21 epidemic was exceptional. The thirty years that had lapsed since the last recorded epidemics of the 1780s probably left the population vulnerable to a fresh outbreak. Like the El Tor cholera which reached India in 1964 and rapidly supplanted the existing strain of the disease, the 1817 epidemic might well have been of a new and more virulent biotype, enabling it to move with great speed and destructiveness from the areas of Lower Bengal where it was (or became) endemic to almost every part of the subcontinent within three years. Subsequent epidemics rarely spanned more than one or two provinces at a time. Lack of immunity combined with exceptional geographical range would lead one to expect high levels of mortality. On the other hand, the most severe of the later epidemics occurred in famine years, whereas famine was almost entirely absent from India in 1817–21.

Certainly, Bengal was badly affected. Statistics collected by James Jameson for the Bengal Medical Board showed mortality in excess of

10,000 in several districts, including Jessore, where the epidemic was first observed in August 1817 and where that number was said to have perished in two months alone. In Calcutta and its suburbs, according to one estimate, there were nearly 37,000 cases of cholera between mid-September 1817 and mid-July 1818, though only 2,382 fatalities. Jameson also noted that towns and districts further up the Ganges valley suffered less than those in Lower Bengal.[11]

In western India the epidemic appears to have been relatively mild. Between August 1818 and February 1819, 24,227 cases of cholera were reported on Bombay island, but only 938 deaths, in a population of some 200,000 inhabitants.[12] South India, as well, does not appear to have suffered the same ferocious assault as Bengal. Cuddapah district lost about 15,000 out of a population of nearly a million (about 14 deaths per 1,000 inhabitants), while in Nellore there were only 3,000 deaths from cholera reported between August 1818 and September 1819, at a rate of approximately 7 deaths for every 1,000 inhabitants. Although reporting was sketchy, for the Madras districts as a whole the mortality during the height of the epidemic appears to have been around 11 to 12 per 1,000.[13] If this figure were applied to the whole of India, with a population of some 120–150 million, the total number of deaths would have been no more than one or two million. This would certainly represent a formidable loss of life, but not on the scale which Moreau de Jonnès and other writers in Europe imagined.

It is significant that opinion in India was itself divided about the scale of the catastrophe. William Scot of the Madras Medical Board, citing a mortality of 27.5 percent among European troops and 38 percent among Indian soldiers, observed that these figures marked the epidemic as "one of the most formidable that has ever afflicted the human race."[14] In Bengal, Jameson thought it "perhaps more destructive in its effects, and more extensive in its influence, than any other recorded in the annals of this country." But although the mortality was "undoubtedly very great," he considered it "vain to hazard a conjecture of its amount." In Calcutta, out of every second or third family, "perhaps one, two, or three, and in some cases, five or six members perished. For many months numerous parties were constantly met carrying the biers of the dead; and the banks of the river [Hughli] were crowded with Hindoos burning the bodies of departed relatives." And yet, perhaps because the fear caused by cholera out-

Table 11. Cholera Mortality in British India, Quinquennial Averages, 1877–1916

Years	Mortality	Years	Mortality
1877–81	288,949	1897–1901	383,294
1882–86	286,105	1902–06	367,160
1887–91	400,934	1907–11	397,127
1892–96	443,890	1912–16	328,593

Source: Report of the Health Survey and Development Committee, 1946, vol. 1, 111.

stripped even its prodigious capacity to kill, Jameson nevertheless concluded that the "sum total of the mortality occasioned by the epidemick fell far short of the rate assigned to it, by the voice of the public, during the season of alarm."[15] A third authority, R. H. Kennedy in Bombay, failed to see any "peculiar malignity" in the disease and thought it scarcely offered "a more distressing image of desolation to our view than what we are in the habit of beholding with philosophic calmness, and ranking among the ordinary casualities of Indian life."[16]

From the 1870s we are on firmer statistical ground. During the last quarter of the nineteenth century, an average of 1.75 out of every 1,000 of the population of British India died of cholera annually. But this relatively modest aggregate masks the enormous yearly fluctuations that were so characteristic of the disease. In 1874, for example, cholera mortality sank to 0.16 per 1,000, and in four other years in the quarter century fell below 1 per 1,000. But in 1877, 1892, and 1906, deaths exceeded 3 per 1,000; in 1900 the total reached a staggering 797,222, or 3.70 per 1,000 (see table 11 and figure 2). The smaller the area, the larger the proportion of deaths appeared. In the Madras Presidency in 1877, 357,430 cholera deaths were recorded (12.20 per 1,000), and in four districts where famine was also rife, between 20 and 25 out of every 1,000 inhabitants perished from the disease.[17] It is nonetheless indicative of the high levels of mortality prevailing in India at the time that even in 1900, the worst cholera year on record, the disease was responsible for only a tenth of all recorded deaths. Between 1896 and 1921, plague caused about 10 million deaths and malaria probably twice that number. The influenza pandemic of 1918–19 swept away 12 to 15 million more.

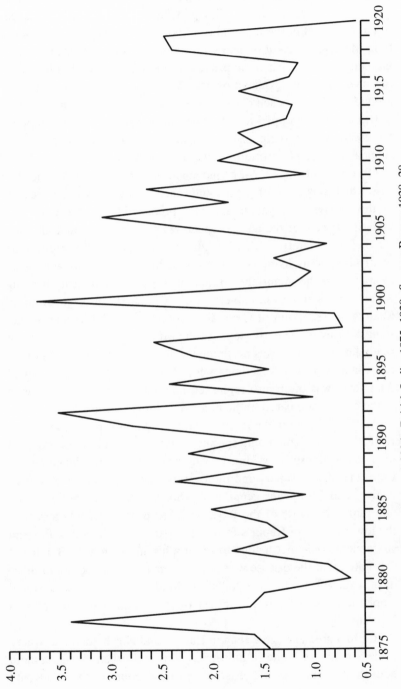

Figure 2. Annual cholera mortality per 1,000 in British India, 1875–1920. *Source*: Rogers 1928, 28.

Cholera mortality began to decline in the early decades of the twentieth century, despite a rising population and with little evidence of improvement in the material conditions of the mass of the population. Medical intervention and sanitary precautions, rather than a rising standard of living or improved socioeconomic conditions, offer the most plausible explanation for this decline. Having hovered at around 4 million in each decade from 1890 to 1919, cholera mortality in British India dropped to 2.2 million in the 1920s and 1.7 million in the 1930s, with a slight resurgence in the 1940s, the decade of the Bengal famine and Partition, to just over 2 million.[18]

Observers of the 1817–21 epidemic noted one feature of the disease which was to be of great significance for the subsequent history of the disease in India: its apparent predilection for the poor and undernourished. Although European residents were at first alarmed for their own safety,[19] India's white elite was partly protected by its relatively healthy living conditions and, by the 1850s, by a growing awareness of the importance of personal hygiene and clean drinking water. The deaths from cholera of Sir Thomas Munro, governor of Madras, in 1827, and of General Anson, commander-in-chief of the Bengal Army in the early stages of the Mutiny in May 1857, were apt reminders that there was no immunity for the privileged and powerful. Cholera, it was sometimes said, "knew no distinction of rank." And yet it was often also remarked how few Europeans succumbed to the disease compared to the number of Indian victims.[20]

Among the poorer classes of India, mortality was particularly high. In 1820 Jameson could only speculate on the cause of the disease and its mode of transmission, but he was struck by its prevalence among Calcutta's slum dwellers and the contrast with the "higher classes of Native, and Europeans generally," who, living in the "better raised and more airy parts of the town, suffered proportionately less than the lower ranks."[21] Reports from other parts of India during this and subsequent epidemics tended to confirm his impression. In Bombay it was noted that the disease was confined mainly to the poor and those most exposed to the elements; in Madras, William Scot stated emphatically that "only the lowest of the common people suffered from this disease."[22]

But to a greater degree than in Europe and North America, where cholera made its home in industrial cities and urban slums, cholera flourished in India as a disease of the rural poor. In the 1860s and

1870s, the largest Indian cities followed the lead of sanitary reform in Britain, particularly with respect to improved water supplies, and these measures had a noticeable effect on urban mortality (though slum dwellers were those least likely to benefit from such sanitary innovations). Calcutta, close to the center of Bengal's endemic cholera zone, suffered between 2,500 and 7,000 deaths from the disease every year between 1841 and 1865. In that year a new sewage system was opened, followed in 1869 by a filtered water supply. Cholera deaths dropped dramatically and, despite the city's rapid growth in the second half of the century, exceeded 3,000 only once (in 1895) between 1870 and 1900.[23] In Bombay and Madras, improved water supplies had a comparable effect, and it was only during famine years like 1877, when the rural poor flocked in from the drought-ravaged countryside, that urban mortality reached its highest levels.[24] But in small towns and villages, without piped water or effective sanitation, cholera remained a recurrent threat.

In the countryside cholera had a double impact. Epidemics alone could cause heavy loss of life, but this mortality doubled or trebled when cholera coincided with famine. The simultaneity of cholera and famine was most devastating during the second half of the nineteenth century, a period of frequent and widespread famines. In Madras in 1866 and 1877, as in Bombay in 1877 and 1900, this lethal combination drove cholera mortality to its highest recorded levels. The absence of major famines after 1908 was conversely an important factor in the overall decline in cholera mortality, just as the Bengal famine of 1943–44 contributed to its temporary resurgence.

There was, however, no automatic correlation between cholera and famine. Epidemics followed seasonal and cyclical patterns of their own, though with a human tally greatly inflated by concurrent famine. In the Madras Presidency between 1869 and 1871, a cholera epidemic resulted in about 100,000 deaths. Cholera deaths sank to 440 in 1873 and to 313 in 1874, but the epidemic cycle then began again with 94,546 deaths in 1875 and 148,193 in 1876. At that stage drought and famine intervened, affecting large areas of the province and giving the epidemic fresh impetus. There were 357,430 cholera deaths recorded in 1877, equivalent to 12.2 per 1,000, "much the highest," Leonard Rogers remarked in 1928, "for any province of [British] India for the last fifty years."[25] Although the famine reached its peak in September 1877, cholera mortality had already begun to fall in February of that year, but deaths from cholera tended to be greatest where famine was most severe. In the ten worst-hit districts in 1877, cholera deaths reached 18 per 1,000, whereas in the six districts least affected by famine, there were only 4.6 cholera deaths per 1,000.[26]

Hot, dry conditions are not normally conducive to the survival of the cholera bacillus, but drought and dearth drove villagers to drink water from wells, tanks, and pools that quickly became contaminated with cholera. Chronic malnutrition might have been a factor in weakening resistance to the disease, though there is no clear medical evidence for this, and the changed patterns of diet and behavior induced by famine were probably more significant in exposing individuals to infection. Hunger led to a desperate and debilitating search for sustenance and relief, and the consumption of roots, leaves, and other surrogate foods often brought on sickness and diarrhea. The mobility of the famine-struck, their concentration in relief camps or in towns and cities, facilitated the spread of the disease, while the collapse of family or community care caused by famine and disease was not compensated by adequate measures of state medical relief.[27]

The close connection with famine does more than account for part of cholera's great mortality. It also underscores the association between epidemic disease and social disruption on a vast scale and points to problems of poverty and hygiene that were too deep-seated for the colonial regime to be able or willing to tackle. Initially, at least, colonialism responded to the challenge of cholera in a far more limited way.

CHOLERA AS COLONIAL CRISIS

It has become so customary to apply military metaphors to epidemic diseases—to speak of their "attacks" and "invasions," of the "devastation" they cause or the "resistance" they encounter, and of their "conquest" by medical science—that one could easily overlook the literal correspondence between cholera and military power in colonial India. The first epidemic of the nineteenth century came hard on the heels of the most decisive phase of British expansion. When cholera erupted in 1817, the East India Company had held control of Bengal for sixty years, but only in the previous twenty had its territorial power been pushed into large parts of the rest of India. In 1817 the war with the Gurkhas of Nepal was barely concluded, and not until

June of the following year was the power of the Marathas finally broken. The arrival of the epidemic in western India in July–August 1818 followed closely the defeat of the peshwa of Pune and thus, the Sikhs of Punjab apart, corresponded with the extinction of sustained military opposition to British rule in South Asia.

The connection between cholera and conquest was not fortuitous. As we have seen in chapter 2, cholera was a leading cause of sickness and mortality among soldiers, especially European troops. Living in crowded and insanitary barracks or lines, surviving during campaigns on whatever food and water they could find, thirsty and fatigued from long marches, troops were particularly susceptible to cholera. Many contemporary reports, perhaps in search of a "native" scapegoat, attributed this vulnerability particularly to Indian camp followers— "always poor, filthy in their habits, and entirely exposed to the varying effects of the weather"—who then passed it on to British and Indian soldiers.[28] On the march or fighting campaigns, soldiers were one of the main vectors of the disease and might carry it with them across vast tracts of rural India. The large-scale movements of troops through northern India from Bengal, cholera's homeland, in 1817–18 facilitated the epidemic invasion of the rest of India, and this pattern was partly repeated forty years later during the campaigns of the 1857–58 Mutiny and Rebellion. To speak of the "invasion" of cholera as if it were an army on the march was thus more than a casual analogy.

In the colonial perception, one of the most perturbing incidents of the 1817–21 epidemic was the outbreak of cholera among troops assembled in Bundelkhand in central India in November 1817 for a campaign against the Pindaris (the scattered bands of freebooters who raided central and eastern India in the wake of the Maratha wars) and against the Marathas themselves. In his account of this episode, James Jameson aptly represented cholera as an enemy force advancing stealthily upon a defenseless and unsuspecting army. After "creeping about . . . in its unwonted insidious manner" for several days among the "lower classes of the camp followers," the disease suddenly, he wrote, "gained fresh vigour, and at once burst forth with irresistible violence in every direction." In a short time there were so many casualties that the medical staff could not cope with them all, and the "whole camp . . . put on the appearance of a hospital." As the death toll mounted, the normal military routine was suspended:

"All business had given way to solicitude for the suffering. Not a smile could be discerned, nor a sound heard, except the groans of the dying, and the wailing over the dead." According to Jameson, the Indian camp followers, having introduced the disease in the first place, now began to "desert" in large numbers, "and the highways and fields for many miles round, were strewed with the bodies of those who had left camp with the disease upon them, and speedily sunk under its exhausting effects." The commander ordered the army to move to a healthier site, but the mortality continued, with 764 soldiers (out of 11,500 fighting men) perishing in a single week. Jameson reported that "hundreds dropt down during every subsequent day's advance, and covered the roads with dead and dying; the ground of encampment, and line of march, presented the appearance of a field of battle, and of the track of an army retreating under every circumstance of discomfiture and distress."[29]

For the next fifty years, cholera kept up its sporadic guerrilla war against British military power in India. For a colonial regime so heavily dependent on European soldiers, especially during the 1857–58 rebellion and in its aftermath, the disease posed a serious military and political threat, and one for which there seemed no ready medical or sanitary solution—apart from retreat to a supposedly more salubrious site. Several senior officers died of the disease during critical stages of the campaigns and sieges of 1857–58, and at times cholera, "that terrible scourge," seemed a more menacing and demoralizing enemy than the rebels themselves.[30] As was pointed out in chapter 2, heavy losses from cholera during and immediately following the rebellion prompted concern for the health of European soldiers in India and made cholera the foremost disease for consideration by the new sanitary commissioners in the 1860s. Between 1818 and 1857, some 5,719 European soldiers under the Bengal command had died of cholera, and a further 3,861 followed between 1858 and 1867, a large proportion of them in the epidemic of 1861.[31]

This continuing drain on military manpower kept alive the idea of cholera as a lurking, dangerous enemy, ever ready to snipe, like the rebellious sepoys of 1857, at white soldiers and their families. While several European officers were castigated for doing too little to save their troops during the 1861 epidemic, others were commended for showing the same bravery in the face of the "enemy" as they had against the recent mutineers and rebels: it was their duty, as on the field of battle, to maintain the morale of their "panic-stricken" soldiery.[32] The slow retreat of cholera from cantonment and camp after 1861 was a significant, if underlying, factor in the increased security of British power in post-Mutiny India.

COMPREHENDING CHOLERA

Many Indians, too, saw a connection between cholera and conquest, but, given the strength of religion in popular perceptions and beliefs, were less inclined to interpret its significance in such secular terms. The episode of the Company's cholera-stricken army in Bundelkhand remained in local memory, too, but bore a sharply different connotation. Villagers believed that the epidemic had begun when, despite a Brahmin's remonstrances, cattle were slaughtered to feed British soldiers camped in a grove sacred to Hurdoul Lal, son of a former local raja. In the popular perception, the British were guilty of a double violation: of a sacred grove and of Hindu prohibitions on the killing of cattle and consumption of beef. The epidemic was accordingly interpreted as a sign of the disorder caused by divine wrath, and Hurdoul Lal was thereafter worshipped and propitiated over a wide area of northern India whenever cholera threatened.[33]

This was not an isolated example. Villagers at Cunnatore in Nellore district of Madras traced the epidemic to the arrival of low-caste soldiers and their camp followers who polluted (in a ritual as well as epidemiological sense) certain sacred tanks nearby.[34] The inhabitants of Ongole in the same district attributed epidemic cholera and small-pox to the residence there of the raja of Gumsur, taken captive by the British during the Gumsur war in Ganjam in 1835. When the imprisoned raja was unable to make his usual offerings to the goddess Mahalakshmi, she vented her ire not only on the British soldiers but also on the residents of Ongole.[35] Moreau de Jonnès reported that Hindus attributed the 1817–21 epidemic in a similar way to the resentment of the deity "Yagatha Ummah" against British rule over India.[36]

Behind these and many other explanations for the origins of cholera lurked a widely shared belief that the British were in some way responsible, whether through the direct violation of Hindu taboos or indirectly through the disruptive effects of their military intervention on the Hindu cosmos. Cholera was the tangible manifestation of some wider disorder. But significantly, the consequences of divine displeasure were more often directed at the Indian population than the conquering foreigners. Cholera appeared more a chastisement of Hindus for failing to resist British incursions and conquest than a form of direct retribution against the British.

Although it became clear during the early nineteenth century that cholera had long been present in India, if not always in such a virulent form, the disease had not, unlike smallpox, been extensively ritualized. There are several possible explanations for this. The symptoms of cholera were less distinctive than the burning fever that signaled an attack of smallpox, and as already suggested, it manifested itself in ways Hindus would regard as deeply polluting. There was no equivalent to the practice of variolation by which to invoke a goddess's blessing. Perhaps, too, cholera had not previously been so widespread and destructive as it became after 1817 and so did not need to feature as prominently in village rituals and Hindu cosmology as the goddess of smallpox. Only in deltaic Bengal, the home of cholera, is there evidence for the worship of a cholera deity, but her title of Ola Candi or Ola Bibi ("the lady of the flux") suggests that she might have been associated with dysenteric and diarrheal diseases generally, and not just with cholera in the form in which it became known to nineteenth-century India.[37] In the absence of an established form of worship over most of India, initial responses to the epidemic were varied. In Bundelkhand, as we have seen, Hurdoul Lal was pressed into service as a male cholera deity. But the dominant response was to represent cholera either as a new manifestation of the powers of an existing deity, like Mariamma or Kali, or as an entirely new deity, known only by such descriptive titles as *jari mari* ("sudden sickness") or *kala mari* ("black death").[38]

But although the identity of the deity was unclear, belief in the power of specific deities to cause or control this disease, like many others, was by no means lacking. One expression of this belief was the appearance of a young woman dressed as the goddess of the disease and worshipped accordingly. Another was the appearance of women claiming to be mediums possessed by the spirit or deity responsible for the disease. Both acted as would-be mediators between the villagers and the gods, voicing the supposed grievances of the goddess of the disease and giving, in return, an immediate focus to local anxieties and alarm. Such mediums and "goddesses" (or *devis*) have been extensively described in the historical and anthropological

literature,[39] but the cholera epidemic of 1817–21 provides some striking illustrations, testifying to the degree of the unease created by this
epidemic in many parts of India.

In January 1818 the Reverend J. Keith reported the appearance of
"an actual avatur or incarnation of Ola Beebee" at Salkhia on the
outskirts of Calcutta. She sat there for two days "in all the state of a
Hindoo goddess" attended by a young Brahmin woman as her "priest-
ess." According to Keith, she was in competition with the priests of
the goddess Kali for the attention and offerings of worshippers
alarmed by the epidemic, but succeeded in "reaping a rich harvest
from the terror she had sown in the minds of the people."[40] A few
months later, in the Bombay Presidency, a woman "declaring herself
to be an Avatar of the fiend of pestilence" was observed at the cantonment of Sirur, about forty miles from Pune. According to Kennedy, she entered the bazaar "almost naked,"

> but her dishevelled hair, her whole body, and her scanty apparel
> were daubed and clotted with the dingy red and ochry yellow
> powders of the Hindoo burial ceremonies. She was frantic with
> mania, real or assumed, or maddened by an intoxication, partly
> mental, partly from excitement from drugs. In one hand she
> held a drawn sword, in the other an earthen vessel containing
> fire (the one probably a symbol of destruction, the other of the
> funeral pile). Before her proceeded a gang of musicians, pour-
> ing forth their discords from every harsh and clattering instru-
> ment of music appropriate to their religious processions. Behind
> her followed a long line of empty carts; no driver whom she en-
> countered on the road daring to disobey her command to follow
> in her train. Thus accoutred and accompanied her phrenzy
> seemed beyond all human control; and as she bounded along,
> she denounced certain destruction to all who did not immedi-
> ately acknowledge her divinity; and pointing to the empty carts
> which followed, proclaimed that they were brought to convey
> away the corpses of those who rashly persisted in infidelity. No
> ridicule, no jest, awaited this frantic visitant, but deep distress
> and general consternation.[41]

A third episode during the same epidemic had a more complicated
story involving a community of Christian Koli fishermen in the village
of Chendnee in Northern Konkan. When cholera struck in 1818,
many of the Kolis died or fell sick, and they appealed to the *sirkar*

(government) for help. When the state's medicine proved ineffective, they asked their Catholic priest to "provide a remedy for the evil," and when he, too, failed to help them, they resorted to a Hindu ceremony, known as *khel*, to which had been added some trappings of Christianity. According to Babington, the judge of Northern Konkan, who described the ceremony as "one of the most savage exhibitions" he had ever seen, the villagers formed a circle round "a number of frantic people, principally females, whose groans and violent gestures were said to indicate that they were under a supernatural influence." They were sprinkled with water and colored earth and "urged to exert themselves to the utmost in a sort of dance by the sound of native music." Once in a trance, the women became mediums for a series of spirit visitors. The first of these was Jesus, who "ordained whatever other Marhatta spirits might appear, as they would do in numbers, we should adhere to them for eight days and afterwards on the ninth day give each his feast and burn two wax lights before him, performing a mass in the Church at the expense of 5 Rupees." The mediums also pointed to certain villagers who were said to have caused the epidemic and who were punished severely. Several Kolis stricken with cholera and placed on litters near a specially erected shrine were miraculously cured "without recourse to medicine, merely by sprinkling earth and water over their bodies." Although these rituals seemed to the Kolis to work when all other expedients and entreaties had failed, they were not well received by their Catholic priest, who refused to allow the people back into his church to celebrate mass or hold their weddings.[42]

Babington, Kennedy, and Keith, like other colonial magistrates, doctors, and missionaries, cited such behavior to demonstrate the primitive, superstitious, and irrational ways of Indians and to commend the superiority of their own medical practices or religious beliefs. In fact, even in their partisan and disparaging accounts one can sense the intensity of the social and spiritual crisis brought on by the epidemic and the strength of the religious fervor it produced. Clearly, the representation of the epidemic in terms of an awesome or avenging deity was a not uncommon one, and for many villagers the collective crisis created by cholera might have been made intelligible or capable of resolution only through the mediation of "goddesses" or spirit mediums. And yet, even if colonial writers sought to dismiss disease "goddesses" and spirit mediums as "disgusting and debasing" examples of Hindu ignorance and superstition, the strength of popular belief could not easily be ignored. The outbreak of an unknown epidemic was also a test of European authority, therapeutics, and faith. The villagers of Chendnee found *sirkar* and padre alike ineffective, and only their spirit mediums and rites were of any apparent use. It was not surprising, then, that the state took the epidemic seriously, feeling its own authority under scrutiny. It was also wary lest the religious "phrenzy" Kennedy and others described should fuel public alarm, spread panic, and greatly increase the disruption that had already occurred in agriculture, trade, and local administration.

Many reports attest to the damage the 1817–21 epidemic caused to the "prosperity of the country," with grain heaps left unguarded as villagers fell ill or fled, as trade came to a standstill and revenue payments faltered or dried up. In areas where the collection of revenue was already difficult, cholera was an unwelcome additional complication.[43] In Madras the government agreed, albeit with some reluctance, to pay Hindu priests to hold propitiatory ceremonies. It did so partly from recognition that this was the customary duty of an Indian state toward its afflicted subjects, but also, pragmatically, as a way of allaying popular alarm and discouraging villagers from deserting their fields.[44]

There was a fear, too, that unless the government was seen to be active, a disturbed populace might turn against the British themselves. At Sirur, where the "detestable delusion" of the "goddess" had begun to have a "serious effect on the feelings of the mob," the *devi* was arrested, put in prison, and her followers dispersed. In a second episode described by Kennedy, at Severndroog in Southern Konkan, where the "same mockery was attempted" and a party of young women "personated the demons of the disease," the authorities acted promptly, having the male attendants unceremoniously flogged in the bazaar. The "goddesses" themselves were arrested, held until they had recovered from their drug-induced "intoxication," ridiculed, and finally released with a warning as a "salutary example" to others.[45] Salkhia's "avatur" met a similar fate. When summoned to the magistrate's office (*kutchery*), she lacked, according to Keith, "sufficient confidence in her own power" not to go. The magistrate berated her for her "imposture" and sentenced her to six months in the House of Correction.[46] Quite apart, then, from any specifically medical response to the epidemic, the British were concerned for the political and financial security of their rule and saw a need to respond promptly and firmly to the religious movements which accompanied the disease.

Apart from appealing to the *devis*, there were many other ways in which Hindu villagers sought to humor or placate the cholera-causing deity.[47] There were enormous local and regional variations in these rites. In parts of southern India, for instance, ceremonies for the goddess who had come to be associated with cholera, whether held annually or in anticipation of an epidemic, commonly included the preparation of an elaborately decorated pot (*karagam*) containing water, coconut, limes, flowers, and other items, which was paraded through the village and honored as a representation of the deity. These rites, performed by a low-caste priest, or *pujari* (from the washerman, carpenter, or barber castes), were often accompanied by the sacrifice of a buffalo or goat. The blood of the sacrificed animal was then sprinkled on rice and offered to the deity before being distributed among villagers or scattered around the boundaries of the village to protect it from the disease. During epidemics, the *karagam* or some other representation of the goddess, sometimes mounted on a small cart, might be taken in procession to the edge of the village. "The villagers of the adjacent villages in their turn carry the karagam to the border of the next village, and in this way the karagam traverses many miles of the country, and the baleful influence of the goddess is transferred to a safe distance."[48] In a variation of this ritual during times of epidemic sickness, buffaloes, goats, or chickens were first dedicated to the goddess, then released at the village boundary and driven off in the belief that the goddess and her pestilence would follow them and leave the village free from disease.[49] Sometimes in northern India a human "scapegoat," such as an untouchable Chamar or a prostitute, was driven out of the village or town to represent the expulsion of the disease.[50]

These practices of disease propitiation and expulsion were among the ways in which cholera, conceived (by contrast to Sitala) as a powerful but undesirable presence, was understood to be amenable to some degree of human control or persuasion. But from the viewpoint of the colonial state, such practices were open to political interpretation, or more often misinterpretation, for there is little evidence of their having had any intentionally political significance. The most celebrated example was the circulation of chapatis from village to village in northern India on the eve of the Mutiny in 1857. In searching after the event for evidence of an organized plot behind the uprising, the British remembered the chapatis and imagined them to have been a kind of conspiratorial call to arms. It is likely, however, that the chapatis were instead a device, similar to those already described, intended to pass on, or in some way afford protection against, the cholera then raging in parts of northern India. But, as Ranajit Guha has argued, it was possible for the chapatis both to have served this specific purpose and at the same time to have given expression to a collective sense of anxiety at the nature of British rule and the anticipation of some impending catastrophe.[51]

Although the use of chapatis for this purpose might have been rare, after the rebellion, when cholera was again at large in northern India, other tokens began to circulate in the countryside. In April 1860, for example, officials in Agra intercepted a *ghura* (earthenware pot) containing 215 *pice* (small coins), 160 cowries, 27 rings, mostly of base metal, and some tobacco. The *ghura*'s progress and the origin of its "mysterious message" were painstakingly traced back through more than ninety villages along the borders of present-day Uttar Pradesh, Madhya Pradesh, and Rajasthan before the trail ran cold. It was thought to have originated somewhere in the state of Gwalior and was passed on, from village to village, between local zamindars by Chamar women, each landholder feeling obliged to contribute to the pot's contents for fear that "otherwise some misfortune might be expected."[52] Officials were eventually satisfied that the *ghura* carried no political message as such and was merely a device (of a kind apparently not uncommon in those parts) to ward off epidemic cholera. But, with thoughts of the recent rebellion in mind, the provincial government directed that such objects, even when seemingly innocent, were to be "narrowly watched, and duly reported."[53]

The judge and magistrate in Bombay's North Konkan district had been similarly concerned in August 1818 at the way in which two buffaloes, "painted in an extraordinary manner," were being driven from place to place by village messengers. A connection was recognized between the current cholera epidemic and this action, but as it came so soon after the defeat of the Marathas and the British takeover, the officials feared that it was "an attempt. . . made by some ill-disposed persons to create an alarm in the district regarding the disorder"— meaning, in this instance, the cholera. The judge and magistrate said they had "no doubt of the wicked design" that lay behind the buffaloes' appearance, but they would have "treated it with contempt" had they "not found that its success upon the minds of the inhabitants has been considerable." They proposed to impound the animals, auction them "to convince the people of the little real consequence we attach to the imposition," and to offer a reward of Rs 300 for information about its originators whom, if found, they would "disgrace in the most public manner."[54] The provincial government considered this response excessive. While agreeing that the buffaloes were probably intended to show that the epidemic was "a visitation of Providence brought on the community for their want of exertion in resisting our power," it thought it unwise to treat the "simple fact of painting the animals" as a crime or to take any action which would draw attention to the buffaloes—unless further attempts were made "to create dissatisfaction."[55]

For British officials and Hindu villagers alike, though often in strikingly different ways, cholera stood for or seemed to presage a wider political or cosmological "dis-order." In particular, either because of their severity or their historical conjuncture, the epidemics of 1817–21, 1856–57, and 1860–61 were to varying degrees identified with conquest and foreign rule. Rituals of disease propitiation seldom, if ever, had a simply anti-British signification, but the secular and political interpretation which British officials placed upon propitiatory devices and actions was not entirely misplaced. Indian reactions to cholera were a reminder of the great cultural gulf that divided the colonizers from the colonized and drew attention to the existence of patterns of rural solidarity and lateral communication over which the state had little control. Although there were sometimes clashes between villages over the unwelcome dumping of cholera offerings or the arrival of someone else's "scapegoat,"[56] more commonly, shared beliefs and mutual self-interest ensured that animals and offerings were promptly moved on from village to village, sometimes—like the *ghura* of 1860—over considerable distances. It was believed, too, that propitiatory ceremonies were ineffective unless the whole village participated in them. For the British, whose own lines of rural communication in India were often singularly deficient and who saw a potential danger to their own power in networks of local solidarity, these were aspects of indigenous society to be viewed with apprehension, even alarm.

THE FALLIBILITY OF THERAPEUTICS

The cholera epidemics of the nineteenth century highlighted the widening gulf between indigenous and Western medicine but also showed the relative ineffectiveness of any medical system when confronted with such a ferocious and yet apparently capricious adversary. At the time of the first epidemics, there was still a certain congruence between the Western and Indian systems of medicine. Early nineteenth-century European doctors remained partly attached to the West's own humoral traditions, as many early descriptions of cholera testify, with their references to bile, phlegm, and disorders of the blood. There was considerable debate, for instance, over the name given to the disease, for "cholera" properly designated a disorder of the bile. According to R. Tytler, the assistant surgeon at Jessore who gave the first account of the "cholera morbus" in August 1817, it was due to a "vitiated state of the bile," as revealed by the patient's thirst, sluggish pulse, yellowish tinge to the eyes, and foul, dry tongue. But other commentators found the name puzzling when cholera in its current form proved to be unconnected with a "morbid flow of bile."[57]

Although the virulence of the early epidemics drove many Indians to seek help in religious ceremonies rather than medical concoctions, *vaidyas* and *hakims* supplied those who sought their assistance with treatments and medicines consonant with their humoral pathologies. Rather than attempting to stop the body's violent evacuations or to deny patients the cool drinks they craved, the physicians administered purgatives, like calomel, to rid the body of its "poison," followed by cooling drinks of rosewater and lime juice, or advised embrocations of turpentine and other fluids to relieve the severe cramps that were such a common and distressing symptom of the disease. The *vaidyas* prescribed medicines composed of black pepper, borax, asafetida, aniseed, ginger, and cloves; some incorporated opium or Indian hemp to dull the pain and relax the body.[58]

During the 1817–21 epidemic in particular, European physicians took careful note of these indigenous therapies in the hope of profiting from the treatment of a disease unfamiliar to them and unresponsive to their therapeutics. In September 1817, soon after the outbreak of the epidemic, the Bengal Medical Board issued instructions for a four-stage treatment of "cholera morbus." The first task was to revive the patient's strength by administering spiritous liquors or, in urgent cases, spirits of hartshorn; then the "irritability" of the stomach and bowels was to be removed to prepare the way for later medicine (for this opium or laudanum was recommended); the third stage was to expel any remaining "morbid secretions" with purgatives such as calomel, epsom salts, or senna; and the fourth, to restore the healthy action of the stomach with tonics and a plain diet free from greasy or "heating" foods.

Apart from the lavish use of spirits as a therapeutic overture, there was not much here of which the *vaidya* or *hakim* could disapprove. Moreover, the Medical Board informed its practitioners that, where Western drugs were not available or seemed inappropriate, local ones could be substituted—such as "watery decoctions" of pepper and other spices and aromatics in common use among Indian doctors.[59] This recourse to local remedies was further encouraged by the fact that "native physicians"—some forty or fifty of whom had already been taken on in Calcutta or dispatched up-country—had been chosen by the board to administer its medicines, and for their benefit the instructions were issued in Bengali as well as in English. The distinction between "Europe" and "Native" medicine, in terms of its practice and practitioners, cannot, therefore, have appeared very great.

Despite this, British doctors often saw significant differences between their own practice and that of Indian physicians. In November 1818, for example, the Madras Medical Board reluctantly agreed to meet two Brahmin physicians from Kanchipuram (Conjeeveram), who had sent a Tamil address to the governor concerning the treatment of cholera—an interesting example of active attempts by *vaidya*s to influence the practice of Western medicine in India. The pandits, Maha Ganapati Sastri and Ramakrishna Sastri, were anxious that the government should treat victims of the epidemic according to their system of Ayurvedic medicine, especially since European medicines containing brandy, opium, and similar substances were offensive to Brahmins. The treatment they proposed consisted of various plant and mineral extracts (including calomel) mixed with honey and administered orally at carefully stipulated intervals. The governor professed himself unable to make any judgment on the merits of their medicines but thought they deserved to be treated with courtesy and respect. The Medical Board was more skeptical, preferring to see a meeting with the Brahmins only as an opportunity to "hold out to the

Natives the strongest proof of the earnest desire of Government to ensure relief to them during the prevalence of the epidemic" and to "open a communication which may lead to the general introduction amongst them of the European practice should it be found of superior efficacy to their own."[60]

Even when conspicuously borrowing from indigenous practice, European doctors remained, like the Madras Medical Board, disposed to believe in the superiority of their own methods and medicines. In Bengal, Jameson discussed Indian doctors' treatments for cholera at some length in 1820 and approved their use of opium, calomel, and other common drugs. But his approval extended only as far as indigenous therapeutics conformed to current Western ideas and practices. Whenever they strayed from that standard they became "frivolous" or "pernicious." The cultural evangelist in Jameson was accordingly gratified when Indians, "even of the highest castes," "saw their superstitions fail them," and "throwing off all their religious prejudices," they applied to European doctors for help. In his view, the epidemic taught them "to place their faith in the only means, which has been yet found, in any measure, adequate to resist the attack"—namely, his own system of medicine.[61]

Whatever their cultural reservations, British doctors in fact borrowed shamelessly from the *vaidya*s and *hakim*s or employed almost identical drugs and treatments. They too prescribed black pepper, calomel, ginger, and asafetida, sometimes mixed, or alternating, with opium, brandy, and arrack. By the 1850s these fiery tinctures had given way (partly in deference to Indian scruples about alcohol or medicines made with "impure" water) to "cholera pills" made from opium, black pepper, and asafetida. More than 140,000 of these were made and distributed at Agra alone during an epidemic in 1856. The local surgeon, John Murray, attributed their popularity to the fact that they were known by Indians to consist of familiar bazaar ingredients. "There is scarcely a [European] gentleman at Agra," he recorded, "who has not reported having saved the lives of some of his servants, or the neighbouring Natives, by the early exhibition of these pills."[62]

Whether prescribed by Indian or European physicians, these putative remedies were not always well received by their would-be patients, especially when they demonstrably failed to save the sick or when religious ritual alone seemed appropriate. One Bombay judge wrote in May 1820 of the "great repugnance" shown by villagers toward any medical measures except from their own doctors, and a similar preference was observed in northern India in 1856.[63] Had the copious bleeding by venesection so earnestly advocated in many early nineteenth-century texts as the "sheet-anchor" of cholera treatment been extensively employed on Indian patients (as it was on many an unfortunate European), the reaction against Western medicine might have been even greater.[64] As it was, the evidence, particularly for the 1817–21 epidemic, shows a great variety of Indian responses—from hostility or indifference to occasional enthusiastic demand.[65]

In the absence of any determined effort by the provincial governments or medical boards to impose Western medicines or hospitalization upon the Indian population, there were few signs of the kind of resistance that marked the far more drastic intervention against plague in the 1890s (see chapter 5). Hospitalization was rare and involved no recourse to coercion. Many of the temporary cholera "hospitals" (in reality mere sheds) that were hastily thrown up in 1818–19 were soon abandoned as useless because very few Indians would come to be treated in them. In Madras, where the Medical Board had set up a number of these temporary "hospitals" in 1819, it was found that Indians "evinced a great reluctance to reside in them even for a day."[66]

The state's own attitude toward medical provision was far from unambivalent. As we have seen, officials were concerned about the effects of the epidemics upon revenue and social stability, and provincial governments were doubtless flattered by being praised for their "humanity" and "generosity" and even saw some political merit in being hailed for their "beneficence." But, as with smallpox vaccination at the same time, the state was less enthusiastic about footing the bill. When the magistrate at Murshidabad to the north of Calcutta rashly suggested in November 1817 that the government's help in treating cholera might be put on a more permanent basis with state-funded dispensaries, he was curtly informed that the government could not possibly maintain the numerous establishments required "without incurring an enormous expense." Institutions of that kind, the secretary to the Government continued, were exclusively supported elsewhere by public contributions "and can only be established and maintained in a similar manner in this country."[67]

Although accounts of the early epidemics speak with remarkable confidence of the success of European medicines and therapies in treating cholera (especially in the early stages of the disease) and saving lives, there were growing doubts among many Western practitioners about the value of their treatments and remedies. In all the voluminous literature generated by cholera in India between 1817 and the 1870s there was no agreement on an effective course of action against the disease. Every physician who rushed into print had his own pet theory, but the disillusionment of one army surgeon, a Dr. Chapman, writing in the 1840s, was perhaps more widely representative of the despair many doctors felt. He had tried venesection, he reported, but gave it up as it appeared only to hasten death, and from none of his patients could he anyway "procure more than a few ounces of black ropy blood." He had tried external and internal stimulants, but, "however powerful," they had no effect, and medicines of all kinds appeared to be "utterly inert" in dealing with cholera. He experimented with different enemata, "but all to no purpose." The disease, he concluded despondently, "set us at defiance, and extorted from us the humiliating confession of our utter inability to contend with such an enemy."[68] William Scot, formerly of the Madras Medical Board, also acknowledged cholera to be a perverse and wily adversary. "In no disease," he remarked in the 1840s, "has the sovereign efficacy of numberless specifics been more vaunted, and in none have the utmost efforts of the medical art been more frequently insufficient, than in cholera."[69]

By the middle decades of the century, with a cure for cholera still eluding them, Western physicians could at least draw solace from the fact that sanitary measures of the kind increasingly being adopted in Britain or in the army in India showed some success in preventing or containing the disease. However, this pointed away from therapeutic intervention, directed at the individual body, and toward greater sanitary policing by the state, directed at the health of the society as a whole. This form of intervention was, in its way, no less problematic.

"THE SQUALID PILGRIM ARMY OF JAGANNATH"

Cholera's Indian origins, and its almost global dissemination through the pandemics of the nineteenth century, made the disease a convenient symbol for much that the West feared or despised about a society so different from its own. One of the strongest expressions of this antipathy arose from the discovery of an epidemiological connection between cholera and Hindu pilgrimage. Vibrio cholerae, a comma-shaped bacillus, enters the body by the oral route, most commonly through drinking water (but sometimes food) contaminated by infected human feces. In India one of the principal modes of disease transmission was through reservoirs and watercourses which provided water both for drinking and for washing and bathing. The mass bathing by Hindu pilgrims in a sacred tank or river, as happened on a vast scale at the *kumbh mela*s, festivals held every twelve years, at Hardwar and Allahabad on the Ganges, and the sipping of water as part of the ritual of worship and religious purification, provided almost ideal conditions for the rapid communication of the waterborne vibrio. The chain of transmission was further extended by pilgrims bringing back Ganges water infected with cholera for relatives and friends to drink. This was particularly ironic, given that water from the Ganges was thought of as especially pure and holy, having special medicinal and protective powers.

Several nineteenth-century epidemics were directly attributed to Hindu festivals and pilgrimage sites. The Hardwar *kumbh mela* of April 1867, attended at its height by nearly three million pilgrims, was the classic case. Only nineteen pilgrims were treated for cholera at Hardwar during the *mela*, but the disease, possibly spread during the mass bathing on April 12, was carried far and wide across northern India by the dispersing pilgrims. The poverty of the pilgrims, the privations they suffered in traveling to and from their destination, and their crowding together in insanitary locations reproduced many of the fatal aspects of the famine conditions in which cholera also thrived. And at numerous tanks and wells along the road the pilgrims left the disease behind them, infecting towns and villages. In the course of the 1867 epidemic, an estimated quarter of a million people contracted the disease, and about half of them died.[70]

Along with Hardwar and Allahabad; the temple of Jagannath at Puri in Orissa and the pilgrimage sites of Nasik and Pandharpur in Maharashtra, Tirupati in Andhra Pradesh, and Kanchipuram in Tamilnadu were all at various times implicated as centers of epidemic cholera. With its reliance upon human vectors (including long-term carriers of the disease) and a waterborne mode of transmission, cholera thrived on the fatal conjunction between its own etiology and Hindu patterns of worship. The distribution of Hindu sacred places across India and the periodicity of major festivals constituted two important determinants of cholera epidemicity in India. At first, colonial reports on cholera made few connections with Hindu pilgrimage. It was noted, without particular comment, that twenty thousand pilgrims probably died of the disease at the Hardwar *mela* of 1783 and that cholera broke out among pilgrims at Pandharpur in 1818, resulting in three thousand deaths.[71] But in 1831 Moreau de Jonnès identified religious pilgrimages and troop movements as two of the main factors in the spread of cholera in India, citing several examples including Puri in 1821.[72]

The discovery of this epidemiological link came at an important historical juncture, for the early epidemics coincided with the opening of British India to Christian missionaries (permitted for the first time in 1813 to preach in Company territory) and their vehement denunciation of Hindu beliefs and practices. The protective stance which the Company had hitherto pragmatically taken toward Hindu institutions and festivals, and the revenue collected from Hindu temples and pilgrim taxes, now came under fire from the missionaries as "state sanction to idolatory." They concentrated their attacks on Puri, believing it to be the "chief seat of the Hindoos" and the place where devotees were said to throw themselves, in an act of fanatical self-immolation, under the huge wooden wheels of the temple car of the god Jagannath. Claudius Buchanan, a Company chaplain who attended the 1806 Rath Jatra (car festival), wrote an impassioned and influential account of the town and the event, which did much to fuel subsequent missionary, and medical, accounts of Puri and its pilgrims. He described the "squalid and ghastly appearance of the famished pilgrims," many of whom, he said, died in the town from "want and disease." His narrative swept in a single gesture of condemnation from the "offensive effluvia" arising from the town to the "obscene" rituals that accompanied the festival, and on to the "magnitude and horror of the spectacle" as the car with its crudely fashioned "idols" was dragged by pilgrims through the streets. "The characteristics of Moloch's worship are obscenity and blood," he declared, echoing Milton. "How much I wished that the proprietors of India Stock could have attended the wheels of Juggernaut, and seen this peculiar source of their revenue."[73]

Sustained pressure from the missionaries resulted in the abolition of the pilgrim tax in 1840, though it was not until 1863 that official involvement in the temple's administration finally ceased.[74] But missionary propaganda had a profound effect on the way Europeans thought about Hinduism, its sacred places, and its connections with disease. Puri epitomized all that was, in Western eyes, obscene, degrading, and epidemiologically dangerous about Hindu India. "Probably no spot on earth," wrote one missionary in 1828, "represents, within so small a compass, such complicated scenes of misery, cruelty, and vice, as are presented to view round the temple of Juggernaut."[75] The Reverend J. Buckley, asked in 1867 for his views on stricter sanitary controls over the pilgrim traffic to Puri, repeated Buchanan's horrific description of sixty years earlier to confirm his own observations of the place. He added:

> All who have any practical knowledge of the subject know perfectly well that the pilgrimage to this detestable shrine has ever been a fruitful source of misery, disease and death not only to the pilgrims themselves, but to the people in the villages and towns through which they pass. The loss of life occasioned by the horrid rite of suttee was trivial in comparison with that occasioned by this wasting pilgrimage.[76]

The linkage Buckley (and indeed Buchanan before him) made between Puri and *sati*, the archetypal barbarity in Western discourse on Hinduism, and with "misery, disease and death," was not confined to missionary polemic alone but also informed much official and medical discussion as well. Indeed, it was common for medical opinion to be influenced by the prevailing Christian view of Puri while further endorsing it with the stamp of its own scientific authority.

The international sanitary conference which met at Constantinople in 1866 to try to coordinate measures to protect Europe from the repeated ravages of cholera pointed an accusing finger at Puri and other Hindu pilgrimage centers (as it also did at the Muslims' hajj to Mecca, seen as the second stage by which cholera was relayed from India to Europe). Taking a strongly contagionist line, the conference stated that "great assemblages of men"—armies, fairs, and pilgrimages—were among the most certain means by which cholera was propagated: "they form great epidemic sources which, whether the people march as an army or scatter themselves, as from fairs and pilgrimages, carry the disease into the country they go through." The conference declared pilgrimages in India to be "the most powerful of all the causes which conduce to the development and to the propagation of epidemics of cholera."[77]

Partly in response to this international indictment, and partly as a result of the recent appointment of provincial sanitary commissioners charged with a special responsibility to investigate the causes of cholera epidemics, the Government of India, now directly under the Crown, instituted inquiries into the sanitary state of Puri and other major pilgrimage and festival sites. The reports produced substantial evidence for a close connection between cholera and pilgrimage, to which detailed accounts of the outbreak at Hardwar in 1867 added further confirmation. But one of the striking features of these accounts was the ease with which they mixed medical observation with moral or religious judgment. In his report on Puri in 1868, Dr. David B. Smith, Bengal's sanitary commissioner, contrasted the pilgrims' view of the town as a holy city, where they would be freed from their worldly sins, with the sanitarian's view of it as anything but "heaven on earth," containing in its many tanks "the waters of death and not those of immortality."[78] In an account which echoed Buchanan, Smith called the temple car "tawdry and contemptible." He found the crudely carved image of Jagannath a "terrible object; terrible in its innate hideousness—yet more terrible in its connection with all the surrounding circumstances." The worship of Jagannath entailed "incalculable misery rather than happiness"; its whole history was "a terrible story of disease and death." "The human mind," Smith declared, "can scarcely sink lower than it has done in connection with the appalling degradation of idol-worship at Pooree." Education was the only "remedy" he could prescribe to save worshippers who were presently

> enslaved by priestcraft, steeped in idolatory, determinedly tenacious of caste, bewildered by frivolous superstitions and legendary fables, strongly prejudiced against education, and content to look forward to their periodically recurring festivals, at which they are despoiled of all they possess.[79]

Smith's report did more than trade in sweeping generalities. It also identified specific connections between disease and religious life at Puri: the disgusting state of the *maha prasad*, the consecrated food eaten by eager pilgrims, the foul nature of the water in which they washed and from which they drank, the dark, disease-ridden lodging houses into which they crowded during the Rath Jatra. But a critical attitude toward Hindu beliefs and practices was never far away. Speaking of the influence of religious rites generally upon disease in Puri, Smith remarked that

> many of the religious forms and ceremonies to which the Ooriyas fondly cling, either involve fatigue, fasting, penance, and pain, or, on the other hand, they lead to fasting, dissipation, sensual excesses, reckless orgies, and great mental excitement. These two sets of influences probably account for much prevailing sickness, and even mortality.[80]

Such damning voices were frequently heard in mid–nineteenth-century reports on health and sanitation, and when it was not the diseased and deluded pilgrims who were the subject of attack, it was the priests, with their selfish pursuit of "pecuniary interest" regardless of the consequences for the public's health, who were charged and found guilty in these sanitary proceedings.[81] Because of the close connection made between cholera and Hindu places of pilgrimage like Puri, the medical and sanitary assault on cholera was also an attack on Hinduism, one which appeared all the more authoritative for its invocation of medical science.

The colonial condemnation of Hindu pilgrimage had a further consequence. It made the pilgrims into a "dangerous class" requiring special measures for their regulation and surveillance. In the existing state of Western medical knowledge, it appeared possible (at least to one section of medical and official opinion) to control cholera only by controlling those most obviously implicated in its transmission. If, in Europe, cholera deepened the propertied classes' fear of the tramping and slum-dwelling poor, so, on an international scale, Europe dreaded Asia's armies of pilgrim poor by whom the disease might be borne on its long march to Europe.

This view was clearly articulated in W. W. Hunter's description of Puri in his history of Orissa published in 1872. He deplored the "homicidal enterprise" which every year at the time of the Rath Jatra turned Puri into a "magazine of mortality" and left ten thousand Indians dead on the pilgrim road to Jagannath. But it was not so much this "yearly sacrifice" and the "superstition of the natives" that incensed Hunter as the thought that the "over-crowded, pest-haunted dens around Jagannath" could become "at any moment the centre from which the disease radiates to the great manufacturing towns of France and England." The pilgrims might "care little for life or death, nor is it possible to protect men against themselves. But such carelessness imperils lives far more valuable than their own." Hunter went on:

> One of man's most deadly enemies has his lair in this remote corner of Orissa, ever ready to rush out upon the world, to devastate households, to sack cities, and to mark its line of march by a broad black track across three continents. The squalid pilgrim army of Jagannath with its rags and hair and skin freighted with vermin and impregnated with infection, may any year slay thousands of the most talented and beautiful of our age in Vienna, London, or Washington.[82]

Europe's ancient and abiding fear of the "Asiatic hordes" found fresh expression—among European writers in India as well as in the West—in this hostility to the cholera-carrying pilgrims of Puri. Like the Huns, the Mongols, or the bubonic plague before it, the "incursions of this Asiatic scourge" called cholera again threatened Europe with death and destruction.[83]

COMING TO TERMS WITH CONTAGION

The identification of epidemic cholera with Hindu pilgrimage, endorsed by much medical and official opinion within India and by several sanitary conferences outside it, might in other circumstances have paved the way for a wholesale assault on the temple towns and pilgrim sites held responsible. In 1867, following the conference at Constantinople and the Hardwar *mela* epidemic, Bengal's sanitary commissioner, Lieutenant-Colonel G. B. Malleson, discussed the need for stricter controls over pilgrimages, including quarantines to protect vulnerable cantonments and municipalities.[84] A committee appointed by the Madras government in February 1867 also urged that the time had come to place pilgrims and pilgrimages under "strict supervision" with quarantines and a pilgrim tax to pay for additional sanitary measures.[85]

In fact, the Government of India held back from such a course for several reasons. One was that the very intimacy of the relationship between cholera and Hindu festivals made the state wary of provoking the kind of religious and political backlash it had experienced in the recent Mutiny and Rebellion. An extensive inquiry into official

and Indian opinion conducted by the Government of India in 1867–
69 resulted in the clear conclusion that Hindu society would not
brook the kind of interference with pilgrimages that would be necessary to extirpate cholera—even though many Indians themselves
dreaded cholera and regarded pilgrims as a frequent source of the
disease.[86] While Hunter claimed in 1872 that nothing less than a
"total prohibition" on pilgrimage to Puri "would put a stop to the
annual massacre," he also believed that "anything like a general prohibition of pilgrimage would be an outrage upon the religious feelings
of the people," "an interdict on one of the most cherished religious
privileges of the people," and, after the promise of religious toleration held out by Queen Victoria's post-Mutiny Proclamation of
November 1858, "a signal infringement of the tenure by which we
hold India." It would be regarded by 150 million of Britain's Indian
subjects "as a great national wrong."[87] For Hunter, Puri was illus-
trative of the wider impasse confronting sanitary science in India.

> In no country does the public health more urgently demand the
> aid of that science. But the ignorance, prejudices, and suspi-
> cions of the people on the one hand, and the vast demands
> upon the revenue for more visibly and perhaps more urgently
> needed public works on the other, do not leave sanitation a
> chance.[88]

Hunter was not alone in urging caution over pilgrimage controls.
David B. Smith, for all his evident antipathy to Puri, thought the prohibition of festivals and pilgrimages impractical and undesirable:
"Better, in my opinion, would it be that India should be devastated
by cholera than subjected to religious persecution."[89] The Madras
government, in reviewing the recommendations of its own cholera
and pilgrimage committee, also concluded that it would not be "politic to take any measures which would have the appearance of the
Government preventing pilgrimages."[90] The Government of India itself decided that pilgrimages had to be tolerated for the time being as
a "necessary evil." In due course, with the spread of Western education and ideas, the problem might resolve itself, as pilgrimages lost
their former appeal and Indians learned the value of sanitation and
hygiene. Meanwhile, all that could in practice be done was to tighten
the existing system of sanitary surveillance at the main pilgrimage
places and fairs.[91]

There were other obstacles to state intervention against cholera. One, as Hunter pointed out, was financial. Stricter controls over pilgrimages and more effective sanitary measures in a host of pilgrim towns and at vast open encampments like those periodically established at Hardwar and Allahabad would be a massive, and hugely expensive, undertaking, and the colonial regime was simply not prepared to commit its resources to such a costly health program. Raising new sources of revenue by, for example, restoring the controversial pilgrim tax—a decision which the Government of India in 1870 delegated to local governments—was open to administrative as well as religious objections.[92]

A further obstacle was the dislike that the Government of India, in common with its superior in London, had for all talk of cordons and quarantines. Although favored by the Constantinople sanitary conference with its strongly contagionist stance, they had long been opposed by the British, who denounced them as an instrument of continental despotism, inimical to free commerce, a source of hardship and oppression to travelers, traders, and residents alike, and, not least, ineffective in preventing the spread of the disease. J. M. Cuningham, the Government of India's long-serving sanitary commissioner (he held the post from 1868 to 1884), whose opposition to compulsory vaccination was noted in the previous chapter, argued strenuously in the 1870s and early 1880s that quarantines and sanitary cordons were unsuited to India. In a country where the police were notoriously venal and vicious, putting them in charge of quarantine measures would simply result in "oppression and hardship to the people." Besides, added Cuningham, who held anticontagionist views, establishing cordons to keep out cholera would be "no more logical or effectual than it would be to post a line of sentries to stop the monsoon."[93] To a government formally committed to laissez-faire and loath to spend more than necessary for its own security on public health, such arguments sounded reassuringly convincing.

But perhaps the greatest single obstacle to state interventionism was the continuing uncertainty within the medical profession in India over the nature of cholera and the manner of its transmission. Reports on the 1817–21 epidemic were generally (though not universally) inclined toward climatic explanations, especially "atmospheric vicissitudes" such as sudden, heavy rain or an abrupt drop in temperature, or else they favored "miasmatic" causes, the "poisonous emissions" and "pestiferous exhalations" thought to emanate from rotting vegetation, crowded habitations, and human "filth" of every kind.[94] James Jameson, "the father of Indian cholera literature," was one of those drawn to atmospheric explanations, but as an "accessory" factor rather than a specific cause of the disease. He doubted that it could be contagious in the sense that person-to-person contact made smallpox a contagious disease. The enduring influence of his work was one reason why many members of the Indian Medical Service clung to an environmentalist view of cholera long after it had become unfashionable in Europe.[95] But just as there were no easy therapeutic solutions for cholera, so was there deep controversy in the 1860s and 1870s about the cause and transmission of the disease. The evidence of pilgrimages, particularly the Hardwar *mela* of 1867, seemed to point strongly in a contagionist direction, but even John Murray, inspector-general of hospitals in the North-Western Provinces, who conducted the most detailed inquiry into the Hardwar episode, was willing to believe that atmospheric conditions precipitated the initial outbreak of cholera, which then spread contagiously among the pilgrim hosts and those with whom they subsequently came in contact.[96]

The contagionist stance of the international sanitary conferences seemed to make the Government of India even more determinedly anticontagionist. It found in J. M. Cuningham a medical officer who, while pleading strict impartiality, took every opportunity to pour scorn on contagionist "doctrine" (and even to deplore "theory" in any form in the sanitary commissioners' reports) and to use his position of authority to stifle the opinions or wreck the careers of officers like Surgeon-Major A. C. C. De Renzy, sanitary commissioner of Punjab, who dared to oppose him.[97] At the end of his long career as sanitary commissioner in 1884, Cuningham was still able to maintain dogmatically that "theories of contagion may be acted on by private individuals if they like, but they cannot be made the basis of any action on the part of the State."[98] And yet, even ten years earlier, he had been ridiculed by the *Lancet* in London for his gross misrepresentation of contagionist theory and for his claim that "because India was the home of cholera, therefore observations made there had a pre-eminent advantage over observations conducted elsewhere."[99]

Although a fresh outbreak of cholera at the 1879 Hardwar *kumbh mela* revived the contagionist arguments of twelve years earlier, Cuningham adamantly refused to accept what he dismissively called "the pilgrim theory." He argued that pilgrims fell prey to cholera only because their fatigue and privations made them "specially prone" to the disease, and not because they carried it with them from place to place. He believed the most likely cause of cholera was an "aerial miasma" (rather like malaria) or thought it was generated by "some particular condition of air or soil, or of both combined." Speaking in effect with the authority of the Government of India, he stated categorically in 1880 that "unless much stronger evidence can be adduced in favour of the pilgrim theory than has as yet been brought forward, such a measure as stopping the [Hardwar] fair would certainly be an unwarrantable interference with the liberty and religious observances of the people."[100]

Anticontagionism seemed to fit some of the observed facts about epidemic cholera better than contagionism, and the wealth of meteorological data and mortality statistics which became available from the mid 1860s onward gave new life to theories that linked epidemic cholera with climatic and geographical phenomena. In 1869 J. L. Bryden, statistical officer to the Government of India's sanitary commissioner, declared his skepticism about the idea of cholera as a waterborne disease as advanced by John Snow in his celebrated investigation of cholera at the Broad Street pump in London twenty years earlier. Bryden denied that human agency was important to the transmission of the disease, claiming instead that the "geographical distribution of an invading cholera is purely a phenomenon of *meteorological significance.*" The prevailing winds, not human intercourse, he said, determined the direction and extent of a cholera epidemic: "The highways by which cholera travels are, in this country, aerial highways, and not routes of human communication."[101]

Bryden's unequivocal claims did not go unchallenged by those far removed from the "Olympian heights of Simla" and with a practical knowledge of cholera. W. R. Cornish, the Madras sanitary commissioner, argued that, at least as far as southern India was concerned, cholera did follow the main lines of human intercourse, and meteorology had relatively little to do with it.[102] But Bryden's arguments enjoyed enormous prestige in India in the 1870s and 1880s, and Cuningham was one of those who expressed his admiration for Bryden's "remarkable work."[103] This was partly because Bryden gave fresh statistical precision and scientific authority to the old idea that it was the elusive but omnipotent forces of the Indian environment which accounted for the bulk of the subcontinent's diseases and their distinctive nature and occurrence.

Subsequent investigations seemed to give added weight to Bryden's arguments. T. R. Lęwis of the Army Medical Department and D. D. Cunningham of the IMS, appointed by the India Office in London to examine the causes of cholera using the latest techniques of microscopy, concluded in 1878 that human agency alone could not explain the peculiar spread and periodicity of the disease and held the opinion that "cholera has as good a claim as malarial diseases to a telluric origin."[104] H. W. Bellew, who conducted his own statistical investigation into cholera in the 1880s, similarly rejected the contagionist view of cholera, seeing instead "a fixed relation between cholera and special climatic conditions."[105]

Even when the German bacteriologist Robert Koch made his critical discovery of the cholera bacillus in a Calcutta tank in 1884 and, in the manner of John Snow thirty years earlier, demonstrated the role of water in the local epidemiology of the disease, many old India hands were disposed to scoff. Cuningham, in his last days as the Government of India's sanitary commissioner, doubted the value of sending Koch to Calcutta to make such "cursory investigations," when, he insisted, "some knowledge of the physical geography of India and of the conditions under which the people live are indispensable for a right understanding of the questions involved."[106] In an era of mounting imperial rivalries, there was patriotic pique as well as professional chagrin that an outsider like Koch should presume to unravel the mystery which had baffled India's own medical service for more than sixty years. But there was also the political and commercial consideration—as Sir Joseph Fayrer, surgeon-general at the India Office Council in London, was quick to point out—that proof of cholera's contagious character would make an irresistible argument for quarantines and tighter international sanitary controls over India's overseas trade. The Government of India and the India Office were, therefore, greatly relieved when a British two-man cholera commission dispatched to Calcutta in 1884 found that Koch's bacillus was innocuous and could not be the specific cause of cholera.[107]

For just over a decade—until the plague epidemic gave the issue fresh force—the British were able to avoid the threat of international sanitary sanctions against India. But subsequent medical research endorsed Koch's findings, and by the mid 1890s the bacillus theory was at last enthroned as the new orthodoxy even in India. Nonetheless, medical writers and researchers in India denied Koch a complete victory over their long-term adversary. They continued to stress that bacteriology was only half the story and emphasized the importance of climate, physical environment, and social behavior as contingent factors in cholera epidemicity.[108] The tenacity with which so many medical researchers and senior medical advisers like Cuningham clung to their anticontagionism can be seen as an indication of how far out of touch they were with advances in medical science in Europe. But they were certainly encouraged by the "ostrich-like" mentality of the Government of India,[109] which preferred for political and commercial reasons to pursue a noninterventionist, laissez-faire policy toward cholera, and by the enduring hold which environmentalist ideas had on the medical imagination in India. Together, these reinforced the "Orientalist" assumption that India was intrinsically different from Europe and the conviction that only those who knew the country well, from long, practical experience, could possibly pronounce upon its idiosyncratic nature and peculiar needs. In their insistence upon the physical or climatic idiosyncrasies of India, the environmentalist school was in curious accord with its contagionist opponents with their eyes firmly fixed not on the heavens or the soil, but on the pilgrim hordes of Hardwar and Puri. One way or another, it was the climate, the soil, the people of India, that were to blame for the ravages of cholera.

However, in India, as much as in Britain, anticontagionism did not necessarily imply complete inertia on the part of the medical profession and the state. Cuningham and his associates declared themselves to be as much in favor of good sanitation and clean drinking water as their contagionist adversaries. But, taken along with the financial and political constraints discussed earlier, anticontagionism undoubtedly strengthened the state's disinclination to treat cholera as an urgent problem and its preference for cautious, piecemeal intervention. By the 1890s, as contagionism finally gained official acceptance, the state began to recognize a greater practical responsibility for the health of its subjects, and medical officers edged their way toward a more active policy with regard to cholera. However, the powerful political obstacles which had inhibited interventionism in the past had not ceased to operate.

In 1892 the Government of the North-Western Provinces took the bold step of breaking up the Mahavaruni *mela* at Hardwar at the end of March. Following an outbreak of cholera among those already assembled at Hardwar, two hundred thousand pilgrims en route to Hardwar were turned back. No physical resistance was reported, but a public meeting at Lahore in July under Pandit Gopinath, a newspaper editor and an advocate for Hindu orthodoxy, passed a resolution protesting against the dispersal of the pilgrims as a violation of the religious toleration promised in Queen Victoria's proclamation of 1858. The British Indian Association, based in Calcutta, also raised its voice in protest, objecting to the "forcible breaking up of the fair, and the oppressive acts connected with the dispersion of the pilgrims." These, it said, had "caused considerable dissatisfaction throughout the length and breadth of the country."[110]

Coming at a time when cow protection riots and the growing force of Hindu militancy were causing the government concern, and when memories of 1857 were still fresh in administrators' minds, reactions to the breaking up of the Hardwar fair were seen as a warning that should be heeded. Lord Roberts, Mutiny veteran, commander-in-chief of the Indian Army, and a self-declared expert on "native sentiments," later observed that:

> Few acts [of the British government in India] have been more keenly resented than the closing of the great Hardwar Fair in the autumn [sic] of 1892. . . . It was looked upon by the Natives as a distinct blow aimed at their religion, and as a distinct departure from the religious toleration promised in Her Majesty's proclamation of 1858.[111]

When draft legislation proposed by the Government of the North-Western Provinces "to put beyond question the power of a Government to disperse fairs and religious assemblies on sanitary grounds" came before the Viceroy's Council for consideration later in 1892, Roberts was among those who thought it ill-advised and provocative. "The spread of cholera," he minuted, "is no doubt a great evil but the awakening of a feeling of mistrust throughout India would be a greater evil still." The viceroy, Lord Lansdowne, drew his own analogy with the recent furor over the Age of Consent Bill, and the proposed legislation was quietly dropped.[112]

As chapter 5 demonstrates, the authorities' caution regarding measures against cholera stood in apparent contrast to their drastic action against the plague epidemic which broke out in Bombay in 1896. But by the 1890s, cholera had come to be seen as a long-established disease and was met with a great deal of official complacency, while plague (backed by the fear of international sanctions) looked new and threatening. The measures that appeared imperative toward the one remained politically unacceptable toward the other. In 1905, Bombay officials responded to cholera at the Pandharpur fair by trying to invoke against cholera the far-reaching powers of the Epidemic Diseases Act, hastily passed in 1897 to combat plague. But they were promptly reminded by the Government of India of the political inadvisability of interfering with Hindu pilgrimages and fairs. The "best protection against an outbreak of cholera at large assemblies is to be found," Bombay was informed, "not in interference with the movements of the people, but in good sanitary arrangements both at the fair itself and on the routes taken by the pilgrims."[113]

The application of new medical and sanitary techniques was similarly inhibited by political considerations. Saline solutions to restore the enormous quantities of body fluid lost by cholera patients were experimented with during the early cholera epidemics but had little apparent success, and their use was subsequently abandoned.[114] Shortly before World War I the practice was revived, or rather reinvented, and it helped reduce mortality among hospital patients to a third or quarter of what it had previously been. As then practiced, however, it was a hospital-based technique and of little use in saving the lives of rural cholera victims remote from modern medical institutions.[115] In the 1890s the Russian bacteriologist Waldemar M. Haffkine pioneered an anticholera vaccine, which he tested experimentally in India in 1893–96. Although he saw the results as very encouraging, the Government of India and its medical advisers remained characteristically cautious. This was partly because of continuing suspicion among the Indian medical establishment about what W. R. Rice, surgeon-general and last of the pre-Mutiny recruits to the IMS, called the "speculations of bacteriologists." But, additionally, as with the banning of fairs and festivals, there was a fear of adverse public reactions, especially if Indians thought that inoculation was to be made compulsory. As a result, before 1914 the use of Haffkine's anticholera vaccine was mainly confined to soldiers, prisoners, and tea-estate workers.[116] As late as 1930 the government rejected the suggestion that compulsory inoculation be used on pilgrims gathering for the Allahabad *kumbh mela*. Again, the objection was political. Locked in bitter conflict with the Congress over its civil disobedience campaign, the administration feared that any attempt to introduce compulsory inoculation would be "deeply resented if not violently resisted" and "entailed risks of an explosion in an already surcharged political atmosphere."[117] It was not until 1936 that compulsory inoculation was introduced (among pilgrims at Pandharpur), and not until 1945 that it was employed as a compulsory measure at the Hardwar *kumbh mela*.[118] Cholera's status as a political disease thus lasted well into the twentieth century.

CONCLUSION

Like any other disease, cholera has no intrinsic meaning. It is only the result of a microorganism, albeit a very potent pathogen as far as human beings are concerned. But in nineteenth-century India, it acquired enormous meaning and significance from its various cultural and political contexts, from the ways in which it infiltrated the lives of the people, from the diverse public reactions it provoked, and from the manner in which it gave expression to the underlying fears and antipathies of the colonized and colonizers alike. With the possible exception of smallpox, no other disease in India was endowed with greater significance by Indians and Europeans or more dramatically illustrated the depth, complexity, and changing configuration of the colonial divide.

For both Western and Indian medical systems, cholera was an exceptionally troublesome disease, unresponsive or resistant to most of the favored therapies of the time. This made cultural and religious interpretations of the disease appear all the more pertinent and attractive; it also added to the British perception that the disease was peculiarly subversive, a disorder which not only challenged attempts to establish the superiority of Western medicine but also emphasized the physical frailty and political vulnerability of colonial rule. Because cholera epidemics were seen to be so intimately bound up with Hindu rites and pilgrimages, even the introduction of sanitary measures and Haffkine's anticholera serum did not resolve the political problems that surrounded attempts to contain cholera. At the same time, divided opinion within the medical profession in India as to the nature of the disease and the mode of its transmission made it more difficult for doctors and sanitarians to press the government to act, easier for the administration to adhere to a noninterventionist policy that favored many of its commercial, financial, and political interests.

Cholera was a disease which seemingly presented an ideal site for the colonization of the body. Its prevalence and its far-reaching military and economic consequences made it an urgent candidate for medical and sanitary intervention; it fueled a powerful, critical discourse about Hinduism and popular religious rites and practices. It made it possible, after the manner of Florence Nightingale, for Western observers to equate sanitation with civilization and find India woefully wanting in both. It was a disease that figured prominently in early public health measures in Britain, an "Asiatic disorder" that aroused the fear of Europe and inspired the holding of several international sanitary conferences. And yet, for reasons this chapter has sought to explain, cholera produced a relatively muted reaction from the colonial regime. Cholera provides a striking illustration of how a political "reading" of a disease, or of the likely consequences of medical and sanitary attempts to control it, could set powerful limits to state intervention against that disease.

5 Plague: Assault on the Body

Between 1871 and 1921, India experienced what Ira Klein has aptly described as a "woeful crescendo of death."[1] A death rate of 41.3 per 1,000 of the population in the 1880s, already high by contemporary Western standards, rose to 48.6 per 1,000 in the decade 1911–21. The causes of this savage upsurge in mortality have been much debated. Some writers have stressed India's increased exposure, through modern systems of trade and transport, to new and invading pathogens like plague and influenza; others see high levels of mortality in India as a register of the ill effects of harsh or deteriorating economic, social, and environmental conditions.

Whatever the underlying causes, an immediate factor in precipitating this protracted crisis of mortality was a series of major epidemics—malaria, cholera, influenza, and plague—occurring against a background of high endemic disease levels. Between the mid 1890s and early 1920s, malaria alone might have been responsible for as many as 20 million fatalities, one in every five deaths recorded. Respiratory diseases—tuberculosis, pneumonia, bronchitis—took almost as heavy a toll, as did dysentery and diarrhea. Although smallpox was beginning to decline, partly under the influence of increased vaccination, this was small consolation while the incidence of cholera remained high, especially in the almost Indiawide famines of the 1890s and early 1900s. Further deadly blows were struck by bubonic plague, which between 1896, the year of its arrival, and 1921 caused an estimated 10 million deaths, and the influenza pandemic of 1918–19, which is thought to have left more than 12 million Indians dead in its wake.[2]

While influenza's impact was both rapid and short-lived, its devastating second wave occupying only a few fatal months, plague took far longer to establish itself as a leading cause of mortality and lingered on as a major killer for several decades. During the first few years, its impact was concentrated in the cities, particularly Bombay, where plague was first officially acknowledged in September 1896,[3] and then in Pune, Karachi, and Calcutta. Within two or three years, it was affecting many smaller towns and reaching out into the countryside, and it was there that most of the later mortality occurred.

In 1901 plague mortality exceeded a quarter of a million deaths; the following year it touched half a million, and in 1904 rose above the one million mark for the first time. Plague deaths remained above this level in 1905 and 1907 but thereafter began a slow and erratic decline (see table 12). Plague lingered on in a few areas of India as late

Table 12. Plague Mortality in Bombay City and India, 1896–1914

	Bombay	*India*
1896	1,936	2,219
1897	11,003	53,816
1898	18,185	116,285
1899	15,796	139,009
1900	13,285	92,807
1901	18,736	283,788
1902	13,820	583,937
1903	20,788	865,578
1904	13,538	1,143,993
1905	14,198	1,069,140
1906	10,823	356,721
1907	6,389	1,315,892
1908	5,361	156,480
1909	5,197	178,808
1910	3,656	512,605
1911	4,006	846,873
1912	1,717	306,488
1913	2,609	217,869
1914	2,941	296,623
Total	183,984	8,538,931

Source: Turner and Goldsmith 1917, 456.

as the 1940s. The full extent of plague mortality, however, could never be determined, partly because of the concealment practiced in an attempt to evade intrusive state medical and sanitary measures. But the areas hit hardest by the epidemic were undoubtedly western and northern India: nearly three-quarters of the 12 million plague deaths recorded between 1896 and 1930 were in the three provinces of Punjab with 3.5 million recorded deaths, the United Provinces (formerly the North-Western Provinces) with 2.9 million, and Bombay with 2.4 million. Southern and eastern India escaped relatively lightly.[4]

But the significance of the plague epidemic lay not merely in its demographic impact, formidable though that ultimately proved to be. The epidemic's political and social impact was felt long before plague mortality had reached its peak. Because of the manner in which it was perceived by the colonial authorities and the nature of the sanitary and medical measures deployed against it, bubonic plague provoked an unparalleled crisis in the history of state medicine in India. The significance of plague for the political epidemiology of colonial India was far greater than that of the concurrent epidemics of malaria or influenza, even though in any given year the mortality they caused might have been considerably greater. Plague, like smallpox and cholera, dramatically restated the centrality of epidemic disease to the colonial state medicine of the period; but it also emphasized the enormous differences in perceptions and response—indigenous and colonial alike—between one epidemic disease and another. One illustration of these differences was the virtual absence of a plague deity, comparable to Sitala for smallpox or cholera's Ola Bibi.[5] A likely explanation is that the state's plague operations often preceded the arrival of the disease itself and were far more distressing. It was the state's motives which provoked a crisis of comprehension, not the activities of an irate or capricious goddess.

The plague epidemic brought to the fore many of the issues that had underlain earlier debates about smallpox and cholera, while presenting them in a new and dramatic light. Plague posed important questions about the place of medical science and the authority of medical practitioners in the colonial order and about the political constraints on medical and sanitary intervention. By contrast with the location of disease within a pathogenic landscape earlier in the century, plague was specifically identified with the human body and thus occasioned an unprecedented assault upon the body of the colonized. Much of the interventionist thrust of the state was directed at this epidemiological moment toward bodily apprehension and control, just as much of the Indian resistance to plague measures revolved around bodily evasion or concealment.

The exceptional degree to which colonial state power was exercised in the service of medicine during the plague epidemic raised questions about the nature and purposes of Western medicine in India and about its reception among Indians of different classes. The early years of the epidemic witness state medicine in uneasy transition from a defensive preoccupation with European interest and physical well-being to a broader, and as yet poorly defined, notion of public health.

A NEW INTERVENTIONISM

Given the caution shown by the state during outbreaks of smallpox and cholera in recent years, the reluctance to provoke public opposition, and the unwillingness to spend more than was absolutely necessary on public health, it is at first glance surprising that in the late 1890s the colonial state launched itself into a series of far-reaching measures against an epidemic of plague which had barely established itself on the shores of India.

At first, it is true, the Bombay government and its medical advisers were loath to acknowledge the presence of so dreaded a disease. Suspicious cases with glandular swellings had been seen by local medical practitioners as early as May 1896, but unfamiliarity with the disease and problems of diagnosis contributed to the hesitancy and delay. Even when on October 1 the government was forced to admit to an outbreak of "true bubonic plague," it tried to minimize the impact of this disclosure by stressing that the disease was of a "mild" type.[6]

But once the admission had been made, the Government of Bombay and the municipal authorities in Bombay city acted quickly and far more drastically than if they had been confronted by yet another outbreak of smallpox or cholera. On October 6, 1896, an official notification extended the already considerable powers entrusted to Bombay's municipal commissioner under the Municipal Act of 1888, authorizing the enforced segregation and hospitalization of suspected plague cases and municipal health officers' right of entry into infected buildings. The municipality simultaneously embarked on a massive, almost comically thorough, campaign of urban cleansing, flushing out drains and sewers with oceans of seawater and carbolic, scouring out scores of shops and grain warehouses (in the vicinity of which many of the first cases had occurred), sprinkling disinfectant powder in alleyways and tenements (spending more than Rs 100,000 on disinfectant alone by the end of March 1897), and, more tragically, destroying several hundred slum dwellings in the hope of extirpating the disease before it could fully establish itself.[7]

But, finding these measures ineffectual in checking the spread of plague from one ward of the city to another and faced with the prospect of the epidemic spreading into the hinterland of Bombay, on February 4, 1897, Lord Elgin gave his viceregal assent to "An Act to Provide for the Better Prevention of the Spread of Dangerous Epidemic Disease," a piece of legislation which had been rushed through his council with exceptional speed and with a minimum of debate or consultation. The act, which applied to the whole of British India and took immediate effect, gave the government powers to inspect any ship or intending passenger; to detain and segregate plague suspects; to destroy infected property; search, disinfect, evacuate, open up for ventilation, or simply demolish any dwelling thought to harbor plague; to prohibit fairs and pilgrimages; to examine and detain road and rail travelers—in short, to do whatever medical and official opinion held to be necessary for the suppression of plague.[8] In Bombay, Pune, Karachi, and Calcutta, responsibility for health and sanitation was taken away from the municipal councils to which it had been entrusted since the 1880s and given instead to small committees of European doctors and civil servants.

In practice, even if not in declared intent, Indian opinion was brusquely brushed aside. Caste and religion were afforded scant recognition except as "superstitious" obstacles to the implementation of essential and scientific sanitary operations. A proclamation issued by P. C. H. Snow, Bombay's municipal commissioner, on October 6, 1896, announced that all plague cases would be hospitalized, by force if necessary. It was not explained that relatives would be permitted to visit the sick, nor that the requirements of caste would be respected in hospital arrangements. A directive from Bombay's surgeon-general two months later, on December 12, openly stated that while caste "prejudices" should be observed as far as possible, they could not be allowed to stand in the way of essential sanitary and medical measures.[9]

What, then, lay behind this unwonted urgency and the far-reaching nature of the state's plague operations? Interventionism was triggered by a combination of domestic and external pressures, by political as well as medical considerations. One factor, as I. J. Catanach has recently indicated,[10] was that the British authorities felt themselves under irresistible international pressure to deal promptly and effectively with plague. Fearing that this disease, like cholera before it, would spread from India to the rest of the world and invade Europe itself, other Western powers threatened an embargo on trade with India unless stringent measures were taken to suppress plague and prevent its transmission to Europe. Strict controls over the movement of sea and rail passengers were, therefore, thought to be absolutely essential if commercial relations with the rest of the world, "on which in the present circumstances of India so much depends," were to be fully maintained.[11] Muslim pilgrimage from (or via) Bombay and Karachi to Jeddah and the exodus of migrant labor to eastern and southern Africa also touched areas of imperial as well as European concern.

In a sense, the ground was already well prepared for such an emergency. The international sanitary conferences that had been held since the 1850s to discuss the threat "Asiatic cholera" posed to Europe provided a ready forum for international action against plague. The tenth such conference, meeting in Venice in February–March 1897, pressed the Government of India to take immediate action and even detailed the kinds of stringent measures that needed to be taken if Indian ports were not to be closed to foreign shipping. Similarly, the regulation of Indian shipping and pilgrim traffic introduced by the Government of India, most recently under the Pilgrim Ships Act of 1895, already provided for the shipboard inspection of travelers. On February 20, 1897, the Government of India went a step further and formally suspended pilgrimage to Hedjaz for the current season, and these restrictions continued intermittently for several years.[12]

Without this international pressure and threat to its overseas trade, the Government of India would have been far more reticent and unlikely to have adopted such draconian measures. Plague had apparently been present in northern India earlier in the century without such extreme measures ever having been considered.[13] It was significant that plague was seen in 1896–97 to be an invading disease (it probably arrived by ship from Hong Kong, where an epidemic had been raging since 1894, though some experts favored a Middle Eastern origin). Unlike cholera, it was not a disease that had originated in India and that, by the 1890s, had long been accepted as part of the epidemiological landscape. As Pune's Municipal Council remarked a little wearily in June 1897, "cholera is what Indian towns are accustomed to."[14]

A second factor behind the extreme measures taken against plague in 1896–97 was that the epidemic precipitated, or perhaps exemplified, a growing crisis of urban control. Cities, especially port cities like Bombay, Karachi, and Calcutta, were the central nodes of colonial power in India. Politically, they represented colonialism in its most visible and tangible forms; commercially and administratively, they were the hub of British enterprise and authority; socially, they were the areas where Europeans were concentrated and where Indian and European life-styles most critically, often most antagonistically, intersected. In these urban arenas, plague posed a composite threat. Of immediate European and governmental concern was trade and hence the prosperity of not only Bombay but also Calcutta, still proudly the first city of Britain's empire in Asia. Indeed, one impetus behind the Epidemic Diseases Act was to protect Calcutta from infection by Bombay, given the close commercial and administrative ties between the two cities.[15] The threat to Bombay's own trade and industry came from the alarm felt among the city's trading communities and the prospect that they would flee to escape both plague and the attempts of the municipal authorities to bring the epidemic under control. Alarm spread rapidly, too, to the city's millhands and municipal scavengers, whose flight, it was feared, would bring the city to a standstill in a matter of days.

In his report on the early plague months in Bombay, Snow, the municipal commissioner, dramatically recounted the effects which a scavengers' strike and mass exodus would have on the running of the city. Before the epidemic, he pointed out, Bombay had been praised by sanitary experts as "the best kept and most sanitary oriental town" they had seen, but its continued well-being relied upon the daily labor of six thousand sweepers—Halalkhors from Gujarat and Marathi-speaking Bigarris, mainly Mahars. "On their presence or absence, respectively," Snow remarked, "depended the safety or ruin of this vast and important City." Since it would be difficult to find any alternative supply of scavengers to keep Bombay in sanitary order, "on these men and their good-will hung the carrying out of every sanitary measure, and even in ordinary times were they all to remove from the town for a fortnight, Bombay would be converted into a vast dunghill of putrescent ordure." There had been strikes in the past; now, Snow feared, if they struck work or fled, "half the inhabitants would speedily follow them, and no single measure could be adopted against the plague either then or thereafter, nor could even the Europeans, Parsis, and high caste natives have remained in the City."[16]

Snow could be suspected of melodramatic exaggeration, but, in fact, out of a population of nearly 850,000, an estimated 380,000 people deserted the city between early October 1896 and the end of February 1897, bringing the commercial and industrial life of India's second largest city almost to a standstill. At the height of the plague exodus, only a fifth of Bombay's millhands remained at work.[17] Calcutta was to experience a similar, if briefer, exodus, in April 1898, when possibly a quarter of the city's residents fled their homes. Ironically, there, too, flight was precipitated more by the threat of plague operations than by the advent of the epidemic itself.[18]

Quite apart from the commercial loss that would result from their departure, the millhands added a further dimension to the difficulties of urban management in Bombay. To Snow and the city's commissioner of police, they had become an "ever-present source of danger,"[19] evidence of the growing turbulence of urban life in Bombay, Calcutta, and other big cities in the wake of industrial development. Their violence—against hospitals, medical staff, and government servants—was influential in escalating the plague crisis in several cities and increasing official sensitivity to popular protest. It was only when the immediate urban crisis had passed and plague had become more widely established in rural areas that the severity of plague measures declined.

It is worth noting that a fear for Europeans' own health and survival did not, in itself, play a particularly important part in inspiring the government's plague measures. By contrast with cholera or typhoid, plague was not a disease that posed much of a threat to European life, though at first there was some uncertainty on this score. A suspected case of plague in a European youth in Calcutta in

October 1896 hastened the formation of a plague committee there, and special cordons were subsequently set up to protect Simla and other European hill stations.[20] But remarkably few Europeans caught the disease and fatalities were extremely rare. This apparent immunity contributed to the popular belief that Europeans were deliberately spreading plague in order to kill off unwanted Indians. Plague was more an inconvenience than a threat to Europeans—as when domestic servants joined in the flight from Bombay and Calcutta or when their *ayah*s were subjected to medical examinations from which Europeans were themselves exempt.[21]

More influential in impelling state intervention was the role of the medical profession. In keeping with their accustomed responsibilities as the principal agents and overseers of the British administration in India, members of the Indian Civil Service were entrusted with overall control of plague operations. One exception to this was in Bombay, where Municipal Commissioner Snow, an ICS officer, was replaced in March 1897 by a plague committee headed by Brigadier-General W. F. Gatacre, partly because troops were by then being used in plague operations in the city and also because it was thought that an army officer would bring military efficiency and determination to a hitherto ineffective, civilian-led sanitary campaign. In Calcutta a special committee was formed in October 1896 under H. H. Risley, secretary of the Financial and Municipal Department, and in Pune the plague committee was headed by another ICS officer, W. C. Rand. It might thus be argued, as I. J. Catanach has done, that "plague was seen as too important a matter to be left in the hands of doctors."[22]

But while the overall authority of the ICS was duly preserved, it is striking how much state policy relied upon medical opinion and personnel during the early months of the plague epidemic. Its medical advisers had initially assured the Government of India that plague would not reach India from Hong Kong and, once it had, that it would not spread much beyond its point of arrival. When both of these assertions proved false, the government still trusted in the claim, made by Surgeon-Major J. Cleghorn as director-general of the IMS, that plague could be effectively contained provided the necessary measures, including the evacuation of inhabitants from infected areas and segregation of suspected plague cases, were rigorously carried out. Cleghorn also assured the government that plague was "only slightly, if at all, either contagious or infectious in the common acceptation of those terms."[23]

Although civilian administrators took the lead in implementing plague measures in Bombay, Calcutta, Pune, and Karachi, they were advised and assisted by committees consisting largely of senior medical officers. Risley's "medical board" in Calcutta, for instance, included the inspector-general of civil hospitals, the provincial sanitary commissioner and his deputy, as well as an Indian doctor, Mahendra Lal Sarkar.[24] As Catanach notes, Rand in Pune was greatly influenced by Surgeon-Captain W. W. O. Beveridge of the Army Medical Service, and it was Beveridge who in February 1897 recommended (on the basis of his recent experience of the Hong Kong epidemic) the adoption of extreme measures to curb the spread of plague, including the use of troops to search out plague suspects. The resulting measures, Rand later observed, were "perhaps the most drastic that had ever been taken in British India to stamp out an epidemic."[25]

Confronted with apparently unequivocal medical advice, ICS officers struggled to translate the new bacteriology of Pasteur and Koch into the more familiar language of administrative command. In attempting to explain why, despite opposition, segregation and hospitalization were necessary in Calcutta, Risley declared in October 1896 that "the whole question turned upon modern bacteriological researches which were extremely puzzling and difficult." He could only inform his audience that "the nature of the [plague] microbe was such that it was highly portable" and "so infinitesimal and so long lived" that it "might come from Bombay at any moment, and propagate infinitely."[26] Given the difficulty of identifying plague in its early stages and local unfamiliarity with the disease, the administration was dependent on the advice of experts like Waldemar Haffkine in Bombay for confirmation that it was indeed bubonic plague that was laying siege to its cities.[27]

Never before in British India had medical science and the medical profession been afforded such administrative authority and been placed in a position to exercise it with such apparent freedom. This in turn reflected a newfound confidence, by no means confined to India, in the capacity of medical science to understand and combat epidemic disease and the willingness of colonial governments, in Africa as in Asia, to listen to the advice of its medical and sanitary experts in tackling plague, sleeping sickness, yellow fever, and malaria, often on a scale even more massive and sustained than the plague operations in India.[28]

At this stage, however, in 1896–98, the etiology of plague was barely understood. The role of rats in its transmission was sometimes speculated upon, if only because their death was such a visible and perturbing sign of impending human tragedy, but rodents were still largely thought of as fellow victims rather than probable disseminators of the disease. The part played by rats' fleas was not conclusively established until around 1908, partly through the research conducted by Glen Liston and W. B. Bannerman in India.[29] Thus, the human body and the conditions of human habitation and sanitation were thought in the 1890s to be primary factors in the spread of the disease. In its report on plague operations in Bombay in 1896–97, Gatacre's committee reported that something more than mere contagion appeared to be necessary for the transmission of plague and suggested that this was "most probably overcrowding, destitution, deficient cubic space, ventilation, and sun-light, and a filthy and generally insanitary condition of person, clothing, habitation, and its surroundings"—of which, not surprisingly, they found an abundance in the poorer quarters of Bombay.[30]

In a summary of current medical opinion and administrative experience prepared for the Government of India in 1898, it was similarly stated that "the primary danger exists in the sick person and his surroundings, his clothing and bedding and other objects that may have been in contact with him, and the room in which he has resided."[31] That human agency, and not merely destitution and dirt, was important to the transmission of plague was suggested by the way in which plague often appeared to move with Banias, Marwaris, and other members of the trading classes. The 1897–98 report of the Bombay Plague Committee commented:

> Banias took the Plague to the Deccan, where it is known as the Marwadi sickness. They carried it to parts of Khandesh, where it is called the Bania disease. Hindu traders, mostly Gujaratis, conveyed the disease to Karachi in November 1896, and to Mandvi in Cutch in April 1897. The Bania is the Plague spreader partly, perhaps mainly, because the Bania is the chief traveller.[32]

The perceived centrality of the human body as plague's source and vehicle was given further emphasis by the difficulty experienced in identifying the disease. It was necessary to physically examine the body to find the characteristic buboes, or swellings; but even a high temperature and glandular swellings might not provide conclusive proof. Many experts, especially in Britain, claimed that postmortems were the only reliable guide. The human body was thus both the presumed vector of the disease and the bearer of its essential diagnostical signs.

It followed that government plague measures concentrated upon the interception, examination, and confinement of the body. This entailed a form of direct medical intervention that—at least until opposition became too troublesome to ignore—swept aside the rival or preferential claims of relatives and friends, of *vaidyas* and *hakims*, religious and caste leaders. The body was treated as a secular object, almost as state property, not as sacred territory; as an individual entity, not as an integral part of a wider community. The body, moreover, was exposed not just to the "gaze" of the Western medical practitioner but also to his physical touch, an intrusion of the greatest concern to a society in which touch connoted possession or pollution.

ASSAULT ON THE BODY

Unprecedented in character and scale, the measures adopted to combat epidemic plague in 1896–98 provoked the greatest upsurge of public resistance to Western medicine and sanitation that nineteenth-century India had witnessed. To judge by the reactions of the Indian press and by official accounts of the riots and disturbances that followed, as well as by the rumors that circulated, the early plague years represented a profound crisis for Western medicine and for the power of the colonial state. The plague episode, even more than the history of smallpox and cholera measures before it, seems to present, almost paradigmatically, a tale of alienation and resistance. The rapid growth of the English and vernacular press in India in the late nineteenth century allows us, moreover, unprecedented access to contemporary attitudes. The character of Indian responses to the antiplague measures suggests how alien and malevolent Western medicine still remained in many Indians' eyes, even in the closing years of a century of growing state intervention and increasing, if gradual, dissemination of Western medical and sanitary ideas. In fact, as will be argued later in this chapter and the next, reaction to the plague measures was more complicated and equivocal than a simple paradigm of resistance would suggest. Nonetheless, the nature of this hostile reaction is too important—to the evolution of state medicine in India, to the history of subaltern protest and middle-class hegemony—to be passed over in silence.

In the first weeks of the plague epidemic in Bombay, the Indian press criticized the provincial government for its apparent inertia and its reluctance to recognize the dangers plague might pose for the welfare of the people of Bombay. The English-language newspaper the *Mahratta*, run by the Pune politician and nationalist leader Bal Gangadhar Tilak, took a characteristically adversarial stance, accusing the government in December 1896 of "criminal indifference" toward plague.[33] However, as the government swung around to a more active and interventionist policy, the Indian press began to express grave doubts about the effects of the new measures and the extent of the coercive power that had been unleashed. In Calcutta, *Bangavasi* remarked that a "law more dangerous and drastic than the Plague Act was never before enacted in this country."[34] The *Mahratta*, at first favorably disposed toward the Epidemic Diseases Act, was soon protesting, especially in regard to plague operations in Pune, that no measure undertaken by the British in India had "interfered so largely and in such a systematic way with the domestic, social and religious habits of the people."[35]

This view was shared by many vernacular and Indian-owned English-language newspapers in the Bombay Presidency. As early as October 1896, the press protested over the segregation of plague suspects and voiced a general repugnance at the way in which hospitalization was being carried out. "Rightly or wrongly," wrote the *Gujarati* of Bombay, "the feeling of the Native community is strongly against segregation." It argued that social customs, religious sentiments, and "the strong natural ties of affection" were all against it. "The very idea of tearing off one's dear relative from those affectionately devoted to him and of his departing from the world without the usual religious ministrations is revolting to the mind of the Native community."[36] A petition from the leading Indian residents of Bombay to the Municipal Commissioner on October 14 expressed a similar view[37] and, along with fear that the sweepers would strike or leave the city, was a factor in persuading Snow to moderate his measures. Nonetheless, the introduction of the Epidemic Diseases Act and the appointment of special plague committees in Bombay and Pune sparked renewed protests at the "indifference and callousness" of the colonial administration and the "enormities committed in the name of sanitary science."[38]

In explaining the extreme unpopularity of hospitals, the *Mahratta* pointed in November 1897 to the difficulty patients experienced in keeping in touch with their families:

> The relatives of the sick man find it extremely difficult even to send word to him, not to speak of approaching him and assuaging his distress by loving attendance and affectionate words. As for attendance and nursing, how effective they might be can well be imagined from the fact that the hospital servants are at best mere strangers, invariably callous and patent mercenaries, and that the sick man, once within the hospital compound, is almost cut off from his private resources.[39]

In Western eyes, a sanitized and healing environment—Gatacre's committee claimed that a plague hospital was one of the safest places to be during an epidemic[40]—the hospital was to many Indians (not least to the higher castes) a place of pollution, contaminated by blood and feces, inimical to caste, religion, and purdah. In April 1897 the *Kesari* (a Marathi paper also run by Tilak) carried the story of a Brahmin who had been forced to live on milk while in hospital because the food he was offered had been polluted by being served by a Sudra. Six weeks later the *Mahratta* complained that caste observances were being violated in Pune's general hospital and protested against the threatened closure of the Hindu Plague Hospital, where, it said, caste had been scrupulously respected.[41] Opposition to state medicine was particularly strong among those Indians who saw in plague a form of divine retribution, a visitation against which medical and sanitary measures were either useless or impious. "We will not go to hospital," declared one young Muslim in Bombay in December 1896. "Our Musjid [mosque] is our hospital."[42]

Although opposition to segregation and hospitalization was commonly expressed in the idiom of male pollution and deprivation, it was the examination and seizure of women and their removal to segregation camps and hospitals that provoked the fiercest resistance and the most vehement opposition. Objections were made on these grounds in Calcutta even during the first discussion of plague measures in October 1896. N. Mukherjee, chairman of the Calcutta Corporation, warned Risley that "people would prefer to die of the plague rather than consent or submit to the removal of their mothers, wives, daughters or sisters to hospital" and that, for this reason, Indian municipal councilors were unlikely to support such procedures.[43] In Bombay in March 1897 a Kazi spoke for many Muslims when he demanded in anger, "How could a husband be expected to tolerate the sight of his wife's hand being in the hand of another man?"[44]

Such strength of feeling lay behind several violent episodes in the early plague years. Nearly a thousand millhands attacked Bombay's Arthur Road Infectious Diseases Hospital on October 29, 1896, after a woman worker had been taken there as a plague suspect—an incident which Snow took to signify general dissent from the policy of segregation and hospitalization.[45] Again, on March 9, 1898, Julaha Muslim weavers in Bombay prevented the removal to hospital of a twelve-year-old girl suspected of having plague. A magistrate was wounded in the resulting fracas, and hospitals and other buildings were attacked and set on fire.[46] At Kanpur (Cawnpore) on April 11, 1900, an attack on the local segregation camp by Chamars, millhands, and butchers was provoked by reports of women being detained there against their will.[47]

The physical examination of travelers and the residents of plague-struck towns and cities also spread alarm and opposition. Because most doctors were male as well as white, their touch was considered polluting or, worse, as tantamount to sexual molestation. This was especially so when, in searching for the bodily signs of plague, doctors tried to examine women's necks, thighs, and armpits. A Sholapur paper, *Kalpataru*, protested in October 1897 that "Native feeling" was "most touchy" on this issue: "Native ladies will prefer death to the humiliation of having their groins examined by male doctors who are utter strangers to them." It saw the appointment of women doctors as the only possible solution.[48]

When the examination of rail passengers began in February 1897, it drew an immediately hostile response. *Gurakhi*, another Marathi paper, angrily denounced the examination of women passengers at Kalyan, a major junction on the lines linking Bombay with Pune, north India, and Calcutta. "That a female should be publicly asked by a male stranger to remove the end of her sari [from the upper half of her body]," it protested, "is most insulting and likely to result in loss of life."[49] Passengers traveling to Calcutta via Khana Junction on the East India Railway were subjected to a similar ordeal. Forced to alight from the train, they were separated into two queues—one for men, the other for women—and made to wait until they were examined, in full public view, by a European doctor. It was only after an outcry in the press had shown the strength of Indian feeling that screens were provided and a few women doctors were found to examine female passengers. But the basic resentment remained. As Moradabad's *Nizam-ul-Mulk* put it in April 1900, "The very sight of plague doctors at the railway station curdles the blood of passengers."[50] The examination of women on the streets of Pune, as much as the frequent and keenly resented house searches, fed mounting indignation in the city and helped provoke the assassination of W. C. Rand, chairman of the Plague Committee, on June 22, 1897.[51]

The physical manhandling of Indians as if they were "mere beasts and as such not entitled to any belief or sympathy,"[52] was made all the more offensive by the use of troops, especially British troops, in Pune and Bombay to carry out house searches. This inevitably invited hostile comparisons with military conquest and occupation.[53] The citizens of Pune, who with some justification felt that they had been singled out for "special treatment," saw the use of soldiers as a crude attempt to punish or intimidate a city which had become notorious for its anticolonial opposition.

But the use of these "white bulls" had a further connotation. In recent years British soldiers had been involved in a series of racial incidents in which women had been molested and raped, villagers had been beaten, even shot at, by soldiers out on hunting expeditions. On one pretext or another—for example, mistaking a villager for a wild beast—the soldiers received only negligible punishments in the courts, a travesty the Indian press bitterly resented.[54] Using nearly a thousand British soldiers to conduct house searches in Pune thus smacked of either gross insensitivity or deliberate provocation. Reports of sexual harassment, insult, and abuse by British troops soon began to circulate in the city.[55] It did not escape comment that when white men or women were attacked, Europeans took a very different attitude. *Moda Vritt*, a Marathi paper, wondered how Indians could be expected to feel grief at Rand's death when Europeans went un-punished for "taking the lives of helpless Natives under the impression that they are monkeys, crows and bears."[56]

Nor was the living body alone subjected to insults and indignities. The examination and disposal of corpses figured prominently in early plague policy. According to Bengal's plague committee in a memorandum of mid-1897, a "plague corpse is a focus of infection." It followed, then, that "all religious rites and ceremonies [relating to the dead] should . . . be curtailed as much as possible."[57] In August 1897 the secretary of state for India, under pressure from medical opinion in Britain, urged that a systematic policy of corpse inspection be instituted as the best means of countering deficient plague registration and as a check to the further spread of the disease.[58] Opinion in India was more equivocal. Civilian administrators were well aware that the issue was extremely sensitive and that corpse inspection was, as Lord Elgin noted in August 1897, "likely to produce great irritation" among Indians of all classes, or as the Bombay Plague Committee put it, "the possible advantages from the practice are outweighed by the certainty of discontent."[59]

The truth of this was amply demonstrated. In October 1896 William Simpson, Calcutta's health officer, caused great indignation by insisting on examining (and taking a sample of blood from) the body of a zenana woman who had reputedly died of mumps, but whom he suspected of having died of plague. "If this is not highhandedness," roared *Hitavadi*, "nothing is. Let the town be cleansed by all means, but let there be no oppression in the name of sanitation."[60] In the Bombay Presidency it was decreed that bodies could not be buried or cremated until they had been inspected by a qualified doctor to ascertain whether plague had been the cause of death. With scores of deaths occurring daily and few qualified doctors available to inspect the bodies, this might entail a delay of many hours before funeral rites could proceed. Twelve, even twenty-four, hours might elapse, complained the *Mahratta* in June 1897, before permission could be obtained for a burial or cremation, even though the "detention of dead bodies in houses for such a long time is condemned both by religion and the science of sanitation."[61] Reports of the government's decision to order the inspection of all corpses was sufficient to create widespread unrest in the Bombay Presidency in March 1898, especially among Muslims. It fueled the riot in Bombay city on March

9, while at Hubli in the south of the province a meeting at the Jama Masjid on March 11 vowed that if any Muslim died from whatever cause, plague or not, "every Muhammadan must collect near the dead body and not allow it to be inspected by the medical officer, nor touched by him, because his touch would defile the corpse." If the doctor tried to persist with his examination, "he should not be allowed to do so even though our lives are sacrificed."[62]

Postmortem examination of suspected plague victims was also fiercely opposed. The practice had to be stopped at Jawalpur, near Hardwar in the North-Western Provinces, after an attack on the plague camp there on March 30, 1898, had drawn officials' attention to the strength of public feeling against it.[63] Interference with customary funeral rites and practices—which in the Bombay Presidency in 1897–98 included the closure of overcrowded cemeteries and a requirement that plague corpses be wrapped in a sheet soaked in perchloride of lime or covered with quicklime—gave rise to several demonstrations of defiance. At the town of Rander in Surat district on March 9, 1897, an order from the assistant collector directing that a plague corpse be taken to a mosque on the outskirts of town attended by no more than fifteen mourners was openly defied. Some three thousand Muslims accompanied the body to the central mosque for the final prayers to be said over it.[64]

The search for plague cases and corpses in Bombay and Pune encountered not only outright resistance but also, more commonly, evasion and concealment. The sick, whether suffering from plague or any other disease that might be mistaken for it, were smuggled out to areas free from search parties or hidden in lofts, inside cupboards, under furniture, or in secret rooms. Corpses were buried clandestinely, sometimes within the house or compound. The British were dismayed that even as "Westernized" a community as the Parsis should resort to such evasion and subterfuge.[65]

Such assaults on the body were not, to be sure, the only cause of opposition to the government's antiplague measures. There was concern, too, for the loss of property and possessions destroyed or pilfered during plague operations. For the poor, hospitalization and segregation meant the loss of wages, possibly of a job. Merchants were resentful of restrictions placed upon their freedom of movement by searches and cordons as well as of the destruction of their grain, cloth, and other goods.[66] Banias and Marwaris, often cited in official reports as agents in the transmission of plague and often among its first victims in a locality, were also among those most resolutely opposed to plague measures, as they were to smallpox vaccination as well. Indeed, they were suspected of deliberately spreading hostile rumors and false reports in order to excite public opposition. Bania resistance might be as influential in its way as that of the subaltern classes. But it was still the actual, threatened, or imagined assault on the body that aroused the greatest fear and anger in the early plague years. And it was this collective fear and anger that found forceful expression in rumor.

PLAGUE RUMORS

Rumor flourished in the atmosphere of uncertainty and alarm generated by plague and, even more, by colonial intervention against it. There are, though, many difficulties in the way of trying to interpret plague rumors as a species of popular discourse. As they have come down to us, the rumors are far from being an uncontaminated source. They were often written down and printed—in the press, in official reports, and memoirs—specifically in order to show the absurdity and naive credulity of the masses, to prove (as one newspaper put it) that "King Mob" was "impervious to reason" or, as Snow averred in Bombay, that the public had been seized by "a wild, unreasoning panic."[67] The wilder the rumor, the better it suited this purpose, the more eloquently it betrayed the part irrational prejudice played in turning the people against operations intended for their own health and security.

Not all rumors were an unalloyed product of the subaltern classes, nor did they circulate exclusively among them. In his report on the Calcutta plague, J. N. Cook, the city's health officer, noted rather despairingly in 1898 that it was "extraordinary how natives occupying a respectable position gave credence to the wildest and most improbable stories."[68] It would also be rash to discount altogether as colonial myth or middle-class prejudice the suggestion made, especially at the time of the Calcutta plague disturbances in May 1898, that some rumors were "set in circulation by badmashes [villains] with the object of frightening people and getting an opportunity of looting them."[69] *Vaidyas* and *hakims* were also suspected—on what evidence is not clear—of spreading alarm in order to discredit Western medicine and promote their own rival practice.[70] But, caveats aside, rumors take us closer to popular perceptions and responses than other sources allow.

One striking feature of the plague rumors, in seeming contrast to many other examples of this form of popular discourse in India, was their preoccupation with the body. It is true that rumors were sometimes of a more general nature. There were, for instance, reports of "absurd rumours" that "the intention of Government was to interfere with the religion and caste of the people" and "to destroy caste and religious observances, with the ultimate design of forcing Christianity on the natives of India."[71] At the time of the Kanpur riot in April 1900, it was said that "the wildest rumours of impending danger to Hindu and Musalman alike" were in circulation.[72] But the overwhelming concern of the majority of reported rumors was with an assault on the body, whether by poisoning, dissection, or other means. The principal themes were these:

1. *Poisoning*. Commonest of all rumors were those relating to the deliberate poisoning of Indians by doctors, hospital staff, and inoculators. One of the first reports to this effect was carried by the *Mahratta* on November 1, 1896, in connection with Bombay city. The *Kesari* of February 16, 1897, also referred to rumors of the "systematic poisoning" of hospital patients. A fuller and more elaborate version was given in the *Poona Vaibhar* in February 1897, which reported that:

> In some villages the people have come to think that the Sarkar [government], finding its subjects unmanageable, is devising means to reduce their number. They say that it mixes poison in opium. They even hesitate to accept the dole of bread distributed in the famine camps under the belief that poison is mixed with the bread. They think that the hospitals are now under the management of new doctors who put poison into the medicines.[73]

In other versions it was the village well or the municipal water supply that had been poisoned; such rumors were rife in northern India in 1900. The *Hindustan* of Kalakankar referred to rumors "to the effect that plague patients are poisoned by doctors, that the waterworks supply has been poisoned by Government to kill the people, and that six bags of snakes and other worms have been ground [up] and dissolved in the water-pipe at Cawnpore to bring on plague among consumers."[74] In the Lahore district of Punjab two years later it was said that the Sirkar had hired the "daktari log" [the doctors] to kill off India's surplus population, and there was "a very widespread impression that doctors or doctors in disguise were going about putting poison in wells."[75]

2. *Cutting up the body: extracting 'momiai.'* A second cluster of rumors concerned the cutting up of bodies, especially in hospitals. A correspondent of the *Mahratta* in December 1896 reported that a man who was told he had plague and would be taken to Pune's Sassoon Hospital said he might as well have his throat cut straightaway. The writer explained that "all the natives have an idea that they are taken to the Hospital and killed in order that the doctors may cut them up." The paper's editor confirmed that hospitals were seen by some Indians as being "so many slaughter-houses for the benefit of human vivisectionists."[76] Similar rumors were evidently circulating in Bombay in October 1896. Snow referred to a "foul brood of fantastical horrors" among which were "extraordinary rumours that the hospitals were torture-chambers and death-traps."[77] After the millhands' attack on the Arthur Road Hospital, *Kaiser-e-Hind* explained that the workers believed that there was "something diabolical" about a hospital "which claimed so many victims." Patients, it was said, were bled to death through the soles of their feet: the hospital was "the very incarnation of the Devil, and the Devil was to be exorcised at all costs and at all hazards."[78]

The purpose behind hospitalization was sometimes seen to be the extraction of an essential oil or balm known as *momiai*.[79] Enthoven attributed the flight of thousands of mill workers from Bombay in October 1896 to the fear that "officials were seizing men and boys with the intention of hanging them head downwards over a slow fire and preparing a medicine drawn from the head."[80] According to F. S. P. Lely, residents of Bulsar in Gujarat would not pass along the road in front of the local hospital because it was "universally believed, or at any rate said, that an oil mill was under every bed to grind the patient into ointment for use on European patients in Bombay."[81] A boatman near Bilimora told another official that the plague inspection shed at the nearby railway station contained a "big machine" for squeezing oil out of passengers' bodies. This substance was then sent to Bombay, where it was "put into other people, and then they get plague too."[82]

3. *Seizing, searching, looting.* Rumors of this class partly overlap with those in the previous categories. They concern the powers said to have been entrusted to doctors, policemen, soldiers, and sanitary officers. In some instances they are barely exaggerated versions of the authority actually conferred upon such individuals. In November 1896 the *Indian Spectator* reported a rumor in Bombay that the police could dispatch anyone they chose to hospital, from which they would never emerge again alive.[83] A common belief, again not without some foundation in reality, was that perfectly healthy men and women were seized and sent to hospitals and segregation camps. It was sometimes said that plague did not exist at all, but had been invented to enable low-paid government servants to plunder the people at will, or that doctors were deliberately spreading plague to drum up business for themselves. At the time of the Calcutta disturbances of May 1898, the police were rumored to carry bottles of poison which they held to the noses of their victims unless bribed to desist.[84]

4. *Inoculation.* The introduction of Haffkine's antiplague serum in 1897–98 sparked off many rumors concerning its nature, purpose, and effects—some of which were elaborations of earlier fears about smallpox vaccination. Despite government denials, rumor was rife in Calcutta that inoculation would be (or had already been) made compulsory. This resulted in several attacks on Europeans and on Indians suspected of being inoculators in the city in May 1898: in one incident, an Austrian sailor drowned trying to escape his pursuers.[85] The sudden appearance of a European accompanied by two policemen at a fair at Varanasi in May 1899 caused immediate speculation that he was an inoculator, and there was "a general stampede."[86] Inoculation was feared because it reputedly caused "instantaneous death" or resulted in impotence and sterility.[87] Inoculation rumors current in the Ambala district of Punjab in 1901–02 included these:

> The needle was a yard long; you died immediately after the operation; you survived the operation six months and then collapsed; men lost their virility and women became sterile; the Deputy Commissioner himself underwent the operation and expired half an hour afterwards in great agony.[88]

When inoculations were performed on Europeans or on prominent Indians without apparent ill effect, it was said that only rosewater had been used, the real poison being reserved for less-fortunate Indians.[89]

5. *Collapse or weakness of British rule.* A rumor of this kind, which moved beyond immediate concern with the body, gave rise to a riot at the village of Chakalashi in the Kaira district of Gujarat in January 1898. According to the *Mahratta*, a local "fanatic" told the people that British rule was over. Lely's version of the story was that locals believed that "the British Empire had fallen in the country south of the Mahi, and that the plague cordon which had been drawn along that river [between British India and the princely state of Baroda] was really for the purpose of preventing the news from getting through to the north." By his account "a new kingdom was proclaimed and preparations made for selecting a Raja"—until the police arrived and bloodshed followed.[90]

A related rumor, touching in another way upon the weakness of British power, circulated in northern India in 1900. This was to the effect that the British were spreading plague deliberately in order to discourage the Russians from invading India. This might be linked to other rumors current at the time about Russian advances into Afghanistan and Kashmir.[91] It was said in Calcutta in 1898 that in order to save British India (from what is not clear), the viceroy had met a yogi in a remote place in the Himalayas "and made a compact with him to sacrifice 2 lakhs of lives to the Goddess Kali." The British were suspected of trying to keep this bargain by distributing poisonous white powders and black pills and by administering lethal injections.[92]

6. *General catastrophe.* A final group of rumors, or in some cases authored predictions (which thus stray beyond the realm of true rumor), concerned a spate of imminent disasters and calamities, of which plague and the famine then sweeping India were but precursors. An earthquake confidently predicted to occur in Delhi in January 1898 increased alarm over the anticipated imposition of plague measures.[93] The month of Kartik in the Sambat year 1956 (November 1899) was expected to usher in an age of general affliction and catastrophe for India and the world.[94] Plague was the harbinger of the great apocalypse.

What significance can we see in these plague rumors? They are clear evidence of how widely and intensely the epidemic was discussed in India at the time and the fear and suspicion with which the state's measures were viewed. "The word plague," reported *Hindustan* in April 1899, "is even in the mouths of children."[95] On the eve of the April 1900 riot in Kanpur, the "plague administration, especially the segregation of the sick, became the common subject of conversation among the better classes of the city," and from them "anxiety gradually extended down to the masses of the people."[96] On April 28, 1898, when Sir John Woodburn, the lieutenant-governor of Bengal, met doctors at the Eden Hospital to decide whether plague had reached Calcutta, rumor rapidly spread. By noon

> the excitement in the town was intense. In business houses and in bazaars, streets and bustees the question was discussed, had the dreaded Bombay plague come at last, were their houses going to be forcibly entered, and their wives and daughters torn away by British soldiers, was quarantine to be established, and were they all to be forcibly inoculated?[97]

In a situation where the government generally failed to take the people into its confidence, rumor had something of a predictive quality. It was an attempt to anticipate and explain what the government was up to, and people took the action—flight, evasion, resistance—that accordingly seemed most appropriate. In Calcutta in April–May 1898, as in Bombay in late 1896, thousands of people fled not just to avoid the plague but also to escape the measures the government seemed intent on imposing on them. Rumor informed action.

The contents of the rumors suggest two basic preoccupations. There was, first of all, a deep suspicion of the nature and methods of Western medicine. As the preceding chapters have shown, this feeling was by no means new. For much of the century, hospitals and such practices as vaccination and postmortems had given rise to fear, opposition, and anger. Some of the plague inoculation rumors, for example, bore a close resemblance to earlier rumors about vaccination. But such doubts and fears were given fresh intensity by the unprecedented scale of medical and sanitary intervention in 1896–1900, by the exceptionally coercive and comprehensive nature of the measures adopted, and by the way in which the body was singled out for attention.

Some of the rumors were garbled accounts of an unfamiliar medical technology: needles a yard long, toxic serums, hospitals that dissected the living as well as the dead. Perhaps even the rumor about snakes in the water supply had its origin in some health officer's slide show about cholera bacilli or other waterborne microbes. But as Indians became more familiar with Western medicine (partly as a result of the sheer scale of medical intervention in the 1890s and 1900s) and as the more coercive plague measures were withdrawn (largely in response to popular protest), inoculation and hospitals lost much of their former terror. As fear abated, the rumors it had occasioned also began to die away.

But it was not only the nature and novelty of Western medical technology that set rumor flying. Plague, and still more the state measures deployed against it, were seen to have a deeper meaning and to reveal the underlying intentions of British rule. In this effort after meaning, rumor pasted together in a vivid collage aspects of the current crisis—plague, hospitalization, segregation, inoculation—along with other disturbing or exciting scraps of news and gossip—famine, war, talk of overpopulation, growing opposition to British rule, Russian advances in Central Asia.

To outsiders it might appear that these fragments were utterly unrelated and were brought together in a completely random and bizarre fashion that showed nothing but the depth of popular ignorance and stupidity. And yet at the level of popular discourse, this association of ideas provided a partially coherent pattern of explanation. It seemed to explain what was otherwise difficult to account for: why, for example, were Europeans immune to the disease unless they had some part in its propagation? Underlying almost all the rumors was an assumption about British self-interest and spite, a readiness to torture Indians and sacrifice their lives in order to preserve British power. As one newspaper pointed out, the rumors gave no support to the idea of the raj as the *ma-bap* ("mother-father") of the people, "that it protects them and redresses their grievances," a belief the British liked to cite as evidence of the paternalistic popularity of their regime.[98] Even the viceroy appeared willing, by popular report, to kill off two hundred thousand inhabitants of Calcutta as the price of maintaining British rule. Here was no kindly czar, no benevolent white queen, to whom an oppressed people could appeal against the tyranny of their masters. European power appeared at this moment of crisis as a monolith, undivided in its malevolence. Such was the apparent British contempt for the bodies and the beliefs of their Indian subjects that it seemed perfectly credible, not some extravagant fantasy, that they should poison wells, administer lethal injections, or grind up people for *momiai*.

It is possible to go a stage further in discussing the importance of rumor as a species of popular discourse. Some of the rumors voiced a suspicion not only of the British but also of those Indians who appeared to be their agents, allies, and collaborators. The rajas and notables who assisted the British in their plague operations or allowed themselves to be inoculated were seen as accomplices in an evil conspiracy to poison, pollute, and plunder. In Calcutta in May 1898, Bengali "topi-wallahs" (those who wore hats in the Western manner) became, along with Europeans, targets of popular violence and were attacked on suspicion of being inoculators or plague doctors.[99] Conversely, the popular credence given to plague rumors aroused antipathy in many middle-class Indians. Tilak, like many other newspaper editors and politicians at the time, and despite his vociferous opposition to the way in which plague operations were carried out in Pune and elsewhere, saw it as his duty as a "leader" to educate the public about Western medical and scientific ideas and to refute the wilder rumors about hospitalization and segregation. "It is true," commented an editorial in the *Mahratta* in March 1897,

> that the masses look upon plague as a providential visitation
> and have little faith in the efficacy of methods suggested by
> sanitary science. But because the masses are ignorant it is a
> mistake to suppose that the leaders and specially the educated
> classes do not appreciate the usefulness of modern sanitary
> measures.[100]

Certainly, Tilak and other newspaper editors were willing, if not actually to endorse public hostility against plague measures, at least to use the opportunity to show the unpopularity of British rule. But there was also real contempt, coupled at times with indignation and fear, in middle-class attitudes toward popular belief and action. The contemptuous language showered upon "ignorant rustics" and the "superstitious" beliefs of peasants and millhands, the criticism of their "filthy habits," and the contrast repeatedly drawn between the "intelligent" or "educated" classes on the one hand and the "foolish and illiterate" peasants on the other cannot have been for the censor's eye alone.[101] This antipathy became even more pronounced when, as in Calcutta in May 1898, the "topi-wallahs" became the targets of popular violence. The editor of *Hitavadi*, previously one of the most outspoken critics of the government's plague policies, angrily decried the actions of the "badmashes" responsible for the attacks. "No one," he fumed, "has the right to kick up a row and create a disturbance."[102] The followers of Ramakrishna in the city were more restrained but issued a statement calling for calm and urging the people not to be misled by "*canards* or bazaar gossip."[103] The desire to lead and educate the "rough people" was partly grounded in a fear of their violent "irrationality."[104]

One final point about plague rumors and British reactions to them: rather like cholera and its association with Hindu pilgrimage in earlier decades, plague and the resistance to plague measures were identified by Europeans with the negative attributes of Indian society. Plague rumors were taken to be indicative of the difficulty of trying to implement an enlightened and rational medical policy in the face of such deep-rooted opposition. Plague rumors conveniently exemplified Indian apathy, fatalism, irrationality. In this way responsibility for the spread of plague, rather like smallpox and cholera before it, was shifted away from the colonial civil servants and doctors and onto Indians themselves. "Orientals," concluded Gatacre's committee in Bombay, were "most conservative," "wedded to many insanitary customs which have been inseparably connected with their life and prejudices for centuries."[105] The Government of India's 1898 summary likewise remarked that "in India the customs and prejudices of the people offer a more or less important obstacle to the adoption of the measures which have been found best adapted to check the disease."[106] Even when the first crisis was over, "fatalism" remained the characteristic most commonly ascribed to Indian attitudes toward plague and administrative attempts to curb its ravages.[107]

"NATIVE AGENCY"

Plague provided a pretext for a second colonial assault—on the growing political assertiveness and leadership of the Indian middle classes. This was most evident in relation to the municipalities of Bombay, Calcutta, and Pune, where it merged with the growing crisis of urban control and where unprecedented powers were given to special plague committees. Of the three, Pune provides the most striking example.

Plague reached Pune, a city of some 160,000 people, toward the end of 1896. The earliest cases, recorded in October, were among plague refugees from Bombay; the first local cases followed in late December. Plague came to Pune at a time when the provincial government, headed by Lord Sandhurst, was already bent on humbling the city's political elite. Through the Poona Sarvajanik Sabha, the political organization founded in 1879, the city's Brahmins, including Tilak, had been persistent in their criticism of British policies, most recently in connection with the famine. If plague provided an opportunity for politicians to step up their attacks on the government, it also gave the administration a convenient excuse to strike back. Tilak was an obvious target. The Sivaji and Ganapati festivals, part of his attempt to promote a more assertive Hindu nationalism among the masses of Maharashtra, were banned in 1897 under the plague restrictions, and he was imprisoned for almost a year for his alleged part in provoking or plotting the assassination of W. C. Rand in June 1897.[108] But the government's counterthrust was not directed against Tilak alone. It was also aimed at the Pune municipal council, of which Tilak was also a member and which British officials saw as Brahmin dominated, politically suspect, and administratively inept.

The issue of the Pune municipality went back to 1885. Lord Reay, the governor of Bombay at the time, decided to meet the demands of the Poona Sarvajanik Sabha and of the municipal councilors themselves by liberalizing the composition of the council. Its membership was raised from twenty to thirty, with only ten government nominees, and the council was given the privilege of electing its own president. This "experiment" was justified as being in the spirit of the local self-government reforms initiated by the Liberal viceroy, Lord Ripon, in 1882 and as reflecting the presence of a "large and intelligent class of educated native gentlemen" in Pune.[109]

By 1898, however, after the new council had been in operation for a dozen years, European bureaucrats had unilaterally decided that Reay's "experiment" had proved a "conspicuous failure," and they seized upon the crisis caused by the advent of plague as further evidence of the council's ineptitude. In May 1897 R. A. Lamb, the collector of Pune, complained to his divisional commissioner, J. K. Spence, that the problems affecting Pune demonstrated what happened to health and sanitation in a large town when entrusted "entirely to native agency." Conservation and sanitation, "as we understand them," he said, are not congenial to the native temperament which prefers to regard the results of insanitation rather as visitations of God than as the inevitable consequence of dirt and filth being inadequately dealt with in thickly populated places. It follows from this habit of mind that sanitation and conservancy, if left wholly to natives, are imperfectly carried out.

Lamb saw this as a matter of particular concern in Pune because the "native" town lay perilously close to the civil lines—"the residence of members of the Bombay Government for 4 months of the year"— and to one of India's largest cantonments.[110] Spence's view was no less damning: "As long as conservancy and sanitation remain under native supervision and control they will remain a farce." A member of the Bombay Government Secretariat further minuted that "the plague has not only strengthened the hands of Govt. sufficiently to justify them before the world in interfering with Local Self-Govt. in the interests of sanitation," but had also "shown the need for this."[111]

In February 1897, shortly before Lamb wrote his scathing remarks, Rand took charge of plague operations in Pune. When he came to write his own report, just before his death in June 1897, he took a similarly disparaging view of how Indians had been running the city, especially its sanitary and medical services. The municipal councilors had, he said, allowed Pune to fall into a grossly insanitary state and done little to check the epidemic when it first appeared. They had shown want of resolution in enforcing hospitalization and segregation in the face of popular hostility and had appointed as health officer a young Brahmin, fresh out of college, who was "quite unfit for the place."[112]

Armed with extraordinary powers under the Epidemic Diseases Act, Rand was able to ignore the municipal council and set up his own three-man committee (known to the *Mahratta* as the "Plague Triumvirate") to run plague operations in the city more as they had been conducted in Hong Kong than as they were currently being carried out in Bombay.[113] His use of European troops to conduct house searches was a clear affront to Pune's Indian elite. Lamb, who fully endorsed these measures, agreed with Rand and Beveridge that since British soldiers were "disciplined" they could be "relied on to be thorough and honest in their inspection," while "no native agency is available, or could be relied on if it were."[114] The only role Rand allowed for "native gentlemen" was "to explain to the public the objects of the search, to act as interpreters between the soldiers and the public and to point out to the soldiers the portions of houses which custom forbade them to enter."[115] That few middle-class residents of Pune would come forward to take up such unpopular and demeaning work was seen by Rand and his committee as further evidence of the uselessness of "native agency." It followed, too, that sanitation in the city would have to remain under European control "for some time to come" if the gains which Rand believed had been made under his direction were not to be forfeited by a return to Indian management. It was conveniently overlooked that the municipal council's earlier attempts to tackle plague had been blocked or ignored by an unresponsive provincial government.[116]

Rand's diatribes against "native agency," shared by other civil servants, such as Lamb, and sanitary officers like Beveridge and his successor, Surgeon-Major Barry,[117] became the basis for a revision of the municipal council. In 1898 the number of nominated councilors was raised from ten to eighteen in order to strengthen official and European control.[118] The irony, not lost on Indian critics, was that the measures so aggressively pursued by Rand and later by Barry, which exceeded those pursued almost everywhere else in India and for which such extravagant claims of success were made, failed to prevent the return of plague in October–November 1897 on a far greater scale than in the earlier months of the year.[119] But although Pune was singled out for "special treatment," bureaucratic contempt for "native agency" was by no means confined to that city. In Calcutta, for instance, there were similar imputations of Indian incompetence, even cowardice, in the face of the plague crisis and there, too, the opportunity was seized to reorganize the municipal corporation, reducing the elected element and thereby weakening Indian control while strengthening the position of European civilian and sanitary officers.[120]

FROM CONFRONTATION
TO CONCILIATION

While racial contempt and political revenge helped inspire the severity of early plague operations, especially in Pune, the political factor also acted, as the crisis deepened, as a constraint on British action, forcing a significant shift in state policy. By late 1897 and early 1898 the administration faced a dual crisis of control. Despite (perhaps because of) intensive operations in towns and cities, the epidemic had continued to spread and was now reaching Bengal, the North-Western Provinces, Punjab, and Hyderabad. Initial attempts to control plague had failed while mortality continued remorselessly to rise. The India Office and its medical advisers in London were pressing for more rigorous measures, including corpse inspection and strict segregation of plague suspects; and a resolution of the Government of India on February 3, 1898, bowing to this pressure, called for the full implementation of antiplague measures.[121]

The resolution proved to be a watershed. There was mounting evidence of the unpopularity of plague measures, and several provincial governments—Bengal, the North-Western Provinces, and Punjab—were doubtful about the political wisdom of attempting to impose them in the face of such clear public opposition. The riot in Bombay in October 1896 was followed by a second in March 1898 and several smaller incidents. There were disturbances elsewhere in the province, including Sinnat in Nasik district in January 1898. In northern India there was rioting against house searches, segregation, and hospitalization at Jawalpur in March 1898, and at Garhshankar in Punjab in April. In the south there was an incident at Srirangapatnam near Mysore in November. But, occurring in the imperial capital itself, the Calcutta disturbances of May 1898 were perhaps the most disquieting of a troubled year. As one Punjab paper wryly commented, if rumors of poisoning doctors and lethal injections could find credence in an "enlightened" city like Calcutta, what hope could there be for plague operations in up-country towns and villages?[122] Deputations of leading citizens, municipal councilors, caste and religious leaders, all urged provincial governments and local plague committees to show greater respect for Indian sentiment and custom while warning of greater opposition and bloodshed if their pleas were not heeded.[123]

If, administrators began to reason, plague operations could provoke such bitterness and resistance in Bombay and Bengal, what would happen when they were enforced against the Muslims and "martial races" of northern India?[124] In February 1898, as if in confirmation of these doubts, anonymous placards appeared in Delhi which drew ominous comparisons with the Mutiny and Rebellion of 1857. One of these, prominently displayed in Chandni Chowk, the busiest thoroughfare in the old city, warned that

People are very much dissatisfied at the issue of notice with regard to the arrangements proposed to be made if bubonic plague breaks out. These would ruin their good name, respect and religion. Is that civilization? We caution Government to excuse us and not to adopt the procedure. We are quite prepared to sacrifice our lives for our religion and respect. We are ready to die. The notice will call emotion equal to that of 1857 Mutiny.[125]

An anonymous "notice" sent to Delhi's deputy commissioner declared:

God forbid that the plague may attack Delhi, but if it does, then the regulations circulated are harsh and unworkable, and the Delhi public shall not be able to carry them out. . . .

As you are responsible for the good government of Delhi, please think over the regulations before putting them in force. The Governor undoubtedly relies on his force, and thinks that he shall have the orders complied with anyhow, but you might bear in mind that where money, women and land are concerned quarrels must ensue. When we will be turned out of the house and our faithful wives will be given over to the Doctors for treatment, there is not the slightest doubt that no Hindu or Muhammadan will sit quietly. . . .

Please bear in mind that although we are poor and are a conquered race, the pure blood of nobility still flows in our veins. How can it be possible that we remain separate and our daughters and wives be in the custody of cruel Doctors?[126]

In such circumstances, the "absolute impossibility of fighting both the epidemic and the people" was becoming clear.[127] In a letter to Lord Elgin on April 29, 1898, Sir Antony MacDonnell, lieutenant-governor of the North-Western Provinces, summed up many administrators' fears and reservations. He claimed that "success"—by which he meant "not only the suppression of the disease, but the prevention of the spirit of discontent"—could be attained only by "working through the people themselves." There must, he wrote, be a compromise. The well-to-do, especially the Muslims of the province, would not put up with "constant domiciliary visits, or the forcible removal of their sick to hospitals." A partial abandonment of isolation and segregation might result in the more rapid spread of plague, but "in the present state of public feeling in the country," he saw "the danger of popular discontent and tumult to be a more serious evil than even the prolongation of the disease."

MacDonnell's letter also drew attention to other factors which militated against attempts to implement plague measures in northern India as rigorously as they had been in Bombay and Pune. One was the enormous cost involved, especially now that plague had spread beyond its urban footholds and was moving inexorably into the countryside. Also cause for concern were the opportunities for extortion and harassment created by the extensive use of police and medical subordinates. "This corruption," MacDonnell believed "was perhaps more oppressive to, and more resented by, the people than even the discomforts of isolation and segregation."[128] Distrust of "native agency" was thus not confined to the Indian elite but (as earlier with smallpox vaccination) extended to the state's own Indian subordinates as well.

The Government of India, at first loath to bow to such conciliatory pressures, was increasingly of the same mind and was beginning to be pushed in that direction by some of its own medical advisers. In an influential memorandum written in mid-April, R. Harvey, sanitary commissioner to the Government of India, acknowledged that "experience is beginning to show that, what is medically desirable may be practically impossible, and politically dangerous." Although such measures as segregation and corpse inspection were unassailable in theory, he wrote, in practice government policy had to acknowledge that the mass of the population in India was "suspicious of innovation, extremely conservative, very ignorant, full of prejudices and superstitions and of amazing credulity." To persist with such measures in the face of public opposition was to risk "grave trouble." Like MacDonnell, he urged a more cautious and conciliatory approach. "Compulsion should be abandoned as causing an amount of opposition which alienates the people and leads them to conspire to defeat our efforts." On the other hand, he argued, "every effort should be made to carry the people with us and to induce them to agree spontaneously to the precautions which experience has shown to be useful."[129]

By the middle months of 1898 many medical officers and civil servants were beginning to doubt that medicine and sanitation could provide the answers so confidently anticipated in late 1896 and early

1897. The flushing out of drains and sewers and the wholesale sprinkling of disinfecting powders—activities so energetically pursued by
Snow in the first months of plague in Bombay—had by now been
largely forgotten, while policies more recently followed—such as hospitalization, segregation, and corpse inspection—had either run into
fierce public opposition or themselves proved ineffective in halting
the spread of the disease. Inoculation still held out some prospect of
success. Haffkine, who had developed his own antiplague vaccine in
Bombay, was convinced on the basis of his early trials that mass
inoculation represented "the only measure known to Science up to
now for combating that disease." Its value, he claimed, had been
established "by accurate observations and measured in an unmistak-
able manner."[130] Haffkine had some support among younger members of the IMS, but the Government of India and Harvey, its sanitary commissioner and later surgeon-general, remained skeptical,
arguing that Haffkine's serum had still to be perfected and that inoculation could not adequately replace evacuation and other sanitary
measures.

There were many reasons why Haffkine did not receive a more
sympathetic hearing from the colonial medical establishment—he was
a Russian, a bacteriologist, and a Jew—but (as with his anticholera
vaccine) one influential objection was political rather than medical.
Fears that inoculation would (or had already) become compulsory
provoked rioting in Calcutta in May 1898 and seemed likely to meet a
similarly hostile reception elsewhere. Political pragmatism dictated
that it could only be introduced slowly, on a strictly voluntary basis,
as part of a larger package of medical and sanitary measures. "The
question," insisted Harvey, was "not one of theory, but of practical
administrative experience." It was "idle" "to dream of an alien Government successfully imposing universal inoculation on the people of
India."[131]

As a consequence of the resistance encountered and the resulting
reappraisal of its political priorities and administrative limitations, the
Government of India made a series of compromises and concessions
in its plague policy in 1898–99. Central to these was the recognition
that the use of force was counterproductive, provoking either outright
opposition or forms of evasion that negated sanitary and medical
measures to such an extent as to render them ineffective. The more coercive and unpopular aspects of plague administration—house and

body searches, compulsory segregation and hospitalization, corpse inspection, and the use of troops—were accordingly abandoned or greatly modified. One consequence of this shift away from compulsion was a greater reliance upon measures which the people were willing to take up for themselves and upon agencies (such as the hitherto despised *vaidya*s and *hakim*s) whom they trusted. The temporary evacuation of villages was one method followed with some success because, it was now argued, once plague was in evidence, villagers were themselves willing to move. Another method was the cleansing and disinfecting of houses in ways that conformed to Indians' customary practices rather than Western medical dogmas.[132]

While denying any intention to make inoculation compulsory, doctors and administrators made every effort to persuade people to accept immunization. In Punjab, where plague had begun to take a tight hold on the countryside as well as the towns, many thousands of inoculations were carried out in the early 1900s. In 1902 the declared aim of Sir Charles Rivaz, the incoming lieutenant-governor, was to rely upon inoculation as the main means of containing plague and to immunize at least two-thirds of the population. The campaign seemed to be gaining momentum when in October 1902 at Malkowal in Gujrat district an infected needle caused the death from tetanus of nineteen villagers. Unjustly, as was later proved, Haffkine's method of preparing the serum in his laboratory in Bombay (which had been altered to meet the enormous demands from Punjab) was blamed for the deaths. It was several years before Haffkine could clear his name, but the Malkowal incident not only cast a long shadow over his career but also rendered even more suspect in public and official eyes the policy of inoculation with which he had been so closely identified.[133]

A further important shift in state policy was the greater reliance now placed upon Indian intermediaries and "leading men," something Tilak and his associates in Pune had long demanded. The British belatedly rediscovered the political and administrative utility of "indirect rule" and the value of trying to annex to their own cause the authority which "natural leaders" had over their coreligionists, caste-followers, and dependents. Although the need for consultation had been cited from the very first months of the epidemic, in practice it had been lost sight of, not least in Pune, in the impatience and distaste shown by doctors and bureaucrats alike toward "native agency." Some concessions had been made in Bombay city by Gatacre's plague committee, and the riot of March 1898 was an important stimulus to consultation and greater reliance upon caste and community leaders. Instead of sending out its own search parties, the government chose "persons possessing personal influence over the inhabitants of their sections" of the city to report plague cases and encourage the adoption of approved medical and sanitary measures.[134] A similar policy was followed in other parts of India in 1898, though often only after popular disturbances had jolted administrative responses. In Delhi, for instance, during the February plague scare the administration enlisted the help of Hakim Abdul Majid Khan ("perhaps the most influential man in the city") to reassure his fellow citizens and quell excitement and alarm.[135] The technique was not infallible. Some "leaders" declined to accept the mantle of leadership or, like Abdul Majid Khan, were abused for their collaboration with the British. Others simply lacked the authority the British wished upon them. In Jawalpur, at Kanpur, and among some communities in Bombay, the administration failed to discover anyone with a controlling influence at all.[136]

In general, then, the British had retreated a long way from Rand's energetic deployment of European troops and his disdain for "native agency." Moreover, the change in policy appeared to bring practical results. Even in Pune, which had been further punished by the imposition of a punitive police force following Rand's assassination, the more conciliatory approach was welcomed and for the first time led to genuine cooperation between civic leaders and plague administrators. In September 1897 the local plague regulations were amended so that the British soldier accompanying each search party remained outside while two Indian soldiers went inside houses to look for plague cases under the direction of an Indian volunteer. This might seem a small concession—force, after all, was still much in evidence—but it was hailed by *Kesari* as providing a "fine opportunity" for Pune's political leaders to show that "Natives are as capable of managing these things as Europeans and that they do possess the organizing and administrative tact."[137] The *Mahratta* also praised the new regulations for being consistent with Indian "self-respect." By contrast, it said, the "excesses in the last campaign," which had helped provoke Rand's assassination, had been "entirely due to Native help and sympathy being despised."[138]

In Calcutta, too, substantial concessions to middle-class protest were authorized in August 1898. Members of families that had been inoculated were allowed to remain in their homes even if a case of plague broke out among them; the compulsory segregation of other occupants of a house in which plague occurred was stopped; and residents of spacious houses were allowed to use their upper stories and roofs as "hospitals" whenever, in the health officer's judgment, this could be done without risk of the infection spreading.[139] When plague did return to Calcutta in February–April 1899 it was not met, as before, with compulsion and the threat of hospitalization and inoculation, and the new approach, according to the municipal administration report, "resulted in a great change in the attitude of the people." Unlike the conditions in May 1898, when there had been "great opposition" to plague measures, "practically nothing of the kind was encountered during the second and far more serious epidemic" the following year.[140]

The Indian Plague Commission, appointed by the Government of India at the height of the crisis in 1898, provided in its report two years later scientific approval for this shift from a coercive to a more conciliatory policy, and though resistance rumbled on sporadically for several years, it became axiomatic that force was counterproductive.[141] It had proved impossible, the Plague Advisory Commission agreed in 1908, to stamp out plague "by the means adopted in European countries in dealing with epidemic disease." In consequence, it had been necessary to substitute a policy of "persuasion and assistance" from the people for the "more rigorous measures" at first employed, even though this meant the continuing spread of the disease.[142] In the end, the gradual decline of plague was probably due less to medical and sanitary intervention than to the natural limits set on its spread by a variety of zoological and ecological factors, such as the geographical distribution of certain species of rat fleas and the growing immunity of rats to the plague bacillus.[143]

CONCLUSION

The early plague years constituted a major crisis point in the history of state medicine in nineteenth-century India. This was not so much because of the scale of sickness and mortality caused by the disease, though over the course of the period between 1896 and 1914 this proved considerable. Rather, the crisis was caused primarily by hostile public reaction to the exceptional measures the government had taken in response to its own political and economic imperatives and to the advice given by its medical and sanitary officers. In many cases, the plague measures anticipated the arrival of the epidemic itself and gave rise to a flurry of rumors about their nature and purpose. The scale and violence of public reaction caused the administration to doubt the political wisdom of persisting with such unpopular measures and brought about a dramatic shift in policy, with senior medical advisers supporting the view that only more conciliatory measures were practical, even though the costs in terms of plague deaths would inevitably be great.

But the opening years of the plague epidemic represent a crisis in a wider sense, too—a crisis of confidence in Western medicine and public health generally. In the slow evolution of public health and state medicine in India, the epidemic marked a critical departure from earlier enclavist attitudes and the narrow preoccupation with European and military health. Clearly, the measures taken in 1896–97, first in Bombay and then in towns and cities across India, involved an unprecedented degree of medical and sanitary intervention, unparalleled in the earlier and more tentative campaigns against smallpox and cholera. And though the intensity of public reactions brought about a substantial retreat from the more assertive policies of the early plague years, these initiatives were never entirely reversed. Rather, they paved the way for later, albeit more cautious, measures and a greater commitment to the idea of public health. Sanitary staff in the cities were strengthened; programs of public welfare and health education were initiated; and the government, still in 1896 largely indifferent to bacteriology and parasitology, accepted the need for new research institutes and a corps of specialist medical researchers.[144]

But the immediate effect of the interventionist measures of 1896–1900 was to stir up a great tide of alienation from Western medicine. Vaccination against smallpox, inoculation against cholera, attendance at hospitals and dispensaries—all these quantifiable indices of the "progress" of Western medicine suffered severe reversals from the fear engendered by coercive plague measures. Even the attempt to overcome the kind of public antipathy and suspicion which provoked the attacks on Bombay's Arthur Road Hospital in October 1896 by setting up "caste hospitals," run by local communities and allowing treatment by Ayurvedic or Yunani practitioners, initially failed to elicit much support, so deep was the prevailing suspicion of hospitals and doctors.[145] Popular rumor revealed how far medicine was associated with the coercive and alien aspects of colonial rule: it was identified with torture and death, not with health and healing. And yet this crisis was perhaps a necessary rite of passage for Western medicine in India. It is remarkable how quickly hospital and dispensary numbers returned to, and then steadily outstripped, their former levels.[146] If there was a single moment when Western medicine in India appeared to have turned a corner, to become something more than just colonial medicine, that moment surely came in the aftermath of the first phase of the plague epidemic.

The reasons for this have much to do with middle-class attitudes, a subject discussed more fully in chapter 6, but they also relate to a belated realization on the part of the government and its medical officers that Western medicine had to change its ways if it were to be effective in India. It had to address itself to the needs and the attitudes of the people while also looking to long-term measures rather than to quick fixes. This change of mind was brought about partly by the strength of popular resistance (though the immediate response was to put that down to "native prejudice" and "fatalism") and by the reassertion of political over medical priorities. But no less significant was the failure of medicine itself to provide any ready answers to the complex problems of disease in India.

In November 1911, at a time when the lessons of the plague epidemic were still being digested by the Government of India, Sir Harcourt Butler presided over the first All-India Sanitary Conference. Butler, who as secretary to the Government of the United Provinces had been closely involved with provincial plague policy a few years earlier, reflected the new pragmatism in relation to medicine and sanitation and also the kinds of political considerations which had prevailed for most of the nineteenth century. Quoting in part from a document recently prepared for the government by the surgeon-general, Pardy Lukis, he told his audience that:

> The basis of all sanitary achievement in India must be a knowledge of the people and the conditions under which they live, their prejudices, their ways of life, their social customs, their habits, surroundings and financial means. . . . The ardent spirits who may think that sanitary measures possible and effective in the West must be possible and effective in India will flap their

wings in vain and set back the cause which claims their laudable enthusiasm.

He declared his commitment to "the slow but sure results of education" as the "forerunner of sanitation," but stressed that "we have to deal with the facts as they are today."

> We have to work out our own sanitary salvation. We have to study the epidemiology and endemiology of our own communicable diseases, the so-called "tropical diseases"—plague, malaria, cholera and dysentery—in order that having ascertained the actual sources and modes of conveyance we may determine scientifically the particular methods requisite for their avoidance, prevention and suppression; and that we may apply with precision those methods which it is possible and politic to adopt. And we cannot do this without the assistance and co-operation of Indians themselves.[147]

That Butler placed plague first among the "tropical diseases" to be tackled reflected the importance of the administrative as well as medical experience of the recent epidemic. In his emphasis upon what was "possible and politic," as well as on the importance of Indian cooperation, Butler was both restating old verities and presenting a manifesto for the future course of Western medicine and sanitation in India. Whether that manifesto could be translated into reality remained, of course, quite another matter.

6 Health and Hegemony

This account of disease and medicine in nineteenth-century India has so far been concerned mainly with Western medicine as an imperial artifact, with the introduction and imposition of an alien and state-oriented system of medical thought and practice, and with the contrasts these presented to Indian attitudes and responses. The hegemonic ambitions of Western medicine have at times been referred to, but more often coercion has appeared as the dominant expression of Western medical activity, albeit greatly qualified by the administrators' fear of a political backlash and by state reluctance to invest in Indian health.

Coercion thus finds an appropriate antithesis either in public resistance or self-imposed state abstinence. But is giving prominence to resistance a form of complicity in colonialism, an implicit acceptance of its negative stereotypes of an unchanging, unheeding Oriental society? Certainly, Indian opposition and the contrary strength of indigenous values were repeatedly cited by the colonial bureaucracy and medical establishment to justify caution or inertia, whether this sprang from fear of political unrest, financial constraints, or a simple lack of interest in Indian well-being. But it has been argued here that resistance was important—as an expression of Indian attitudes and a measure of the cultural and political gulf Western medicine revealed, but also as a formative influence on the ways in which Western medical ideology and practice were formed and presented in colonial India. This is not to suggest, however, that Indian attitudes were uniform and unchanging, nor that Western medicine served only to articulate imperial needs and colonial authority. Any account of Western medicine in India before 1914 has also to recognize its hegemonic attributes and ambitions and its value to Indian elites as well as to British rulers.

It would be difficult in a single chapter to do justice to the many and various ways in which aspects of Western medicine came to be accepted and internalized in Indian society. In India's vastness there were inevitably great variations across time, class, and region. But during the nineteenth century, and more especially from 1880 to 1914, health and medicine (as the West conceived them) crossed a cultural threshold in India and became an active ingredient in indigenous rhetoric and social practice. In part this reflected the cumulative effect of state medicine and public health on the major towns and cities. It also showed the growing prestige Western medicine was acquiring and its implication in the evolving concerns and changing outlook of many Indians, especially of the urban, middle classes. Health and medicine were integral to an Indian drive for "improvement" and for a redefinition of "self." They informed attempts to mediate between the demands and conventions of the domestic and the public spheres of life, between indigenous values and a beckoning or threatening colonial order. If they formed part of the perceived benefits of Western civilization and science, they also gave grounds for criticism of British rule and its wanton neglect of the Indian people. The cultural rhetoric and political authority of Western medicine had by 1914 become too powerful for India's elites to ignore. It represented not only an immediate domain of health but also a wider realm of cultural and political hegemony. Terms and images plucked from the colonial language of medicine and disease began to infiltrate the phraseology of Indian self-expression, to become part of the ideological formulation of a new nationalist order.

HEGEMONY

The term *hegemony* is subject to so many different meanings and interpretations that its use here calls for some explanation. In his *Prison Notebooks* in the 1930s, Antonio Gramsci gave a new and challenging meaning to an old concept. He suggested that political leadership could be based upon consent rather than coercion and that such consent might be secured through the diffusion of the world view of the ruling class.[1] There have, however, been differing interpretations of what exactly he meant. Does hegemony arise of its own accord from the prestige and authority of dominant groups, or is it contrived through ruling-class manipulation and indoctrination? Joseph Femia, for instance, contends that hegemony "is attained through the myriad ways in which the institutions of civil society operate to shape, directly or indirectly, the cognitive and affective structures whereby men perceive and evaluate problematic social reality."[2]

But other writers have placed greater stress on the purposive nature of hegemony, seeing in it a calculated enterprise by the ruling (or aspirant ruling) classes to exercise control over subordinate or subaltern groups. In one of the most emphatic statements of this view, Christine Buci-Glucksmann calls hegemony "a strategy for gaining the active consent of the masses" and sees it as being consciously organized in the interests of class domination.[3] But this element of deliberate intent and conscious manipulation seems at odds with Gramsci's own political and philosophical position. At one point in the *Prison Notebooks*, for instance, he describes hegemony as

> the "spontaneous" consent given by the great masses of the
> population to the general direction imposed on social life by the
> dominant fundamental group; this consent is "historically"
> caused by the prestige (and consequent confidence) which the
> dominant group enjoys because of its position and function in
> the world of production.[4]

The prominence given here to "spontaneity" (itself a problematic concept) suggests something voluntary and emulative, though it leaves unexplored the question of the means by which ruling-class prestige is relayed and represented to the masses. Gramsci does not appear here to be presenting hegemony as merely an exercise in self-legitimation. The consent of the subordinate classes is seen to arise naturally, perhaps even unprompted, from the prestige and power of the hegemonic class and its commanding position within the "world of production."

A second issue arising out of the Gramscian concept of hegemony concerns the relationship between force and consent. Some writers have tried to wrench hegemony from the rest of Gramsci's writing and make it an autonomous concept—independent not only of his Marxian understanding of socioeconomic structure but also of the dialectical interplay between hegemony as "consent" and the state as "coercion." Gramsci himself saw the state in terms of "hegemony protected by the armour of coercion" and used the Machiavellian image of the centaur, half-man, half-beast, to characterize the duality of political power and its reliance upon *both* coercion and consent.[5] Where hegemonic "consent" is absent or has worn thin, where there is no agreement as to how society should be organized, coercion becomes more necessary for the survival of the ruling group. But even in this extreme situation, coercion by itself is unlikely to be effective without some degree of hegemony to sustain it, just as hegemony alone could not entirely supplant coercion in the armory of the state and the ruling class.[6] This duality, this paradox, in Gramsci's thought—between manipulation and "spontaneity," between coercion and consent—provides some clue to the labyrinthine ambiguities and contradictions of medicine and public health in colonial India.

British India might appear, on the face of it, to be unpromising territory for the operation of any system of hegemony. Colonial rule in India has often been depicted—not least in nationalist and Marxist historiography—as a coercive domain, founded on conquest, governed by greed, and sustained by the strength of its army and police, its courts and jails. This does not appear to be a society which allowed much room for the gentler arts of persuasion and consent seeking. The cultural, social, and administrative gulf between the British and the mass of the Indian population has often seemed to scholars so vast as to have been unbridgeable. Indeed, one trend in the recent historiography of India has been to deny that colonialism had much capacity to regulate or transform indigenous society and that real power continued to reside with elites, magnates, and intermediaries of various descriptions. British rule appears as a "limited raj"—weak, alien, ill informed, often blunderingly ineffectual—and hence an improbable candidate for Gramscian hegemony.[7]

Even apart from the prominence of coercion, there are undoubtedly other difficulties in applying Gramsci's concept of hegemony (born out of the study of a very different historical process) to India under colonial rule. One of the central motifs in Gramsci's prison writings is the distinction drawn between political society (identified with the state and its coercive agencies) and civil society (represented by trade unions, schools, churches, voluntary associations etc.), which, while not formally part of the state structure, helped to extend the authority of the ruling classes and to socialize the masses into quiescence. But if by civil society in India we were to mean European society, then we are presented with something notoriously introverted, cut off by racial aloofness and even by physical distance from Indians of almost every class. In India the authority and prestige of Western medicine and public health—such as it was—emanated directly from the state and not from white civil society.

There were, of course, some possible exceptions. For instance, medicine was an area in which Christian missionary societies were particularly active. As early as the 1830s, the London Missionary Society in southern India had taken up medical work in the belief that it could "open a wide and effectual door into the hearts and minds of the natives," if only because medical aid was "one of the very few forms of help which the Hindu is at liberty to receive."[8] This evangelizing strategy later gave rise to the zenana missions—the Church of England Zenana Missionary Society began in 1880—and their attempts to bring health and education (as well as Christianity) to the secluded women's quarters of Indian households. But the extent to which missionaries were successful disseminators of Western medical ideas and practices in India remains, for the present, a matter of speculation as it has yet to receive serious scholarly attention.[9]

There has, however, been something of an academic consensus that the impact of Western medicine upon Indians' ideas, life-styles, and experiences was very limited, at least before 1914. On this issue there is a remarkable measure of agreement between the critics of imperialism who assert that the British provided little by way of medical care for the Indian population because they were basically uninterested in the health of their subjects, and the writers more favorably disposed toward the colonial episode who argue that Indian opposition prevented the wider adoption of Western medicine and sanitation. The implication is either that the British made little effort to exercise their hegemony in the sphere of medicine and public health or that, if they had such an objective, they singularly failed to achieve it. Either way, the practical results would appear to be much the same.

When charged with the complaint that they were doing too little for public health in India (an increasingly frequent criticism by the 1890s), colonial officials were wont to argue that the size of the problem was so great and the resources at their disposal so small that it was impossible to make any greater progress. In addressing the Seventh International Sanitary Science Congress in 1891, Surgeon-

Colonel R. Harvey of the IMS (shortly, as sanitary commissioner to the Government of India, to be in the thick of discussions over anti-plague measures) answered the critics of medical policy and performance in India by claiming that the government had "already done a great deal," but faced two major obstacles. One was a lack of money: there was never enough to meet India's enormous health needs and, when it came to a share of state funds, sanitation was often "crowded out in the scramble for Government allotments." But if this could be seen as a mild rebuke of the state's financial priorities, Harvey's second and seemingly more substantial point was the "ignorance, apathy, and prejudice of the native population," who had "for the most part no idea of the benefits of sanitation, nor of the dangers which result from its neglect." "What was good enough for their fathers" was "good enough for them," and whenever any innovation was proposed the cry of "religion in danger" was "invariably raised." Except for patiently trying to educate the Indian public in "modern ideas of sanitation," the state and its servants could do little to overcome this. "A government," concluded Harvey in a phrase that anticipated his position when plague policy went awry seven years later, "and especially an alien government, cannot offend the root-ideas of its subjects."[10]

A willingness to blame Indian indifference or hostility for the shortcomings of public health under British rule was not confined to colonial officials alone. It can also be found, for instance, in Hugh Tinker's account of local self-government in colonial India and Burma first published in the 1950s. To be fair, Tinker is not uncritical of colonial policies and attitudes: he refers on more than one occasion to the inadequate provisions made by the state and condemns the narrow-mindedness and obstructionism of many colonial bureaucrats. But an equal, perhaps even larger, share of responsibility for the relative failure of public health is allotted to the indigenous population. In India, Tinker states, "the public was not much interested in the promotion of public works and sanitation: unfamiliar western methods seemed to be opposed to all the teachings of religion and custom." As a result, "public health services were developed only because officials fostered them. Almost the whole range of municipal services was evolved in response to pressure from British officials rather than as a result of the desires of the people." Elsewhere he speaks in similar terms of the "barrier of custom" insulating "the ordinary Burman or Indian from the aims of the civil engineer or health officer." Here as in much colonial discourse, a stark contrast is repeatedly drawn between West and East, between technology and science on the one hand and religion and custom on the other. "Public feeling was very seldom in accord with the technical and scientific standards of western social services," and there was a "lack of harmony between [Indian] social habits and the techniques of the West."[11] However well-intentioned some British policies might have been, they failed by this account to win much conviction or commitment, to elicit much more than the most inert or involuntary consent.

One can contrast this line of argument with the nationalist and leftist critique of the colonial public health record. We have already seen (in chapter 2) Radhika Ramasubban's argument about the enclavist nature of colonial medicine in nineteenth-century India and the general lack of interest in health needs beyond the army and the white community. To this might be added an earlier view. Writing in the 1930s, and warmly anticipating the day when Indian politicians would assume responsibility for the nation's health, N. Gangulee asserted that British commitment to a policy of noninterference with Indian beliefs and customs had led to a serious neglect of public health, even though individual medical and sanitary officers might have seen it as one of the main duties of an "enlightened government." He found this attitude "not unnatural" in "an alien government" but still chastised the British for failing to use their "prestige and power" to win over Indian opinion to public health.[12] Gangulee did not deny that Indians were often resistant to Western medicine and sanitation (a matter on which Ramasubban is singularly silent) but believed the British had a responsibility nonetheless to educate the public and develop its sanitary awareness—in other words, to take a more active and assertive leadership role.

But these views represent only part of the story, and it is necessary to consider rather more closely how far and in what contexts Western medical ideas and practices had gained acceptance by Indians before 1914. As this is potentially a vast subject, the present discussion is confined to five case studies: hospitals and dispensaries, midwives and women doctors, patronage and leadership, municipal government, and ideas of race and nation.

HOSPITALS AND DISPENSARIES

Hospitals for European soldiers and civilians in Calcutta, Bombay, and Madras date back to the seventeenth and early eighteenth centuries. They were enlarged or rebuilt during the course of the nineteenth century, but generally kept their exclusively colonial character.[13] Sometimes a dispensary was also established for the treatment of the "native poor" or a police hospital erected to accommodate the sick and destitute who flocked into the cities in times of drought and famine. The establishment of medical schools was a further stimulus, creating a demand for teaching hospitals, where the cases of Indian patients could be observed and followed by medical students. But beyond these basic institutions the colonial authorities were reluctant to commit themselves, and it was left to public subscriptions and individual philanthropy to provide a substantial part of the funds for new hospitals and dispensaries.

The fate of Calcutta's proposed Fever Hospital in the 1830s and 1840s was indicative of this generally negative state attitude. Following a proposal made by J. R. Martin, a committee was convened in 1836 to investigate the possibility of establishing a fever hospital for the city. This in turn became part of a wider urban improvement scheme, intended to benefit Indian as well as European inhabitants. For the time it was a rare attempt to extend the bounds of Western medicine, to make it more attractive and accessible to Indians of all castes and communities. After taking evidence from British and Bengali residents, the eight-man committee (which consisted of equal numbers of Indians and Europeans) concluded that Indian "prejudice" against hospitals had been "greatly overrated" and that a fever hospital would be widely welcomed. But a greater obstacle was the attitude of the government itself. Lord Auckland welcomed the scheme but regretted that it should rely so heavily upon state support. He contrasted the situation in India, where the generosity of only a small number of "Native gentlemen" could be relied on, with Britain, where similar projects were "founded, and warmly adopted, and permanently supported by the liberality and under the operation of the humane sympathies of individuals."[14] If financial obstacles were thus seen to be the greatest difficulty, that in turn reflected the government's own lack of commitment. As a result the fever hospital never materialized, and the funds collected, amounting to Rs 52,000 in 1844, were used to build a hospital for the new Medical College.

It was only in the second half of the nineteenth century that the number and distribution of medical institutions began to grow and to serve a wider public purpose. An important factor in this development was the spread of dispensaries rather than hospitals. The relative merits of hospitals and dispensaries had been hotly debated in connection with the Fever Hospital proposal of the 1830s. Lord Auckland was among those who, following the precedents of Britain and Ireland, believed dispensaries the best way of distributing medical assistance as widely and as cheaply as possible. In his view they might ultimately be the principal means of "improving such habits amongst the people as are most injurious to health."[15] By contrast, the city's medical establishment, led by J. R. Martin and Assistant Surgeon Duncan Stewart, forcefully disputed this claim, arguing that dispensaries were effective only in the alleviation of disease and did not assist in its study or cure. They offered few facilities for the close observation and systematic treatment of acute diseases, and so failed to provide the practical training medical students required. They also failed to remove the sick from the environment in which their diseases were contracted and in which they might continue to infect others. The "ablest and most experienced" physicians could not afford the time and energy needed to attend dispensary outpatients. In a hospital, however, patients were concentrated in one place, under a carefully controlled regime, and could be given the best possible attention.[16]

Despite the medical profession's preference for hospitals, dispensaries began to flourish in India, though they hardly began to meet the increasingly evident health needs of the Indian population. In the 1850s the three sprawling presidencies of Madras, Bombay, and Bengal had fewer than ninety dispensaries among them. By 1880 there were some twelve hundred public hospitals and dispensaries in British India under government control, and by 1902 around twice that number, but that still amounted to only one dispensary for every 330 square miles.[17]

There had been dispensaries in the Madras Presidency from early in the century. One of the first was located at Chintadripet in Madras in 1829; a second followed in Black Town in 1837. In 1842 there were only eight dispensaries in the whole presidency, including the two in Madras city: together they treated 13,252 patients, but a mere 212 were inpatients. In 1852, a year in which only 859 European and Indian patients were admitted to the General Hospital in Madras, the city's four main dispensaries saw nearly 42,000 patients. By 1860 there were 46 dispensaries in the province, visited by more than 300,000 patients a year, including 13,000 inpatients.[18] By 1900 the number of dispensaries in the province had risen to 267, and along with the 197 hospitals they treated nearly 4.5 million in- and outpatients during the year. But, partly because the government was unwilling to put more resources into local services, the number of institutions remained small compared to the size of the population and the scale of its needs. In 1900 there was estimated to be only one hospital or dispensary for every 71,428 people in the province. In a relatively wealthy district like Thanjavur, which could afford to support 39 hospitals and dispensaries, mainly from local and municipal funds, this ratio fell to 58,823, and if on average 10,000 people visited each of these institutions every year, this might mean that 1 in every 5 or 6 people had some experience, however fleetingly, of a hospital or dispensary. But in other districts, like poor and famine-prone Cuddapah, with only 19 hospitals and dispensaries, the ratio plummeted to one medical institution for every 111,111 people. It would be easy to conclude from such statistics that the overall pattern of illness and mortality, especially in rural areas, can have been only marginally affected by the presence of medical institutions.[19]

Apart from the slow increase in their number, two further factors impeded the growth of the dispensaries and hospitals. In the early decades, hospitals and dispensaries were visited in disproportionate numbers by the poorer Europeans and Anglo-Indians (including European sailors in the ports). Only with the growth in the number of institutions, particularly in the smaller towns, and with increased Indian attendance, did the proportion of patients coming from these minority communities shrink in significance. In 1855 the dispensaries in the Madras Presidency were attended by 1,577 Europeans and 9,739 Anglo-Indians (equivalent respectively to 0.86 and 5.29 percent of the total number of patients). In 1900 8,215 Europeans and 47,025 Anglo-Indians attended the civil hospitals and dispensaries of the province, but their share of the total had fallen to 0.19 and 1.06 percent respectively. Interestingly, the proportion of Hindus (at around 73 percent) and of Muslims (moving from 15.70 in 1855 to 12.2 in 1900) remained fairly constant over the period.[20]

What these figures do not clearly reveal (except perhaps in the category of "other classes," which amounted to more than half a million patients in 1900) is the extent to which these institutions also attracted disproportionately heavily from the lower sections of Indian society. While the higher classes of Hindus and Muslims had strong religious and social objections to visiting European hospitals and dispensaries, the lower social strata apparently had few such objections or became patients less from choice than from desperation or because the police or their European employers sent them there. In calling for a fever hospital for Calcutta that would both serve as a teaching institution and be attractive to high-caste Hindus, David Hare remarked in the 1830s that the patients currently admitted to the local police hospital consisted "for the most part of wretched objects, pilgrims, beggars, and criminals, the very dregs of society, who seldom claim admission to the establishment until they are reduced to the last extremity either by poverty or sickness."[21] In 1866, a year of dearth, the apothecary in charge of Berhampur dispensary in Ganjam district noted that the inpatients there consisted "almost entirely of the mendicant class and prostitutes; the former seek a home, food, and shelter in the Institution, while the latter come simply to be cured as speedily as possible."[22] In garrison towns such as Secunderabad, Bellary, and Madras, the presence at dispensaries of prostitutes brought in by the police for the treatment of venereal disease was said to offend "poor but respectable females" and discourage them from attending. Other would-be patients were deterred by the visits the police themselves made for treatment.[23]

The extent to which dispensaries became "asylums for the destitute" and places where prostitutes or the European poor went for treatment created a dilemma for the colonial medical establishment. Although it was thought necessary for them to cater, as semicharitable institutions, to the poor and needy, the stigma which resulted from the identification of European medicine with the lowest and most-polluting classes, with the "very dregs of society," was far from welcome. As a result, attempts were made, more often on an ad hoc and local basis than as part of any concerted government strategy, to compromise with high-status communities—by building separate visiting rooms for high-caste patients (for instance, at Palayankottai in the south of Madras Presidency where Brahmin and Sudra patients were kept strictly segregated[24]), by attending to caste requirements with respect to diet, accommodation, and even the choice of acceptable medicines and treatments, and latterly by constructing hospitals and dispensaries expressly for the needs of high-caste and purdah women. In a manner suggestive of this wider process of accommodation, the assistant surgeon in charge of the Chittoor dispensary wrote in 1852 that:

a careful and conciliatory manner is observed to all applicants, and the prejudices of castes as far as may be sedulously observed; brahmins especially when required to be furnished with liquid medicines, are allowed to bring water in their own vessels for its preparation, and I have found all these little concessions duly appreciated.[25]

This type of colonial accommodation of indigenous values (or of what were taken to be indigenous values) was thought to be an important part of the growing acceptability of these institutions. It was another example of the way in which Western medicine in India found it expedient to Orientalize itself in order to gain cultural and social respectability.

The increasing popularity of the hospitals and dispensaries owed at least as much to surgical as strictly medical work. A large part of the work of the Madras dispensaries, for instance, was given over to setting broken bones, excising tumors and cancerous growths, amputating diseased or crushed limbs, removing cataracts, or dealing with other ophthalmic cases. One reason for the apparent success of this side of dispensary and hospital work might have been its relative neglect by indigenous practitioners. Surgery was shunned by Ayurvedic doctors and left to low-caste barbers. In Lal Behari Day's novel, *Bengal Peasant Life*, a local *kaviraj* admits to the "superiority of English to native doctors in surgery," but in his opinion "surgery formed no part of the functions of a medical man." Surgical operations "belonged, properly speaking, to the province of the barber."[26] The prestige and popularity of Western surgery was also remarked upon by W. R. Cornish, the surgeon-general in Madras in 1881. He had "no doubt that the people of India estimate European medical treatment more by what they see of the skill of our surgeons than by any professed faith in the value of our treatment of internal disease." After forty years of dispensaries, the battle for a medical monopoly was, in his view, far from won:

> To this day physicians have to compete with old women and exorcists, and have not yet so demonstrated to the native mind the superiority of their practice, that they can command implicit faith in it. In surgery, however, the native population do admit the advantages and superiority of European methods.[27]

As their reputation grew, dispensaries also treated malaria, rheumatism, respiratory diseases, cholera, dysentery and diarrhea, venereal complaints, ophthalmia, ulcers, skin diseases, and worms. But, in many instances, patients turned to Western medicine and surgery only when the *hakim*s could no longer help them. As the assistant surgeon at Rajahmundry complained in 1852, "the native practitioners are still trusted till disease puts on a severe type."[28] Dispensaries were often left to cope with patients already far advanced in disease or incurably ill. They served as "curers of last resort," not a role they relished or which enabled them to display their skills in a favorable light. "The prejudice of the Natives against the use of English medicines," wrote J. Appavoo, a hospital assistant at Hospet in 1869, was shown by the fact that "almost every case treated in the Dispensary has attended after the Native Hakeem's remedies have failed."[29]

While many Indians might have remained skeptical about the value of Western medicine as practiced in the hospitals and dispensaries, there were apparently few doubts of its imminent or increasing success in the eyes of its own apostles and practitioners. As early, one might say as prematurely, as the 1850s the Madras Medical Board saw evidence not only of the "increasing usefulness" of the dispensaries under its charge but also of the impending triumph of European medicine over its Indian adversaries. "In almost every quarter of the Presidency," wrote A. Lorimer, the board's secretary, in 1854, "the superiority of European over native medicine and surgery is acknowledged, even by the Hakeems." As a result, he enthused, of "well-tested practical observation, not only as to ordinary diseases surgical and medical, but also of some happy cures in desperate cases abandoned as utterly hopeless by the native doctors," the "native mind" had begun to free itself from its "natural prejudice" against European medicine.[30] Three years later, Lorimer was even more ecstatic. Writing in his 1856 report, he remarked that the "onward progress of these institutions must be highly satisfactory to the Government; in their working, truth has prevailed over error to a great degree. . . ." He detected a great change even over ten years earlier, such that "the native community now see and have become thoroughly convinced of the superiority of European medicine over the system of their own hakeems." The speed and reliability of European cures had, he boldly declared, made them "universally acknowledged."[31]

Because of their increasing number, and the professional preference of European doctors for hospital and city postings, dispensaries were one of the few medical arenas where Indians were employed in significant numbers and entrusted with some individual responsibility. They became, in their turn, enthusiastic propagandists for Western medicine, an evangelical role for which many Europeans believed them well suited. S. Jesudasen Pillai, an Indian Christian in charge of the dispensary in Black Town, Madras, worked hard to build up Indian attendance and support. His services, he reported in 1857, had been largely employed by wealthier Hindus,

> and I have found them generally willing to submit to any instructions I gave them which were necessary for their recovery. There are it is true still a good number of families who will not submit to all that is required of them; but these are generally persons who have not kept pace with the times, who from want of an enlightened education have not been able to enfranchise themselves from the yoke of their ancestral customs and prejudices. I endeavour as much as possible to humour their failings, with a view to inducing them eventually to adopt the right course.[32]

The following year Jesudasen Pillai confidently announced that European medical science continued to "gain ground, and to diminish the influence of ignorant hakeems and vitheyams [Hindu practitioners]"; but he regretted that the "peculiar nature of Hindoo etiquette" denied him greater access to Indian women. "[T]he only means available to me for communicating to them a knowledge of physiology and hygiene, are the visits I pay them as their medical adviser, when I endeavour to explain to them the general principles of physiology and how to preserve health." The rest of the population he addressed through a series of public lectures on "popular anatomy, physiology, and hygiene" held at the Madras Young Men's Literary Institute. According to Jesudasen Pillai, these were "well attended by the most respectable members of the native community, and they seem to listen with a lively interest, while they examined the skeletons and diagrams with admiration."[33]

Nor was Jesudasen Pillai an isolated case, even in 1858. In the Triplicane quarter of Madras, with its large Muslim population, Moodeen Shereef was said to be gaining the confidence of his community for Western medicine, while in Cuddapah district another native surgeon, Iyaswamy Pillai, had begun a vernacular class on the "first principles of midwifery" (though this lasted only a year before folding).[34] It is not hard to see in the work of these dispensaries a hegemonic enterprise in which Indians trained in Western medicine were as actively involved as their European colleagues and were arguably more influential.

WOMEN AND MEDICINE

Women's health occupies a special place in the history of Western medicine and colonial hegemony. From a present-day perspective, it is striking how little consideration was given to women's health in colonial India before the 1860s and 1870s, but it is also remarkable how rapidly thereafter it assumed a prominent and emblematic position in debates over the nature and authority of Western medicine.

In the early nineteenth century, in an essentially male-oriented and male-operated system of medicine, women appeared only as adjuncts and appendages to the health of men. The primary arenas of state medicine in the first half of the nineteenth century—the army, the jails, even the hospitals—were primarily male domains in which women played little part. Even when they were present—as prisoners, as soldiers' wives and daughters—their specific needs were largely ignored. Sickness and mortality among the wives of European soldiers were duly noted in the sanitary commissioners' annual reports from the 1860s onward, but with scant comment, and the declining number of British Army wives in India (there were barely three thousand by 1890) strengthened the almost exclusively male orientation of military medicine. Indian soldiers' wives received hardly a mention in the sanitary reports. The one state medical measure before the 1880s which did have a direct bearing on women was the Contagious Diseases Act of 1868, but this was clearly designed to address the problem of venereal disease among British soldiers rather than the health of prostitutes (or soldiers' wives). There appears to have been no serious discussion of venereal disease as it affected women in India before the 1920s. The diseases that preoccupied colonial medicine in the nineteenth century were epidemic diseases, the communicable diseases of the cantonment, civil lines, and plantations, the diseases that threatened European lives, military manpower, and male productive labor.[35]

When women were mentioned in early nineteenth-century medical texts it was either in a gesture of exclusion—remarking how little European doctors knew about the diseases of Indian women because of the physical inaccessibility of females in purdah—or, if they were European women, they were incorporated in the environmentalist paradigm which had such a powerful hold over European conceptions of health and disease at the time. Within this paradigm, women served as markers of the rapid and destructive effects of a tropical climate on European constitutions.

As far back as 1773 John Clark described the effects of India's climate as being that it "relaxes the solids, dissolves the blood, and predisposes to putrefaction." He found these effects most evident among European women, whose "lively bloom and ruddy complexions" were "soon converted into a languid paleness; they become supine and enervated, and suffer many circumstances peculiar to the sex, from mere heat of climate and relaxation of the system."[36] William Twining in the 1830s similarly dwelt upon the greater physical hardships Western women endured in India, numbering among these the problems attending menstruation and childbirth, the frequency of miscarriages, and maternal mortality. The converse of this assumption of European vulnerability was a belief that Indian women were more attuned to their environment. Twining, for instance, thought hysteria rare among Indian women because of "the modified scale of sympathies" between body and climate which saved Indians from many of the complaints which afflicted Europeans.[37]

As the century progressed, there were subtle shifts in European attitudes. There was a declining (though certainly not negligible) sense of European vulnerability, and the seemingly more secure health status of women was one perceptual marker of this. The development of hill stations, well under way by the 1860s, was a form of disease evasion and environmental adaptation thought especially advantageous to women's and children's health. The old language of constitutions and exoticism gradually gave way to a more confident belief in the value of personal hygiene and sanitation. With the growth of the European community in the second half of the century (and the increasing number of white women) Western doctors sought to be reassuring about the prospects for European survival—and safe childbearing—in India. But, significantly, women's health was still not seen to be a state responsibility. It was left to a host of medical manuals and family health guides to inform and instruct—occasionally, as in 1871, with a government prize as an incentive to their publication.[38] Attending white women in labor might have been one of the more common and lucrative parts of a civil surgeon's private practice (and perhaps a reason why they did not welcome the idea of women doctors for India), but it was not seen to be the responsibility of state medicine as such.

However, Indian women were by no means irrelevant to the emerging discourses and evolving practices of colonial medicine. Their very elusiveness was an implicit challenge to the hegemonic ambitions of Western medicine. Moreover, Western medicine could claim little success if it was effectively shunned by half the indigenous population. Equally, women in India—as elsewhere—were taken to represent a society's true nature and worth. As has often been pointed out, this gender agenda was set early in the century by James Mill when he remarked in his *History of British India* that "the condition of women is one of the most remarkable circumstances in the manners of nations. Among rude people, the women are generally degraded; among civilized people they are exalted." He added, in case his reader should be left in any doubt, that "nothing can exceed the habitual contempt which the Hindus entertain for their women."[39] The campaign against *sati*, the suppression of female infanticide, and the later debates over widow remarriage and the age of consent were all powerfully informed by this equation of Indian—more especially Hindu—society with barbaric behavior toward women.

Nor were the women themselves the only focus for this critical attention. Another was the zenana, the women's quarters in Hindu and Muslim households. This, provokingly, was "uncolonized space"—in Western eyes an abode of ignorance and superstition, a place of dirt, darkness, and disease.[40] From the 1860s, Christian missions were established with the aim of penetrating the zenana, using women missionaries to enter where no male outsider would be allowed, and employing education and health as the means of gaining access to the hearts and minds of secluded women. For Western medicine the zenana became a battlefield, increasingly implicated in resistance to Western medicine and a site where disease and ignorance about health and hygiene needed urgently to be defeated—not just for the benefit of the women themselves but also for the health of their children and husbands. As Western medicine and public health crossed the threshold and entered the Hindu home, so "new" diseases, like neonatal tetanus and tuberculosis (seen very much as a zenana disease by the early twentieth century), came to the fore.[41]

One of the most striking examples of the growing attempt to incorporate women into a colonizing medical discourse and practice were moves to replace or reform the traditional Indian midwives, or *dais*. Attention began to be drawn to them from the 1860s and 1870s as European women doctors and missionaries learned more about their crude and often dangerous techniques and as the scale of infant mortality in India began to be recognized. The *dais*' activities were freely labeled "barbaric." Thus, in the course of an appeal for funds to provide medical aid for the women of India in 1890, Lady Dufferin referred to "the condition of those women, who debarred from all skilled medical relief, are subjected to the barbarous practice of ignorant midwives."[42] The journalist Mary Frances Billington, who visited India in the 1890s, wrote in similar vein:

> That infant mortality is very high, is not on account of evil intent, but is due to the appalling ignorance of the *dhais*, . . . whose methods of treatment are simply barbarous, and, indeed, viewed in the light of our scientific knowledge, seem as if they would be enough to kill every unfortunate victim upon whom they practiced.[43]

R. J. Blackham, in his guide to *Indian Home Nursing* published in 1913, stated that

> When the *dai* is sent for to a case, she usually changes even her ordinary working clothes for filthy rags, and the delay is a fortunate thing, as, if she reaches the woman in the first stage of labour, so much the worse for the patient. She makes her run about the room, lift heavy weights, or squat on the mud floor; and if these efforts fail to produce sufficient progress, she places heavy weights on the abdomen, or inserts a vaginal plug of dirty rags. The results of these manoeuvres are often to precipitate delivery, with injury to the child, haemorrhage, and of course, rupture to the perineum.[44]

One colonial response to the horrors perpetrated by the *dais* was, as with the *tikadars* and variolation, to seek to oust the traditional specialists and replace them with "modern" agents and institutions. Women were encouraged to give birth not in their own homes (in darkened rooms and squalid outhouses) but in lying-in or maternity hospitals, like the one opened in Madras in 1844. But, in one of those characteristic inversions which aligned what was most esteemed in Western medicine with what was most impure and degrading in

Hindu society, such practices ran counter to the Hindu perception of birth as a highly polluting state and, indeed, to the seclusion of women practiced by many high-caste Hindu families and by Muslim purdah women. Although the Lying-in Hospital in Madras was open to all, in practice it catered either to low-class Europeans and Anglo-Indians (who occupied a separate ward) or, in greater numbers, to the local "Pariahs," or Untouchables, who showed few apparent objections to it on caste or religious grounds. In 1858, 833 "Pariah" women were admitted to the hospital compared to 87 "East Indians" (Anglo-Indians) and only 19 Hindus and 18 Muslims.[45]

High-caste Hindu and purdah Muslim women shunned the hospital entirely, and the tendency for their hospitals and dispensaries to be seen as "low-caste" institutions, out-of-bounds to the higher castes and communities, was one of the greatest problems confronting European women doctors throughout this period. Even when the Victoria Hospital for Caste and Gosha Women was opened in Madras in 1890 in an attempt to overcome this cultural resistance, it at first attracted very few inpatients because "respectable caste people still look upon a residence in any hospital as a degradation."[46] The general reluctance of women to enter hospitals had not greatly changed by World War I, even among the middle classes. In 1913 some 3,687 births in Madras city took place in hospitals, but this represented less than a fifth of registered births in the city.[47] In rural areas there were hardly any comparable facilities at all, even if women and their families had been willing to use them.

Attempts were also made to recruit a new kind of midwife among women who were not from the same lowly background as the traditional *dais* and who had some education and medical training. But the number and impact of these approved midwives remained small before the 1920s. In Madras in 1913, where Western midwifery had made greater headway than in cities in the north and east of the country, 220 women were known to practice midwifery, but of these only 17 had received formal training. Of the remaining 203, the majority were women from the barber and washerman castes, who, according to the local health officer, "know nothing of the art and practice of midwifery."[48]

In the Madras Presidency, local government boards provided scholarships and subsequent employment for trained midwives. In 1891 there were 208 midwives working under local authorities in the province, but they attended only 11,703 cases—an average of only 56 cases per midwife in a year. In one district, Cuddapah, the 14 midwives saw a mere 387 cases, barely 2 a month. Such was the reported "prejudice" against Western-style midwives that only in extreme and difficult cases were they called in instead of *dai*s from the barber caste.[49] By 1900 the number of midwives attached to hospitals and dispensaries had risen to 321 and the number of cases attended to 25,793, but that still amounted only to just over 80 each per year, scant evidence for the triumph of Western midwifery over the "uneducated and dangerous dhai" that some enthusiasts claimed to be imminent.[50]

An alternative strategy, as with the *tikadar*s of Bengal, was to co-opt the existing specialists and try to convert them to Western ideas and techniques. Rather than ditching the *dai*s, it made practical sense to recognize that they already existed in virtually every Indian village, they were cheap, and they were trusted. However, whereas a strategy of co-option had a fair degree of success with *tikadar*s, it made little headway with *dai*s. They were middle aged or elderly, illiterate, and understandably suspicious of attempts to coach them out of their old ways. A pioneering scheme to retrain *dai*s was begun in Amritsar in Punjab in 1866 by the civil surgeon, Dr. Aitchison. It then passed to a missionary's wife, Mrs. Clark, and Aitchison's successor, Dr. Taylor. In 1886 the project was taken over or revived by Miss Hewlett, a medical missionary of the Church of England Zenana Missionary Society. The involvement of women missionaries in this branch of medical work among women was a further indication that women's health was still not seen as a matter of state concern.[51] Within its modest limits, the Amritsar Dais' School appears to have been fairly successful, but progress was slow and the number of *dai*s willing to come forward for training remained small. Similar attempts, some using the Amritsar school as a model, were made in the following decades, and with the expansion of existing medical schools and the opening of new ones, courses in midwifery were more widely instituted. In 1890, for instance, Lahore Medical College awarded a diploma in midwifery after a two-year course of part-time instruction, while at the medical colleges in Madras and Calcutta about fifty women were taking midwifery classes.[52]

Dissatisfied with these piecemeal endeavors, in 1903 the vicereine, Lady Curzon, established the Victoria Memorial Scholarship Fund to provide training scholarships for *dais*. It was hoped to enable them to "carry on their hereditary calling in harmony with the religious feelings of the people, and gradually to improve their traditional methods, in the light of modern sanitation and medical knowledge."[53] During the first ten years of the fund, 1,395 *dais* underwent training, though across British India as a whole, with a population of more than 100 million women, this amounted to a proverbial drop in the ocean. Moreover, without adequate supervision and inspection of their work after training (an important element in the Amritsar program), there was little to prevent *dais* from reverting to their earlier practices.[54] As long as "traditional" *dais* continued to be employed in preference to Western-trained midwives, they had little incentive to attend schools and acquire diplomas. Moreover, whereas *dais* were expected to perform various menial tasks in return for their modest fee—such as washing soiled clothes, burying the placenta, and attending the mother during the period of ritual pollution—the midwife, conscious of her professional status and perhaps of her caste, would refuse to do such demeaning work.[55]

WOMEN DOCTORS FOR INDIA

A series of separate initiatives was launched in the 1870s and 1880s to provide women doctors for India. One of the earliest of these came from Mary Scharlieb, the wife of an English barrister in Madras. Reacting to what she learned of the *dais* and their methods, she had herself trained as a midwife but, feeling that this was not enough, persuaded the provincial surgeon-general, Dr. Edward Balfour, to allow her to attend classes at the Madras Medical College in 1875. Perhaps not surprisingly, Scharlieb ran into considerable opposition from a skeptical and resentful male medical establishment in India. The *Indian Medical Gazette*, the unofficial voice of the IMS, did not disguise its strong views on the matter. It claimed, first, that there was no proven demand for women doctors in India and, second, that while women were "physically, mentally and morally fitted for the profession of nursing," they were quite unsuited to the demands and skills required of doctors. As far as the *Gazette* was concerned, opening medical education in India to women was a dangerous and wholly unwarranted experiment.[56] Nonetheless, Mary Scharlieb succeeded in qualifying and, after further medical training in England, ran a successful medical practice in Madras for five years before ill health forced her to return to England.[57]

In 1881 the maharani of Panna sent a message to Queen Victoria, through a missionary doctor, Elizabeth Bielby, asking that more be done to provide medical help for Indian women. Dr. Frances Hoggan (one of the first British women to qualify as a doctor) followed up this plea by proposing that a medical department be set up in India run exclusively by and for women. She argued that the IMS had failed to provide the medical services needed by India's women and that only women doctors could overcome their objections to being examined and treated by male surgeons and physicians. In her view, the "shrinking" of women patients from male doctors was not a "prejudice" to be disregarded; it was a "natural" attitude which "religion and custom alike consecrate." It was the "right of Indian women" to expect this sentiment to be "respected and not outraged."[58]

Hoggan's plea drew no public response from the IMS, but it made such an impression on George A. Kittredge, an American business-man in Bombay, that he began to raise funds among his Indian ac-quaintances to bring two or three trained female physicians from Europe or North America. Kittredge believed "that to be successful in this country, women must be recognized as the equals of men in the medical care of their own sex. This recognition could never be gained by those who had taken a partial medical course and an inferior degree at an Indian University."[59] Like most of his contem-poraries, Kittredge thought of women doctors as uniquely suited for the "medical care of their own sex," but not for medical work in gen-eral. In this respect there was a broad compatibility—one might say complicity—between the professional roles allowed to Western women in India and the restrictions imposed by female segregation and purdah. It was possible for women doctors to "colonize" this social and professional space precisely because it was largely inacces-sible to male physicians, and though the latter were (as the editorials in the *Indian Medical Gazette* attest) initially hostile to the develop-ment, there seems to have been a more ready acceptance than in Britain at the time that women had a distinctive role to perform.

With help from Sorabji Shapurji Bengali, a wealthy Parsi, Kit-tredge was able to collect Rs 40,000 in two months, and the initiative gained further momentum when another Parsi, Pestonji Hormusji

Kama, offered Rs 150,000 to establish a hospital for women and children—provided the government made available a site for the building and met maintenance costs and salaries. At first the Bombay government was reluctant to give its financial support and opposed the idea of allowing women to run a hospital without male "instruction and guidance."[60] But in 1883 Kittredge persuaded Dr. Edith Pechey to come from England to Bombay as the new hospital's senior medical officer, and she was joined in 1884 by an assistant, Charlotte Ellaby. Pechey was one of the five women, led by Sophia Jex-Blake, who went to Edinburgh University to study medicine in 1869, only to run into a wall of male abuse, obstruction, and prejudice. Ultimately, Pechey obtained her M.D. degree from a Swiss university in 1877. Although she had not previously been to India, she presumably saw it as a chance to escape from the hostility she and other women doctors continued to encounter in Britain and to show that women had the ability to run a major hospital.[61]

By the time the Kama (or Cama) Hospital opened in August 1886, Kittredge and his associates had scored a further victory in their campaign to provide female doctors for India: Grant Medical College opened its doors to women, and this set a precedent for women's medical education elsewhere in India. Having thus achieved much of what it had initially set out to do, the Medical Women for India Fund was dissolved in 1889. By 1908 the hospital had a hundred beds and treated two thousand inpatients and eight thousand outpatients a year. The brief career of the Bombay Fund was a demonstration of how much (but also how little) could be achieved through private action and with minimal official support. As Kittredge commented, the Bombay government had shown "as little faith in the abilities or capabilities of medical women as could be found anywhere. India would have waited many years for women doctors, had she depended on Government."[62]

The state's own initiative, when it eventually came, was characteristically half-hearted. On hearing of the medical needs of Indian women (from Mary Scharlieb and others), Queen Victoria urged the new vicereine, Lady Dufferin, to do what she could to promote medical aid for India's women. A fund was duly established in 1885, commonly called the Dufferin Fund but formally known as the National Association for Supplying Female Medical Aid to the

Women of India. Its main objectives were to provide medical instruction, including teaching and training in India, for women as doctors, hospital assistants, nurses, and midwives; to organize medical relief for women and children, including the establishment of hospitals, dispensaries, and wards under female superintendence; and to supply trained female nurses and midwives.[63]

In recent years the Dufferin Fund has been either eulogized or derided. It has, for instance, been described as "a lucid example of British paternalism in India" and cited as evidence of the general failure of "imperial reform initiatives" in women's health before the 1920s.[64] But it would be foolish to ignore the considerable impact the fund had on women's health and medical education, just as it would be reckless not to see its practical limitations and its political significance within an expanding colonial order. The increase in the number of women (and, with them, of children as well) attending hospitals and dispensaries in the first years of the fund represented a significant widening of the bounds of Western medicine, often through the creation of hospitals and dispensaries solely for women and children.

In the Madras Presidency, the number of women attending hospitals and dispensaries virtually doubled in ten years—rising from 374,439 in 1883 to 710,493 in 1893. In Bengal there was an even greater increase in women patients from 180,072 in 1888 to 517,858 in 1899. By 1907 more than 2 million women a year were being treated at institutions wholly financed or partly funded by the Dufferin committees.[65] It was thus no idle boast for the joint secretary of the fund's Central Committee to say in 1907 that "all credit" was due to the Dufferin doctors "for popularizing Western medical science among the female population of this land."[66]

Nonetheless, it is necessary to look critically at the nature and significance of the Dufferin Fund. The history of the fund reveals deep contradictions in state attitudes toward women's health. At the level of imperial rhetoric, the work of the Dufferin Fund was proudly acclaimed for bringing the benefits of Western civilization to Indian women and, as Lord Curzon put it in 1899, lifting the veil of purdah "without irreverence."[67] An earlier viceroy, Lord Lansdowne, speaking at Agra in November 1890, described the work of the fund as one of the most important "experiments" to have been attempted by the British in India. He continued:

we have to overcome the dislike of going to hospitals, the old aversion to Western medical and surgical methods and all the prejudices which, till now, have caused this particular branch of the medical profession to be degrading and to be relegated to persons of the lowest caste.[68]

And yet, for all the viceregal rhetoric, it is indicative of the secondary importance that was actually attached to medical work for women that it was left to wives of viceroys and governors, that the Dufferin Fund operated through a series of volunteer branch committees with only a weak central structure, rather than being taken up as official business. The government offered its goodwill but would not take up the work itself. It believed that if it did so private subscriptions would dry up, the burden of administration would fall upon its already overworked officials, and it would be obliged to carry the additional burden of pay and pensions for women doctors. And yet without that commitment, the activities of the Dufferin Fund were difficult to sustain and unable to command wide public support. As Lord Wenlock, governor of Madras, told a branch meeting in December 1895, the Government of India had always made clear that while providing "general medical aid," it would keep itself "studiously. . . aloof" from schemes designed to give "special benefit for any particular class." However, as the governor also told a meeting earlier in the year, because the Dufferin Fund was not an official body, it could not always count on the support of officials, and "Unless we have officials supporting us as we ought to be supported, it is almost impossible to do any good work."[69]

Moreover, the Dufferin Fund faced the same dilemmas as Kittredge's fund had earlier in Bombay. Was it better to invite qualified women from Britain and elsewhere to work in India or to promote the medical education of women within India? In the short term, the Dufferin Fund's Central Committee saw no alternative but to pursue the first course. The progress which had recently been made in women's medical education in Britain and North America made it possible to recruit women doctors abroad without having to wait several years for India to produce its own. But their availability had its price. They could only be persuaded to come to India if suitable pay and living quarters were provided for them: this was a heavy strain on the fund's limited resources (amounting to an income of only about Rs 30,000 a year by 1910) and meant that it was unable to employ as many women as it would have liked. On the other hand, it was even more difficult for women than men to set themselves up as independent medical practitioners. Women's medicine thus remained particularly dependent upon the employment opportunities created by the state or its underfunded surrogate, the Dufferin Fund. In addition to the lack of promotion prospects and the distrust and condescension they encountered from male colleagues, the female practitioners found working eleven months of the year in an Indian city to be "a severe trial to the health of most English women." Many left India because of ill health or found more conducive, or more remunerative, employment elsewhere.[70] Some provincial committees, however, followed a different course. The Madras branch, for instance, believed it better to invest in the training of Indian women and to build up confidence among women patients through dispensaries than to spend meager resources on appointing foreign women to expensive hospital posts.[71]

Again, although Hoggan and others claimed that women doctors were naturally best suited to practice among members of their own sex, this gender-before-race argument ignored the fervent politicization of women's bodies in late nineteenth-century India. In an age of Hindu revivalism and nationalist self-assertion, debate over such issues as the Age of Consent Bill of 1891 (which aimed to raise the permissible age of sexual intercourse within marriage from ten to twelve) brought the "women's question" firmly within the domain of Indian, especially Indian male, political discourse.[72] European women doctors were walking into a minefield. Some, like Edith Pechey in Bombay, took a defiant position, lecturing the Hindus of Bombay in 1890 on the evils of child marriage, a practice, she warned them, "so barbarous in its immediate effects and so disastrous to you as a race in its remoter action that it should at once be put a stop to."[73] Others, more unwittingly, became a target for accusations of racial arrogance and cultural ignorance; some were suspected of being undercover agents for the evangelizing work of the Zenana Missions (indeed, the Dufferin Fund found it difficult to distance itself from the activities of missionary women doctors).

It did not help that newly arrived women doctors rarely had any knowledge of the "languages, customs and habits" of the people among whom they were to work, and it was not until 1890 that the Central Committee of the Dufferin Fund recognized the importance of doctors' knowing enough of a local language to be able to communicate directly with their patients rather than through interpreters.[74] Hindu newspapers in Bengal in the 1890s launched a sustained attack on the Dufferin Fund and white women doctors, denouncing zenana hospitals as an insult to the Indian traditions of childbearing and dismissing the doctors themselves as "half-educated good-for-nothings."[75] How far the sentiments voiced by male newspaper editors reflected the attitudes of women themselves is more difficult to assess, but in a society where men controlled women's access to health care, male hostility had obvious implications.

The plague epidemic of the 1890s and early 1900s was in this, as in many other respects, a critical episode. The unprecedented nature and extent of state medical and sanitary intervention led to Indian demands that women doctors be appointed for such sensitive tasks as the physical examination of female rail passengers and the inspection of zenana quarters. As we saw in chapter 5, many of the riots and violent clashes which occurred in Indian towns and cities during the early plague years—in Bombay in 1896 and 1898, in Kanpur in 1900—revolved around the forcible dispatch of women to plague hospitals or segregation camps. But even when the state responded to these demands (often inadequately because of the paucity of women doctors and nurses), there were fresh complaints that Western women behaved arrogantly or did not understand Indian ways, being ignorant, for example, of the ritual impurity attached to menstruating women.[76]

In Calcutta, it was clear from the start that men of the *bhadralok* ("respectable" middle class) would not allow their women to be carted off to hospitals, and here the government agreed to a compromise whereby the spacious houses and compounds of the well-to-do were officially regarded as hospitals where the sick and suspect could be segregated and nursed without being sent elsewhere.[77] This avoided further conflict, but it also illustrated the way in which women's bodies might form the centerpiece for men's resistance to intrusive state medicine and, indeed, to colonial authority in general.

The recruitment of Indian women also presented problems for the Dufferin Fund. Women medical students had to battle against opposition from family and friends, against the low-caste and polluting associations of the medical profession, and the problems of finding suitable accommodations and transportation in unfamiliar cities. The difficulty of attracting and keeping high-status, especially Brahmin, women as medical students was frequently remarked upon in the reports of the Dufferin committees. In fact, the first medical graduates from Bombay, Calcutta, and Madras were an eclectic mixture of castes and communities, including Indian Christians, Anglo-Indians, Jews, and Parsis. Only gradually did medicine become a "respectable" profession for women.[78]

By 1910 the Dufferin Fund was in deep crisis. In some respects, it had proved highly successful, with 13 provincial branches, 140 local committees, 160 hospitals, wards, and dispensaries to its credit. But the very progress made by the movement had drawn attention to needs the fund was financially and administratively incapable of satisfying, and this problem was exacerbated by the discontent caused by the poor pay and uncertain prospects of its doctors. In 1908 the Central Committee asked the Government of India to help with an annual grant of Rs 50,000. The secretary of state for India declined to meet the request, though he did agree to give an amount that matched the fund's recent income from donations and subscriptions. These, however, had already sunk to such a low ebb that the amount of assistance offered was too small to meet the fund's basic needs.[79]

Meanwhile, the struggle was resumed for a women's medical service on an equal footing with the IMS. Soon after her arrival in Bombay in 1885, Edith Pechey revived Frances Hoggan's proposal for a separate medical department to provide women surgeons and physicians for India's hospitals and dispensaries. But the government of Lord Dufferin, while professing to have the "greatest sympathy" for the movement for women doctors with which his wife's name was so closely identified, refused to admit women even as uncovenanted members of the IMS.[80] In 1911 Dr. Mary Scharlieb and other medical women in London again proposed a Women's Medical Service for India. They asked for the state to provide a women's hospital for every district with a woman doctor in charge, with status and pay equal to that of male civil surgeons. They called for a two-tier service, run like the IMS, with inferior and superior grades, headed by a woman deputy inspector-general responsible to the Government of India for the internal management of the service.

After lengthy deliberation, in 1913 the proposal for a state-run Women's Medical Service was rejected, but the government agreed to sanction Rs 150,000 for the Dufferin Fund to set up and administer a service of its own.[81] The new service was inaugurated in January 1914 and by 1928 had a staff of 41 women doctors. At that date there were in all about 400 qualified women doctors in India. In addition to 57 in the Women's Medical Service and its junior branch, there were about 90 attached to the provincial and local governments, 150 with missionary societies, and about 100 in private practice.[82] The colonial reluctance to see women's health as a state responsibility endured well into the twentieth century.

But the training of midwives and the appointment of women doctors was only one of the ways in which changes in Indian attitudes and practices came about. Meredith Borthwick's study of the *bhadramahila* (women of the *bhadralok* class) of Bengal between 1849 and 1905 reveals an additional process at work. This was a drive for self-improvement among middle-class households, beginning, often enough, with male householders concerned at the death of their infant children or anxious that their sisters, wives, and daughters should reflect their own appetite for Western education and science. From mid-century a new genre of family medical guides and marriage manuals appeared, generally written in Bengali and sometimes directed toward women themselves. Commenting on the production of books on child care in particular, Borthwick remarks that their publication and use reflected "a desire on the part of educated Bengalis to benefit from modern scientific knowledge, and a growing humanitarian concern for the welfare of mother and child."[83] Partly because of the high fees they charged and the cultural and social barriers involved, European doctors, whether male or female, were only occasionally resorted to, and hospitals (as the plague epidemic of the 1890s forcefully demonstrated) continued to be shunned. Moreover, Western medicine did not acquire an exclusive monopoly even in educated households but had to compete with homeopathy and an Ayurvedic revival. This was one illustration of the way in which Western medicine was gradually gaining a wider influence, but not necessarily on its own "colonizing" terms.

PATRONAGE AND LEADERSHIP

It would be all too easy to assume that the initiatives behind medicine and public health came almost entirely from the British side and (as the colonial literature repeatedly suggests) that Indians were merely unenthusiastic recipients or outright resisters. While it is certainly important to recognize the extent to which Western medicine in India relied upon state action for its propagation and to take into account the influence of Indian resistance on its development, it is also necessary to appreciate the role of Indian leadership and indigenous strategies of accommodation and appropriation in this process. One largely neglected aspect of this wider process is the role of Indian patronage.

Medical patronage and philanthropy in India took many forms and sprang from a variety of motives. One of these, which placed philanthropy clearly within the colonial field of force, was the kind of benefaction that resulted directly from interaction with the British, often as a result of pressure from the colonial authorities. The British looked to the leaders of Indian society, as they saw them, to take up colonialism's hegemonic project. Part of the inspiration for this lay in Britain's own social history in which private philanthropy and public charity had played a major part in the founding of hospitals, dispensaries, and medical schools. The great wealth of India's merchant classes and ruling chiefs made them—in British eyes—obvious candidates for a similar role. But there were other motives, too. As we have repeatedly seen, the colonial power took a narrow view of its own responsibility for the health and welfare of the bulk of the Indian population and, until well into the second half of the nineteenth century, tried to restrict its financial and administrative commitments to those areas of immediate concern or inescapable involvement—like the army and the jails. It was therefore expected that Indians should bear at least part of the cost of their own medical provision, and individual philanthropists were pressed to fund the establishment of hospitals and dispensaries.

The dispensary system in Bengal began in this way in the early nineteenth century, with the government asking local donors and subscribers to contribute to the basic expenses while it provided the medical staff and help with the cost of medical drugs.[84] A similar procedure was followed in Madras. In 1861 the provincial government resolved to cut back on its own expenditure on dispensaries (amounting by that date to more than Rs 200,000 a year) by encouraging wealthy Indians and other local inhabitants to take up part of their operating costs. Donations were soon forthcoming from zamindars, merchants, and Indian government servants (the latter, one suspects, under official duress). By 1865 roughly a quarter of the costs of dispensaries in the Madras Presidency were met by subscriptions, and by the 1890s the share directly contributed by the government had fallen to below ten percent.[85] In the relatively wealthy district of Thanjavur between 1857 and 1880 private subscriptions from landlords, merchants, and members of the former Maratha ruling house helped fund two municipal hospitals, a medical school, and three dispensaries.[86] Substantial though these contributions were, they seldom matched colonial expectations. On the contrary, there were frequent complaints that promised donations never materialized, or that, with characteristic cultural perversity, Indians gave more money for the care of sick animals than for needy humans.[87]

Farming out responsibility for medical patronage and funding had its place, too, on the political agenda. In India's hierarchical society, where tradition and community were presumed all-powerful, it was seen to be advantageous to the promotion of Western medical science if Indian leaders and notables could be associated with this most public project, who, by their participation, would dilute the more obviously alien and coercive aspects of colonial medicine and public health. At this point, however, the colonial project was often taken over—one might say hijacked—by Indians, particularly the new urban elites, and made part of indigenous networks of patronage and authority. One influential factor here, which owed nothing directly to colonialism, was India's strong cultural tradition of philanthropy and charitable works: from feeding and giving alms to the poor to building rest houses for pilgrims and travelers. It was not surprising that these traditions of charity and religious duty continued and found fresh outlets under colonial rule.

But medical philanthropy was also part of a strategy of accommodation. It was a means of buying influence, prestige, even political recognition, from the colonial regime. Individuals advanced their personal standing with the British by giving money to hospitals or the Dufferin Fund. The reward might be a personal message of thanks from Queen Victoria, the award of a title or some other honor in the state's gift, or simply the good offices of the local Collector or Resident. Medical patronage might serve as a public celebration of an individual's successful association with the ruling power, as when Sir Dinshaw Manekji Petit of Bombay decided to set up a scholarship for women students at Grant Medical College on the occasion of his knighthood in 1889.[88] Although many of the patrons of the Dufferin

Fund were men (an example of the way in which the cause of women's health and education might serve patriarchal power), it also provided a rare opportunity for maharanis and begums to help strengthen the princely alliance with colonial rule. The enthusiasm with which the Dufferin Fund was initially taken up by the princes and zamindars of India partly reflected the knowledge that it was a cause close to the queen-empress's heart—and might be correspondingly rewarded. But, in addition, it came at a time when the British, eager to consolidate their position in post-Mutiny India, were seeking a closer association with India's old ruling and landed elites: the Dufferin Fund, like the durbars, was part of this declaration of mutual support.[89] In practice, though, such heavy reliance upon princes and zamindars proved a poor long-term strategy, alienating or ignoring middle-class sentiment and providing an inadequate financial basis for the development of health services for women.[90]

Acts of philanthropy often served an immediate and personal purpose in helping to perpetuate the memory of the donor and his or her family, but they also strengthened community ties or enhanced the prestige and reputation of an individual within the community. While many hospitals and dispensaries were intended for the benefit of the population as a whole or for the "native poor," it was not uncommon for special provision to be made for the patron's own community. In the Jamshedji Jijibhai and Kama hospitals in Bombay, for example, a ward or wing was set aside for the exclusive use of Parsis. Medical scholarships and prizes were not infrequently stated to be primarily or exclusively for members of the donor's community.[91]

For the Parsis of Bombay, medical philanthropy had a particular value. As a numerically small community, initially very dependent upon British favor and overseas trading connections, the Parsis found that funding hospitals and dispensaries was a way of cementing a close and mutually beneficial relationship with the ruling power. It was no accident that Sir Jamshedji Jijibhai, a major beneficiary of Bombay's China trade and the first Indian to be knighted, should have responded to requests from the East India Company to help fund the hospital that came to bear his name and for which he gave Rs 164,000 in 1843. The hospital's cornerstone duly recorded the donor's "unmingled respect for the just and paternal British Government in India."[92]

His example was quickly followed by others. The Sir Kavasji

Jehangir Ophthalmic Hospital opened in 1866 with nearly Rs 100,000 given by Sir Kavasji Jehangir Readymoney, who later also gave half of the Rs 60,000 needed for a new hospital building. In 1874 the Jehangir Nasarvanji Wadia Dispensary was formally recognized at Mahim, and in 1885 the Nasarvanji Petit Charitable Dispensary was opened. As we have seen, a donation of Rs 164,300 by Pestanji Hormasji Kama made possible the Kama Hospital for Women and Children, which opened in 1886. In 1890 Bomanji Edalji Albless gave the money for an obstetric hospital which bore his name, and the following year another Parsi magnate, Framji Dinsha Petit, gave the money for a medical research laboratory attached to Grant Medical College.[93]

The value of this association with Western medicine was evident in other fields, too. Although Parsis had originally been lukewarm toward smallpox vaccination, by the 1860s and 1870s they were among the citizens of Bombay most favorably disposed toward it. Parsi philanthropy had a role here, too: donations from Sir Kavasji Jehangir in 1869–70 helped Bombay to pioneer the development of bovine lymph in India.[94] When plague struck the city in 1896–97 Parsis were among those who sought to evade the government's sanitary measures, but Parsi patrons were also prominent on the committee set up in December 1896 to inspire public confidence in antiplague measures. Parsis set up their own plague hospital, and of the first eight thousand residents of Bombay to be inoculated against plague with Haffkine's serum, forty percent were Parsis. Leadership as much as life-style may help to explain why Parsis suffered relatively lightly from the plague epidemic.[95]

The example of the Parsis stimulated Bombay's Hindus and Muslims to a kind of competitive civic philanthropy, which representatives of the state, like the governor, Sir Bartle Frere, in the 1860s assiduously encouraged.[96] Acts of Hindu philanthropy included the Gokuldas Tejpal Native General Hospital (opened in 1865 with a donation of Rs 150,000 from its patron) and several smaller establishments like the Dwarkadas Lallubhai Dispensary for women and children.[97] Among Muslims, the Aga Khan, head of the Ismaili community, contributed to the fund for a new leper asylum in the 1890s and urged his followers to carry out the government's plague measures and take up inoculation against the disease.[98]

Encouraged by community leadership and by the resulting proliferation of medical institutions, Western medicine became more familiar and accessible to the people of Bombay. Between 1880 and 1908 the number of hospitals in the city rose from five to nine, and the number of dispensaries reached twenty. In this period, the number of beds in hospitals and dispensaries went up from 764 to 1,883 (still a tiny figure for a city of 850,000); the number of outpatients rose from 61,280 to 162,410, and inpatients from 9,522 to 18,906.[99] This growth occurred despite the plague epidemic of the late 1890s and the deep public suspicion of hospitals it aroused. Perhaps it was partly because the popularization of Western medicine through indigenous patronage and leadership appeared to be advancing so rapidly and successfully in Bombay that the authorities were so shocked and surprised by the violent dissent against their antiplague measures in 1896–98.

If the work of Parsi and other patrons and philanthropists seemed both to serve their own interests and to further the spread of Western medicine and public health in a manner the British approved and encouraged, there was less apparent compatibility between colonial intent and the kind of assertive Indian leadership that was emerging in the late nineteenth and early twentieth centuries. As has already been shown in chapter 5, the plague epidemic marked an important stage in the growing indigenous challenge to Western medicine and attempts to assert the right of Indians to be leaders rather than colonial errand boys and interpreters. For Tilak, in particular, the medical and sanitary issues involved in the plague epidemic were secondary to the question of leadership.[100] In an editorial in the *Mahratta* in April 1897 entitled "Do the Educated Lead the People?" he roundly condemned those members of Pune's elite who, for all their professed patriotism, had fled the city at the first sign of plague. It was, he insisted, their duty to help the poor—the main victims of the disease—by securing for them adequate medical attention and educating them out of their worst "prejudices" and "superstitions" about plague and the medical and sanitary measures being used against it. It was also the responsibility of the educated classes to protect the "common people" from the excesses of state action and, through their intercession, force it to recognize the people's legitimate needs and just apprehensions. The colonial state had to be made to see that, as an alien regime, it could not hope to exert direct authority (except by force) over the mass of the people. To be effective, British medical and sanitary intervention must first acknowledge the authority of India's own leaders and then work through their guidance and mediation.[101]

Popular resistance against the antiplague measures thus provided a critical site for intervention by the nationalist middle classes and enabled them to assert a rival leadership of their own over the subaltern classes. And yet, paradoxically, there still existed a degree of compatibility between the respective positions of the colonial state and the aspirant Indian elites. Because of the political conflict generated by the plague episode, the British were forced to accept the claims of the middle classes to more privileged treatment, as the adjustments made to house inspections and other aspects of plague policy in Pune in late 1897 indicated.[102] Conversely, in claiming to speak for the interests and physical well-being of the masses, for the body (both literally and metaphorically) of the people, the middle classes were announcing their own hegemonic intentions. But there was a powerful contradiction in this bid for ascendency. While condemning British rule as alien and remote from the masses, the "leaders" also displayed their own contempt for the ignorant masses and a real fear of the violent propensities of "the mob."[103] Although they were willing to use subaltern protest to wrest concessions from the British, the middle classes were also ready to modify or abandon their protests once their own objectives had been secured. Leadership had its limits.

MUNICIPAL ARENAS

Health and sanitation were among the principal responsibilities entrusted to India's fledgling local government boards in the late nineteenth century. "The most important duty of the Municipality is to look after the public health," declared Chhotalal Ranchhodlal in December 1883 shortly after becoming Ahmadabad's first nonofficial municipal chairman.[104] Sanitation, observes Hugh Tinker, was the "basic function of municipal government"; in Veena Talwar Oldenberg's view, it was its "raison d'être."[105] Conservancy, the provision of piped clean water, sewerage, and drainage, the maintenance of hospitals and dispensaries, vaccination, the regulation of markets, slaughterhouses, burning *ghat*s, and burial grounds—all these were among the basic tasks of Indian urban government, whether it was Ahmadabad or Allahabad, Lucknow or Calcutta.[106]

The municipalization of public health owed much to precedents in

Britain, for there local authorities were given a large share of responsibility for the health of the rapidly expanding urban population. In India the trend was encouraged by the fact that the cities were the main centers of European residence. One of the unwritten assumptions about municipal government was that it existed to protect Europeans' health and to provide the kinds of civic facilities (from filtered water to metaled roads) they demanded. In this way, in a divided city like Allahabad, the requirements of the civil station, where the Europeans lived, almost invariably took priority over those of the more populous and needy "native town."[107]

Concern for European health was one factor contributing to a strictly functional view of municipal affairs. Municipal committees and corporations could be judged by their efficiency, or lack of it, in supplying potable water and keeping the streets clean. But the Liberal viceroy Lord Ripon, in his resolution on local self-government in May 1882 posited a second possibility: that municipalities should serve as academies for the education of the ablest and most intelligent Indians, fostering a "responsible spirit" among them and giving them the opportunity to contribute to the running of their own towns and cities, even though this might mean some temporary decline in efficiency.[108] At one level, such devolution was attractive to colonial bureaucrats, as it shifted part of the burden of government—including levying unpopular local taxes—onto Indian shoulders. Perhaps, too, it was a reflection of the bureaucrats' basic unconcern for Indian well-being that such a large measure of responsibility for urban health and sanitation was thus transferred to underfunded municipalities. This effectively downgraded public health, and the plight of the municipalities was made worse by their lack of trained staff and sanitary expertise and by the need to go cap in hand to the provincial government for grants and loans to pay for major health and sanitation schemes.

The inadequacy of this system was often remarked upon. One of its most trenchant critics was W. J. Simpson, health officer for Calcutta in the 1890s and something of a rarity in not being a member of the IMS. In December 1895 he declared the urgent need for a "sanitary service" for India. At present, he explained, responsibility for urban sanitation rested with municipal councilors who were "wholly unacquainted with the principles or practice of preventive medicine." Civil surgeons were expected to act as their sanitary advisers, but they had no authority to enforce their recommendations or see them carried out. The effect of delegating power in sanitary matters to local authorities, without at the same time devising "an efficient and strong local and central agency to guide and control these authorities," was, in Simpson's view, to bring discredit on local self-government while seriously impeding much-needed sanitary reform.[109]

Barely a year after Simpson's article appeared, the plague epidemic broke upon India and found its municipalities ill prepared for such a momentous crisis. Criticism of local government grew sharply, while the increased demands on urban health and sanitary services threw many municipal authorities into debt and disarray. As the liberal nationalist G. K. Gokhale argued in 1905, at the height of the plague crisis, a system of municipal government which suited the wealthy cities of the West had proved far from appropriate for the needs of urban India.[110] Moreover, as was pointed out in the previous chapter in connection with Pune municipality, the colonial bureaucracy was resentful of the powers that had been taken away from it by Ripon's local government reforms. It seized the opportunity plague provided to denigrate Indian administration in the municipalities and to claw back some of the control reluctantly surrendered in the 1880s. By the early years of the twentieth century, the plague-driven "efficiency" argument again took precedent over Ripon's educational "experiment."[111]

The bureaucracy did not have everything its own way, but it was sufficiently powerful to thwart Indian attempts to reform municipal health. Across British India as a whole, doctors were not present in very significant numbers in local government before 1914. This is not surprising, since there were few Indians in private practice outside the provincial capitals, and the doctors who sat on municipal councils were more likely to be nominated than elected members. Tinker notes that in 1894, doctors formed only four percent of Bengal's municipal councilors, the same percentage as schoolteachers, but far behind government servants, landlords, and lawyers.[112] But from the time it was reconstituted in 1878–79, doctors formed about ten percent of the council of the Madras Corporation, and they included elected Indians as well as nominated Europeans. By far the ablest and most articulate medical member was Dr. T. M. Nair, who entered the council in 1904, seven years after returning to India from medical training in Edinburgh.[113] As a Western-trained doctor, Nair was highly critical of the way in which the municipality and its health services were run. In a municipality where the (European) president and the executive health and sanitary officers were beyond the control of the elected councilors, this assault was necessarily largely polemical and, to Nair's intense frustration, had little practical effect.

At a council meeting in April 1905, Nair attacked the city's emigration depots, where emigrant laborers were housed while awaiting ships to take them to Mauritius, Natal, and other destinations. These, he said, had been the source of recent outbreaks of disease, including bubonic plague. In proposing to relocate the depots outside municipal limits, he showed little sympathy for the "tramps, vagabonds, indentured coolies and others of that class" who had flooded into Madras in a famine year, seeing them rather (from a middle-class perspective) as a threat to the city's health. But his main criticism was directed against the emigration agents, the British firm Parry and Co., whose interests on the council were defended (successfully on this occasion) by two IMS officers, one an Indian, the other a European.

At subsequent meetings in August and September, and with outbreaks of plague and cholera threatening, Nair and his allies returned to the attack. When K. C. Desikachariar described the depots as a "hotbed of epidemic disease," the European and IMS councilors retaliated by calling them "islands of disciplined and almost perfect sanitation in a sea of insanitary surroundings"—in other words, shifting the blame from the emigration agents to the Indian population of Madras. A vote at the September meeting resulted in a tie, but the president cast his vote in favor of Nair's proposal. When the Madras government declined to accept the resolution and move the depots, there was a further angry debate in the council chamber. Criticism of emigration from the Indian side was met by allegations about the "filthy" state of the city, particularly its *parcheries*, or Untouchable slums, by Europeans on the other. In a vote which divided the council along racial lines, Nair's resolution to have the depots moved was again put to a vote. This time it was narrowly defeated.[114]

In the following year, 1906, Nair initiated a debate about vaccination and revaccination in the city, and this time there was greater division among the Indian council members. Where some of his fellow councilors were skeptical about the practical value of vaccination or had strong cultural reservations, Nair was resolutely in favor of it. He believed that vaccination, when performed properly, was safe and effective, but he recognized that there were problems with the way in which it was currently administered in Madras. Following a government resolution urging the corporation to promote revaccination against smallpox, Nair went a stage further and moved that revaccination be made compulsory in the city and, since many of those attacked by the disease were outsiders, that vaccination be made compulsory in the surrounding suburbs and villages as well. The council supported a proposal that primary vaccination be made compulsory throughout the province but referred to a subcommittee, which included Nair and the president, the question of what could be done to encourage revaccination in the city.

At the council meeting in October 1906 vaccination came in for severe criticism from several quarters. P. Tyagaraya Chetti claimed that vaccinators were making scratches six inches long on children's arms, so that, as he put it, "the cries of these infants is a most horrible sight." A second councilor spoke of vaccinators "hacking to pieces" children six to ten months old. In this heated debate, Nair's was the voice of moderation, defending vaccination in general but condemning the employment of unqualified vaccinators who made "scratches on the arms which appear like a ploughed field. This is cruelty and ought to be put a stop to tomorrow." He urged that trained medical men be employed to supervise the vaccinators and that the calf-to-arm technique, in his view the most effective and least painful, should be used in preference to preserved lymph.[115]

In addition to his participation in council debates, Nair also kept up his criticism of the corporation's president and its health and sanitary officers through the pages of his medical journal *Antiseptic*. In an article entitled "Sanitary Play-acting in Madras," he launched a scathing attack on the corporation's health record, including the state of the water supply, drainage, conservancy, vaccination, the inspection of food and milk, and the incidence of malaria, typhoid, and dysentery. In a resolution moved at the council meeting in May 1909, a fellow doctor, U. Rama Rau, quoted Nair's indictment at length and castigated the corporation's sanitary and health officers for their ignorance and neglect. Like another middle-class politician of his day, Rama Rau stressed the importance of indigenous leadership in a society where the majority was uneducated and illiterate.

Our people being ignorant, [he declared] are always against
sanitary improvements. They cannot understand the usefulness
of sanitary precautions. So what our sanitary authorities ought
to do is to popularise the sanitary methods by convincing the
people of their necessity. Instead of that, our Health subordinates exercise their authority and frighten people with different
motives. . . . [But] if we convince our people of the necessity
for improvement, they will obey.[116]

The response to this attack was predictable. Rehearsing an old
argument, a European councilor retorted that Indians were themselves to blame for not being willing to court electoral unpopularity
by raising taxes to pay for better sanitary services. The president,
E. S. Lloyd, ICS, added an equally familiar jibe: "It is not the fault
of the Health Department if Madras is dirty, it is the fault of the
people. Madras will not improve for another hundred years if the
people do not improve." When a motion to set up a committee to
investigate defects in the Health Department and to improve the
city's sanitation was overwhelmingly defeated, Nair gave vent to his
mounting anger and frustration. "The President," he said, "has remarked that the people are dirty. If the people are dirty it's the duty
of the Sanitary department to put them right. . . . Poor people are
dirty in all countries and it is the principle of proper sanitation to
make them better." Health Department officials, he continued,

do not understand nor have they the capacity to understand
how to deal with the defects and yet you turn around and say
that the people are dirty. The Health department are inefficient
and have no sanitary knowledge, and it is the inefficiency of the
Sanitary department that stands in the way of improvement.

Whenever complaints were made, the response was to ask the critics,
"Do you want to be the executive?" Yes, Nair declared, he was willing to head the Health Department himself if that were necessary to
prove his point. But he believed the government had no genuine interest in sanitary reform: it played hide-and-seek with the municipal
rules to prevent anything substantial from being done. "Time after
time we attempted to bring up defects and criticise the officials; but
we are ruled out of order." If the government were serious, it would
give councilors effective control over the executive. Otherwise, Nair
concluded bitterly, the whole thing was "a farce."[117]

Although T. M. Nair remained on the corporation council for a few more years and continued to harry the executive on issues of health and sanitation, bitter experience had already taught him that little could be achieved by elected councilors in the face of European disdain and official obstruction. Here, rather in contrast to the arguments presented by W. J. Simpson or by Hugh Tinker, was a case in which pressure for change came from informed Indian council members, while the Europeans dragged their feet or uttered fatalistic platitudes. These heated exchanges in the Madras council chamber show how the rhetoric of health and sanitation could be turned against the colonial regime which had deployed it so authoritatively in the past and could become part of an unfolding challenge to British rule, as part of a bid, albeit before 1914 a largely ineffective one, to seize the hegemonic initiative.

HEALTH, RACE, AND NATION

Just as there were few doctors among the municipal councilors of early twentieth-century India, so were they few among the Indian political leaders of the time. But while it may be true to say, as Roger Jeffery has done, that medical practitioners exercised little influence on Indian politics and on the development of the Indian National Congress,[118] Western medical ideas had a far greater impact on political movements and social ideas than such a comment suggests. This is not to say that Western medical ideas held undisputed sway even over the Western-educated middle class, but they had begun to infiltrate and inform public debate and political language to a quite remarkable degree.

The discussion of race and nation points up this trend. It was not surprising that imperial ideas of race and latterly of social Darwinism had a profound impact on India in the late nineteenth and early twentieth centuries. Not only were they part of an assertive ideology of imperial expansion and domination but they were also extensively used in social and political discourse within India itself. On the one hand, there was the praise lavished by the British on the "martial races" of India for their fighting prowess and "manly physique," juxtaposed with descriptions of the weak, cowardly "effeminate babu."[119] On the other, there was a renewed assault on Indian social institutions, particularly child marriage. Although the government itself was reluctant to act in such a controversial matter, British doctors contributed their own strong and seemingly authoritative opinions about the resulting enfeeblement and degeneracy of the Indian people. Mention has already been made of Edith Pechey's address to the Hindus of Bombay in 1890, roundly denouncing the practice of child marriage in medical and racial terms and concluding that Hindus' attachment to it was "one important factor in the predominance of the Anglo-Saxon race."[120] This was by no means an isolated example. "As regards race," declared Dr. Kenneth McLeod of the IMS in the same year, "there can be little doubt that the marriage of children, often with aged males, tends to physical deterioration of the human stock, and physical deterioration implies effeminacy, mental imperfection, and moral debility."[121]

In an address given at Madras Medical College later in the year, Surgeon John Smyth asked why the medical profession should interfere in this sensitive issue. His reply was that

> we know more about it than anybody else; that we are the recognised and responsible protectors of the persons of our neighbours; that our unique relations with our neighbours have unfolded to us a state of affairs hostile to the welfare of our race, and we feel morally responsible to do our best to remove this source of danger to the persons of our neighbours as we do to run and arrest a haemorrhage that would otherwise prove fatal.

He impressed upon his audience the seriousness of the "canker of child-marriage" which affected the health not only of individuals but of an entire race. And he ridiculed a Hindu who had told him that India's climate would forever keep it "in the rear of the rest of the nations of the earth." Environmentalist explanations might have been acceptable in the 1830s, but they were not to Surgeon Smyth in the 1890s:

> Poor fellow! His small rotund figure and childish prattle were clearly incompatible with the accomplishment of much in this "struggle for existence"; but these conditions were by no means attributable to climate. His mother was 13 years old at the time of his birth and his father 17! His little mother and little father and himself prattled away happily enough maybe—but it was impossible that a man should be the outcome of it all. The impossibility was intensified. . . by the fact that childishness was to him a hereditary condition transmitted through many ages.[122]

It was not surprising that this racial assault, at its height in the 1880s and 1890s and backed with all the confident authority of medical science, found its reflection and response in Indian debate and polemic. When the Parsi social reformer Behramji Malabari launched his crusade against Hindu child marriage in the mid 1880s, many local organizations endorsed the view that the institution was, as the doctors claimed, a cause of physical and moral degeneracy. The Indian Association of Jessore, for instance, held that "early marriage weakens the physical strength of the nation; it stunts full growth and development, it affects the courage and energy of the individuals, and brings forth a race of people weak in strength and wanting in hardihood."[123] As president-elect of the Indian Social Conference in 1889, Dr. Mahendra Lal Sarkar of Calcutta told his audience that "the Hindu race consists at the present day . . . by virtue of this very blessed custom [of child marriage], of abortions and premature births." It was not surprising, he added, that the people of such a weak nation had fallen victim to every tyrant that had chosen to trample on them.[124] Fifteen years later, when G. K. Gokhale addressed the National Liberal Club in London, he spoke of the "continuous dwarfing or stunting of our race that is taking place under your [British] rule," and though his immediate reference was to the spiritual and moral diminishment of Indians through the denial of political rights and responsibilities, his earlier remarks about the "frightful sum of human misery" evinced by India's high death rate and the physical frailty of its people, gave his remarks a literal as well as metaphorical meaning.[125]

This sense of racial decay seems to have been particularly powerful in Bengal. Speaking in November 1912, at the Second All-India Sanitary Conference, Motilal Ghosh, editor of the Calcutta newspaper *Amrita Bazar Patrika*, gave an extended account of Bengal's decline under British rule, an account in which disease and race were again closely linked. He claimed, on the basis of his own childhood in Jessore, that sixty years earlier the Bengali countryside had been remarkably free from disease. After the autumn rains people might have been attacked by fever, but by fasting or following a "low diet" they were quickly cured. Enteric fever was rare; cholera practically unknown. Smallpox occurred intermittently, but the *tikadars* treated it "with wonderful success." "What a pity," lamented Ghosh before an audience of doctors for whom the battle against variolation was barely over, "that this race of specialists has now become extinct and that their treatment is lost to the world." In those days, he continued, the "pick of the nation" lived in the countryside. Villages had "an excellent system of drainage" and tanks were full of clean drinking water. No people on earth "were more cleanly: they rubbed their bodies with mustard oil and bathed at least once during the day." Food was abundant, and villages "teemed with healthy, happy and robust people, who spent their days in manly sports," untroubled by "the bread question or the fear of being visited by any deadly pestilence."

But those idyllic days were over, and "those fine specimens of humanity are now rarely to be found in Bengal." Citing official reports and statistics, Ghosh dated the "deterioration of the race" to the outbreak of "Burdwan fever" (malaria) in the 1860s. "Within the last sixty years malaria and cholera have swept away tens of millions of people from Bengal. Those who have been left behind, generally speaking, are more dead than alive." Where once prosperity, health, and happiness had reigned, now there were deserted villages, chronic malaria, and common misery. To stop the people from "dying like flies from malaria" the state must confront the problems of poverty and disease through a comprehensive program of rural sanitation before it was too late. Reminding his audience that the recorded birthrate for Bengal had sunk below the death rate, Ghosh concluded: the "Bengali race is. . . dying out, and it must ultimately disappear like the old Greeks, who also fell a prey to this fell disease [malaria], unless vigorous steps of the right sort are promptly taken to save them from extinction."[126]

Not all contemporary commentators drew such extreme contrasts between an idyllic past and current misery, but there was much in common between this account of Motilal Ghosh and many others written by Bengalis at the time, stressing the weakness of the race and internalizing many of the brutal judgments the British had made about them over the course of the past half-century and more. Ghosh looked to the British government in India, and more especially to Western sanitation and science, to provide answers to this problem of physical and moral decline. But others among his contemporaries looked to Indians themselves to recover their physical prowess or reassert the value of their own cultural traditions as a way of reversing their decline and re-creating pride in their own race.

Swami Vivekananda, one of the most influential Hindu reformers of the period and again a Bengali, provides an interesting illustration of this latter trend, for he showed in his speeches and writings a familiarity with Western medical science, while at the same time seeking to contrast the crass materialism of Western civilization with the virtues of India's spiritual legacy. In an article entitled "The East and the West," first published in 1901, Vivekananda began with a striking description of the way Westerners saw India, in which disease played a significantly conspicuous part.

> Devastation by violent plague and cholera; malaria eating the very vitals of the nation; starvation and semi-starvation as second nature; death-like famine often dancing its tragic dance; the Kurukshetra of malady and misery; the huge cremation ground, strewn with the dead bones of her lost hope, activity, joy and courage . . . —this is what meets the eye of the European traveller in India.

Similarly:

> A conglomeration of three hundred million souls, resembling men only in appearance; crushed out of life by being downtrodden by their own people and foreign nations, by people professing their own religion, and by others of foreign faiths; patient in labour and suffering, and devoid of an initiative, like the slave; without any hope, without any past, without any future; . . . full of ugly, diabolical superstitions which come naturally to those who are weak and hopeless of the future; without any standard of morality as their backbone; three hundred millions of souls such as these are swarming on the body of India, like so many worms on a rotten, stinking carcase,—this is the picture concerning us, which naturally presents itself to the English official!

Against this unrelenting picture of vice and misery, of disease and oppression, Vivekananda contrasted the Indian's view of the Westerner as the "veriest demon":

> lustful; drenched in liquor, having no idea of chastity or purity, and of cleanly ways and habits; believing in matter only; . . . addicted to the aggrandisement of self by exploiting others' countries, others' wealth by force, trick and treachery; having no faith in the life hereafter, whose Atman [soul] is the body, whose whole life is only in the senses and creature comforts.[127]

Vivekananda saw error and ignorance on both sides. Europeans judged India only on the basis of their contacts with the servant class, just as Indians judged Westerners by superficial impressions—their neglect of caste distinctions, their fondness for liquor, their brazen attitudes toward women. Vivekananda conceded that in some areas, such as health, "westerners are far superior to us" and that there were many things Indians could learn from them. Westerners lived longer: they lived in a better climate, but also they did not marry at an early age like Hindus. "In point of longevity and physical and mental strength," therefore, "there is a great difference between the Westerners and ourselves." But he also asked why it was that, despite so much "misery, distress, poverty and oppression," the Hindu race had not died out centuries ago: "If our customs and manners are so very bad, how is it that we have not been effaced from off the face of the earth by this time?" His answer was that India had a "national idea, which is yet necessary for the preservation of the world." India was "still living" because "she has her own quota yet to give to the general store of the world's civilisation."

Vivekananda met the assertive universalizing of Western materialism and science with an equally universalistic but, in his view, superior notion of spirituality. The two ideas were represented in opposing (but to Vivekananda not entirely irreconcilable) concepts of cleanliness and purity. Westerners might have a scientific and medical understanding of what constituted pure or clean water. This was not invalid, but Indians possessed, and could give to the world, a sense of spiritual health and purity which transcended any strictly medical or materialist definition.[128]

In the early years of the twentieth century, M. K. Gandhi went even further than Vivekananda in seeking to detach Indians from what he saw to be the harmful influence of Western civilization and to link ideas of health with India's *swaraj* (literally "self-rule"). In his youth Gandhi appears to have been attracted to the medical profession. At one stage he wanted to go to England to train as a doctor but was stopped from doing so by his brother, who said that "we Vaishnavas should have nothing to do with dissection of dead bodies."[129] Nonetheless, as Bhikhu Parekh has aptly observed, the adult Gandhi's language and thought were "suffused with medical images. He thought that the Indian 'body politic' had become 'weak' and 'diseased' and unable to resist the attack of 'foreign bodies.'" It was the self-appointed task of "Dr Gandhi," as Parekh dubs him, to be India's "national physician" who diagnosed his country's ills and "knew how to restore it to health and build up its strength."[130]

Gandhi's medical and sanitary "experiments" began during his years in South Africa. In a series of gestures which on a personal level rolled back the swelling tide of Western medicine and, like the successive changes in his dress from English suits to homespun *khadi*, marked stages in an individual but highly emblematic decolonization of the body, Gandhi acted as midwife for his last child and refused to allow Western doctors to attend his son Manilal when he was close to death from typhoid and pneumonia. At Tolstoy Farm, the community he established near Johannesburg in 1910, medicinal drugs and doctors were banned, and Gandhi pursued various health cures of his own. Unlike some Indian nationalists, he found no inspiration in Ayurveda and the traditional healing arts of India, developing instead his own eclectic ideas and practices. But above all, Gandhi saw health as an integral part of his spiritual and physical quest for self-discipline, for *swaraj* in its widest, as well as most intimate, sense. For Gandhi, good health did not mean having the services of a good doctor but rather, by being able to control bodily desires, to prevent disease and nurture one's spiritual well-being.[131]

Perhaps Gandhi became so obsessed with health and sanitation because he recognized the extraordinary authority Western medicine had acquired by the 1890s, an authority which had to be confronted and contested if India were ever to free itself from its colonial bondage. Possibly health and sanitation assumed such importance for Gandhi in South Africa because of the accusations made by whites that Indians were "filthy in habit and a menace to the public health." These accusations seem to have stung Gandhi's growing pride in his own race and civilization, a civilization which, after all, regarded purity and cleanliness as supremely important values. He seems to have internalized these racist jibes by assuming a scrupulous attention to personal sanitation and hygiene, while hurling back at the West a biting critique of its spiritually corrupting and physically deleterious civilization.[132]

The clearest statement of Gandhi's linkage of health with nationhood was made in *Hind Swaraj* ("Indian Home Rule"), first published in 1909. In the course of a rather cumbersome dialogue between the Editor, whom one takes to represent Gandhi's views, and the Reader, doctors are implicated along with lawyers and railways as being responsible for the decline of India under British rule. In a familiar simile, Western civilization is likened to consumption, a disease that does not seem to cause much "apparent hurt" but which, below the surface, progressively undermines health and strength.[133] When the Editor turns to doctors in the course of his diagnosis of the "condition of India," Gandhi reveals that, although he had once been "a great lover of the medical profession" and had intended "to become a doctor for the sake of the country," he now sees doctors in an unfavorable light and understands why traditionally India's *vaidya*s did "not occupy a very honourable status."

But it is Western doctors and Western medicine that are the main target of Gandhi's attack. "The English," he declares, "have certainly effectively used the medical profession for holding us." They have done this in a literal sense by using their professional position with "Asiatic potentates" for political gain, but in a more general sense they have done so by undermining Indians' capacity to rule their bodies as well as their country. Disease is the result of indulgence, of overeating or "vice." Doctors cure their patients, but take a fee for themselves (exploiting suffering for material gain) and allow the patients to return unrepentant to their old vices and indulgences. "A continuance of a course of medicine must, therefore, result in loss of control over the mind" as well as the body. If the doctor did not intervene, the Editor insists, "nature would have done its work, and I would have acquired mastery over myself, would have been freed from vice and would have become happy." Hospitals, the principal temples of this vicious cult, are "institutions for propagating sin. Men take less care of their bodies and immorality increases." European doctors are "worst of all." In a deft inversion of Western medical claims and racial stereotypes, Gandhi declares that doctors "induce us to indulge," with the result that "we have become deprived of self-control and have become effeminate. In these circumstances, we are unfit to serve the country. To study European medicine," he concludes in a memorable phrase, "is to deepen our slavery."[134]

Gandhi's critique was as rare as it was radical. Not many Indians of his time were prepared to go so far in rejecting not just British rule but also Western civilization as a whole. Some, like Vivekananda, looked for a way in which the East could both learn from and subsume the West; others, like Dr. T. M. Nair, wholly endorsed Western medicine but were critical of the British for not doing more to give—or allow—India the benefits of science and sanitation. But if Gandhi's views were far from being representative, they were nonetheless, by the very ferocity of their exposition, a demonstration of the hold which Western medical ideas and practices had begun to exert on Indian society and the extent to which what had once been the hallmark of an alien presence was fast becoming part of India's own ideology and leadership.

CONCLUSION

In 1887, when medical services in India were threatened with drastic retrenchment, the *Indian Medical Gazette* thought it timely to remind the colonial government of the inestimable value of Western medicine to British rule. The journal argued that doctors represented "the agents of the humanity and charity of the Government." It might be tempting to effect retrenchments at their expense, but it was doubtful whether this was politically wise:

> Ever since the arrival of the English in India, the services of medical officers have been recognised by the military and civil authorities as extremely valuable in rendering the yoke of foreign domination more easy to be tolerated by the people and in popularising English rule.[135]

The IMS had professional and political reasons of its own for claiming that Western medicine performed an important hegemonic role in India. The government did not always share this view, or it wanted hegemony without the expense and without the risks of a political backlash. As a result, its practical concern for Indian public health was often lukewarm, its commitment to the spread of Western medical ideas and practices half-hearted or hedged about with many administrative and financial reservations.

But it would be a mistake to judge the impact of Western medicine as a hegemonic force in terms of state policy and expenditure alone. Doctors—Indian as well as European—had their own evangelizing agendas and were confident that their practical successes would bring increasing recognition of the superior efficacy of Western medicine and the benefits of colonial rule. To an extent that even mid–nineteenth-century doctors and surgeons had not anticipated, Western medicine began to gain in popularity and authority and to make colonizing inroads into new areas of Indian society: even the secluded women of the zenanas began to feel its force. But in the course of its expansionist career, Western medicine also set up opposing currents and countereddies.

Outright resistance might be one expression of this, but so were varying degrees of accommodation and appropriation. What had once seemed an ideal vehicle for colonial hegemony could be annexed to the prestige and ambitions of India's own leaders. The glowing rhetoric and the deficient reality of Western medicine and public health in India could be turned against the colonial power and used as a critique of its niggardliness and want of common humanity. Western ideas of health and hygiene could be unhitched from the colonial wagon and made to serve a new Indian sense of self and nation. In the works of a writer like Vivekananda, Western medicine could be weighed and found wanting when matched against the values of India's own civilization. And it could be invoked, as it was by Gandhi, to represent all that was most insidiously destructive of Indians' capacity for self-rule. The effects of the growing diffusion of Western medical ideas and practices were far more diverse and complex than simply to popularize British rule and render more tolerable "the yoke of foreign domination."

Conclusion

Western medicine has a long history in India, and a complex one. Unlike many colonial territories in Africa and, indeed, in other parts of Asia, Western medicine did not arrive abruptly in India as part of the "new imperialism" of the 1880s and 1890s, but had an active history stretching back into the eighteenth century and even earlier. During the course of the nineteenth century (and extending that period up to 1914) it is possible to see reflected—sometimes weakly, sometimes aggressively—many of the momentous changes that were taking place in Western medicine at the time. Some developments, such as vaccination against smallpox in the 1800s or the Contagious Diseases legislation of the 1860s, passed rapidly to India. Others, like the public health movement or the germ theory of disease, though slower to find a footing, were eventually able to establish themselves. In some instances, such as the investigations into what increasingly came to be thought of as "tropical diseases," India had a pioneering role and played a significant (and as yet undervalued) part in the more general evolution of Western medicine.

These medical transferences and exchanges illustrate one part of the colonizing process in which medicine was implicated. They show the ways in which colonialism facilitated—at times dictated—the movement of ideas, practices, and practitioners between two societies thousands of miles apart and, more especially, from Britain, as the politically dominant partner in this relationship, to South Asia. In this rather restricted sense, Western medicine in India was self-evidently a "colonial science," moving mostly from metropole to colony and reinforcing the institutional and technical dominance of the colonizers over the colonized. But we need to advance our understanding of medicine as a colonial science beyond this narrow conceptualization.

We can do so in several ways. One is to judge Western medicine by its ideological dynamics and not just by its rather meager demographic effects. While it is largely the case that Western medicine had its greatest impact before 1914 on certain "enclaves" (especially the European community and the army) and tended to neglect the health of the Indian population at large, this enclavism can easily be overstated. Western medicine in India was never content to be confined to a white ghetto: it was too restlessly ambitious merely to minister to sick civil servants and ailing generals, even had it been deemed practical to draw a neat dividing line between European and "native" health. Although there were some who aspired to create sanitary enclaves and "oases," the history of medicine and disease in nineteenth-century India offers repeated reminders of the indivisibility of the colonial process. It does not neatly divide like a chocolate eggshell into two self-contained halves—one European, one Indian—but constantly feeds upon the interaction between the two. A colonialism, such as some recent writers seem eager to discover, which has no effective purchase upon an indigenous society and whose ways and works are not in turn shaped by that society, is barely recognizable as colonialism at all. Thus, medicine needs to be understood as an influential and authoritative vehicle, not just for the transmission of Western ideas and practices to India but also for the generation and propagation of Western ideas about India and, ultimately, of Indians' ideas about themselves.

For a host of reasons—because medicine was an applied and not an abstract science, because epidemic disease presented such a formidable challenge to European survival and the viability of colonial rule, because the state's physicians and surgeons were entrusted with so many practical administrative duties and responsibilities, and because they were among the few scientific observers and advisers British India could muster—the medical profession had a profound influence upon the way in which the colonial power investigated, understood, and ultimately attempted to manage indigenous society. This is not to say that doctors were all-powerful: colonial India was not a medicocracy. Indeed, even within such seemingly secure professional havens as the army and the jails, where one might assume that their authority ran broad and deep, the doctors' urgent advice often went unheeded, and they were obliged to recognize the practical and political limitations of their trade. Yet these setbacks did not altogether diminish their authority, which in general grew as the century advanced and arguably reached its apogee in the 1890s. Moreover, medical discourse seldom confined itself to the specifics of disease and health alone. It was grounded in the body, its principal professional and political site, but gave itself license to range expansively across religion and society, climate and topography, education, labor, and diet.

Through their voluminous studies of medicine and illness, doctors and surgeons helped to form and give a seemingly scientific precision to abiding impressions of India as a land of dirt and disease, of lethargy and superstition, of backwardness and barbarity—images which have remained so powerful even in the contemporary understanding of India—and to contrast this Orientalized India with the cool-headed rationality and science, the purposeful dynamism, and the paternalistic humanitarianism of the West. This was a message too powerful—or too convenient—for others to ignore. The colonial establishment took it up as part of its own imperial credo, and the missionaries incorporated it into their evangelizing, while the critics of empire either pointed to the crude discrepancy between rhetoric and reality or identified Western medicine not with liberation and well-being but with subjugation and "slavery." That medicine spoke with all the authority of science and in universalizing utterances made it all the more attractive to espouse, all the more difficult to contradict. If Western medicine's close association with state power brought it scorn in some quarters, in others it excited envy and a thirst for power. Moreover, by the later decades of the nineteenth century there were enough evident successes—in the falling death rates in the army, in the increasing impact of smallpox vaccination—to carry conviction.

The colonizing force of Western medicine has to be understood as more than a crude device of imperial self-legitimation, a mere "tool of empire." Medicine also marked out a ragged arena full of unresolved issues, a contested space as well as a colonizing one. Thus, medicine strove to grapple with an abiding contradiction between universalizing and Orientalizing. While adhering resolutely to medical science as a universal boon and a universal truth, while it sought to exclude its rivals and establish its monopolistic authority over the body, Western medicine was forced to recognize that, if it were to have any tenure in India beyond the immediate constituency of the Europeans themselves, it had to be more than a mere carbon copy of medicine in Europe. It had to fashion its own compromise, negotiate its own passage, between the laws laid down in the scientific metropolis and the practical possibilities and priorities determined by colonial rule over an "alien" society. In a sense, even the environmentalist paradigm, which gave such elevated importance to the climate, the soils, the landscape of India, was itself a vast metaphor for an ineluctable otherness—of people as well as places—that European science and medicine found in India and could never entirely gainsay. Disease *was* different in India—though there were various preferences and fashions as to how that difference could be defined—and medicine and the attempts to control or suppress disease had to recognize that cultural and political fact.

Paradoxically, too, Western medical discourse, which seemed in many ways to add a new luster and a more authoritative dimension to colonial rule, also set firm limits to its own practical capabilities and responsibilities. It did this not least by privileging indigenous resistance. Again, one can identify several reasons for this—because it could thus contrast its own dynamism with the idiosyncratic perversity of its Oriental clientele, because resistance relieved it of greater administrative and financial commitment, or because medical and sanitary intervention seemed to provoke actually or potentially explosive political unrest. Whatever the precise cause—and the reasons necessarily varied—the upshot was to make medicine more than ever answerable to politics and to a cautious pragmatism that tended to contradict the sermonizing rhetoric. But the convenience of this approach was that Indians could be seen to be vetoing their own advancement, confirming the negative stereotypes colonialism had thrust upon them, and salving the imperial conscience about having apparently achieved so little.

Indian resistance was real enough, though it sprang from a multiplicity of causes. In some instances, it arose from a very different cultural understanding of the nature of disease and the appropriate manner of its containment and control. At other times, it expressed a preference for a different system of medicine or for one that proceeded from the people themselves and not from the good offices—or the coercive agencies—of the colonial state. Resistance thus needs to be disentangled, not homogenized, if its real cause and objects are to be effectively understood and evaluated. But, even then, resistance must form only part of the picture, for it was a further characteristic feature of colonial medicine in India that it was always a site of some Indian negotiation and participation. India might be present in texts or personal informants, in the form of subordinate agency or of elite patronage. Increasingly, it was present in the form of Indian practitioners, participants in state medicine or in private practice. Although that India was often one which Europe summoned up, perhaps from its own imaginings, there can be no doubt that Indians were often active, and not just passive, participants, and their participation did much to diminish the perceived foreignness of Western medicine, to integrate it with indigenous cultural values and political structures.

Paradoxically, a system of medicine which often proclaimed its intentions of sweeping away custom, caste, and superstition often ended up quietly negotiating for its own acceptance. Just as it did not want to be merely the white man's medicine, so it also aspired to be more than medicine for the half-caste and the Untouchable. Western medicine craved status and respectability, and India, for all its political subordination, exacted a price for this cultural acceptance. The practitioners of colonial medicine might not have believed in caste, but they participated in the creation of caste hospitals. They certainly doubted the efficacy of indigenous medicine, but were obliged even in the 1900s to make some room for the *vaidya* and the *hakim*.

Thus, the colonizing processes of colonial medicine could never find their fulfillment in colonial hands alone. In the end (and that end was already foreshadowed by 1914), the future of Western medicine in India lay not with Europe's colonizers but with India's emerging elites. They had their own political programs and professional agendas to pursue, their own course to steer between "cosmopolitan" science and subaltern society. While some sought to tear down Western medicine along with the crumbling edifice of colonialism itself, many were beginning to see a more active, a more public-oriented, role for state medicine than colonialism had ever thought politically expedient or financially desirable. In the years after 1914, they were to take up Western medicine as part of their own hegemonic project.

Notes

INTRODUCTION

1. *Statesman*, 30 June 1908, in Home (Med), 96, Aug. 1910, NAI.
2. Ibid.
3. C. P. Lukis, 31 Aug. 1908, "Note on the Self-Constituted Medical Schools of Calcutta," ibid.
4. Notes to Home (Med), 117–32A, July 1913, NAI. For the issue of medical registration in India, see Jaggi 1979, chap. 4. An All-India Medical Registration Act was introduced by Sir Pardy Lukis in 1915 and became law the following year.
5. Note by A. Earle, Sec, Home (Med), 1 Sept. 1910, Home (Med), 37–55, Dec. 1910, NAI.
6. *Thacker's Indian Directory, 1900*, 376.
7. Marriott 1955; Ramasubban 1988. See chapter 2 below.
8. Guerra 1963; Fanon 1970, chap. 4; Doyal 1979; Turshen 1984.
9. Dubois 1905, 73–74.
10. Yang 1985, 108–27.
11. *Centenary of Medical College, Bengal* 1935, 13; Gupta 1976, 370.
12. Cook, "Report on Plague in Calcutta," 31 Aug. 1898, in Bengal, *Report of the Epidemics of Plague in Calcutta. . . . up to 30th June 1900*, 8.
13. Foucault 1976; 1979; 1980.
14. Nandy 1983, 1–2.
15. In this respect I see this study of medicine and disease as complementing my earlier study of the Indian police (Arnold 1986). For further discussion of the relevance of Foucault to colonial medicine, see Vaughan 1991.
16. Foucault 1980, 73, 158.
17. Eliot Friedson, cited in Leslie, ed., 1976, 6.
18. Cf. Sontag 1983.
19. Said 1978.

CHAPTER 1

1. Crawford 1914, vol. 1; Patterson 1987; de Figueiredo 1984.

2. Ramasubban 1982, 1988. For a critical commentary on this argument, see Jeffery 1988a, 100–2; and below, chapter 2.

3. Marriott 1955, 241.

4. Gupta 1976, 369–70; Balfour and Scott 1924, 126–41; India, *Report of the Health Survey and Development Committee* 1946, 1:22–24; Arnold 1987.

5. For example, alongside Western allopathic medicine, homeopathy had a considerable impact on India, especially in Bengal: see Bhardwaj 1981.

6. For an outline of the "modernization" of India's medical systems, see Leslie 1974.

7. Headrick 1981.

8. Basalla 1967.

9. Twining 1832, xxiv.

10. Johnson 1813, ix, xii.

11. Annesley 1828, 1:vii.

12. *TMPSB* 1 (1838): ii.

13. *TMPSC* 1 (1825): iii.

14. Ibid.: iii–v. A third provincial journal, the *Madras Quarterly Medical Journal*, appeared in 1839 with a similar prospectus. On medical societies and journals in India, see Neelameghan 1963.

15. *TMPSC* 1:v–vi. Ironically, much the same complaints were to be made by Ronald Ross about his experience in the Indian Medical Service a half-century later: Ross 1923.

16. Crawford 1914, vol. 2, chap. 29.

17. *TMPSC* 1 (1825); cf. *Centenary Review of the Asiatic Society of Bengal* 1885, section 3.

18. Cited in Crawford 1914, 2:125.

19. *IMG* 1899, 34:259; Cantlie 1974 2:217–30. One indication of the wider influence of Indian medical literature is its frequent citation in August Hirsch 1883 (see especially the entries for smallpox, malaria, cholera, and typhoid).

20. Martin (1796–1874) served as a Company surgeon in Bengal from 1817 until he retired in 1840. On his return to London, he served as a member of the Royal Commission of Enquiry into the Sanitary Condition of Large Towns and Populous Districts in England and Wales (1843–45) and on several other boards and committees including the Royal Commission into the Sanitary State of the Army in India, which reported in 1863. He helped set up the military hospital at Netley, and his revision of James Johnson's *The Influence of Tropical Climates on European Constitutions* established him as one of the leading authorities on tropical diseases and medicine in Britain at the time. He was knighted in 1860. See Fayrer 1897. Edmund A. Parkes (1819–76) served as an army assistant surgeon in India, 1842–45. Back in England, he was appointed to investigate the causes of the 1848 cholera

epidemic in London and in 1864, while professor of military hygiene at the Army Medical School, published *A Manual of Practical Hygiene*, which established him as "the founder of the science of modern hygiene." See Pelling 1978, 70. A former Company ship's surgeon, Neil Arnott (1788–1874) was an associate of Edwin Chadwick and an influential sanitary reformer in Britain. See Flynn 1965, 34. For details of these and other careers, see Crawford 1930.

21. Hunter 1804: 1.

22. Martin, ed., 1838, 1:vii–x. For Buchanan's other interests, see Vicziany 1986.

23. Annesley 1825, 255. The importance of statistics to colonial medicine in India is discussed in chapter 2.

24. Crawford 1914, 2:166, 247; Fayrer 1897, 59.

25. Martin 1856, 99.

26. Ibid.

27. Ibid., 103–4.

28. *IMG* 1866, 1:178.

29. Zimmermann 1987.

30. Martin 1856, 35. For the influence of Montesquieu and environmentalist ideas, see Marshall and Williams 1982, 136–39; Guha 1963, chapter 2.

31. Riley 1987, 36–48.

32. For the concept of scientific paradigms, see Kuhn 1970.

33. E.g., India, *Leprosy in India* 1893; but cf. the discussion of goiter in M'Clelland 1859.

34. Fayrer 1882, 154.

35. This is not to say that such diseases were entirely neglected: e.g., for beriberi, see Malcolmson 1835a.

36. Ballingall 1818, 18.

37. Annesley 1825, xv.

38. MacGregor 1843, vii; Mackinnon 1848, 6; Martin 1856.

39. Morehead 1856, 1:viii–x.

40. Johnson 1813, xi, 11, 80–81, 232–50, 460; cf. Balfour 1925; Sheridan 1985.

41. Curtis 1807, xvi–xvii.

42. Johnson 1813, 26.

43. Hegel 1956, 142; Archer 1980; Archer and Lightbrown 1982.

44. Burton 1851, 1.

45. Strong 1837, 9–10.

46. Taylor 1840, 322, 329–30.

47. Johnson 1813, 59.

48. Annesley 1828, 1:83.

49. Twining 1832, 1–2; cf. Ballingall 1818, 40.

50. Twining 1832, 566–67.

51. See chapter 4 on cholera; also Macnamara 1880; Fayrer 1882. Louis Pasteur, the great proponent of the germ theory of disease, is reported to

have said on his deathbed, "The microbe is nothing; the terrain is every-thing," but this was not the view that subsequently prevailed in Europe: Learmonth 1988, ii, 11–12.

52. Clark 1773, 267.

53. Johnson 1813, 19–24, 265; cf. Martin 1856, 32.

54. Clark 1773, 3–4.

55. MacGregor 1843, 3–4.

56. Annesley 1828, 1:xi.

57. Johnson 1813, 160.

58. Morehead 1856, 1:206–16; Twining 1832, 347; Martin 1856, 157; Russell 1955, 99–100. For similar practices elsewhere, see Curtin 1964: 190–94.

59. Annesley 1825, 312.

60. Johnson 1813, 1–5, 79, 83–86.

61. Annesley 1828, 1:7; cf. Livingstone 1987.

62. See also Lind 1808, 146. Despite the new tropical medicine of the 1890s and the greater protection it promised to give Europeans in the tropics, it was still argued in India that since climate was a major cause of "tropical deterioration," it remained an obstacle to white health and settlement: *IMG* 1898, 33:456–57.

63. Johnson 1813, 105, 417–60; Curtis 1807, 280.

64. Twining 1832, xxii–xxiii; 1835, 2:417–38.

65. Twining 1832, 123–25.

66. Mackinnon 1848, 1. The extension of the environmentalist paradigm to include social and cultural variables was also common to Europe's own medical discourse at the time: see Jordanova 1989, 25.

67. Martin 1837, 49.

68. Rankine 1839, 26.

69. Ibid., 52; cf. Elliot 1863.

70. Cited in Kopf 1969, 152.

71. Cited in Mukhopadhyaya 1923, 1:4–5.

72. Ainslie 1826, 2:v, vii.

73. Wise 1860, i–ii, v.

74. Ibid., iii, xix.

75. Drury 1873; Crawford 1914, 2:148–52. For the arguments for substituting Indian drugs for imported ones, see the Report of the Committee on Indian Drugs, 1853, in Madras, *Medical Reports Selected by the Medical Board* 1855.

76. Ainslie 1826, 1:x.

77. O'Shaughnessy 1844, iv–v; cf. Waring 1860, 1897.

78. Playfair 1833, iii.

79. Ibid., 5–6, 189.

80. Ibid., 12–13, 22–23; cf. Irvine 1848: 2.

81. Wilson 1979.

82. For Sen, see Mittra 1880.

83. Wilson 1825, 2, 4–7, 25–26, 44.

84. Wise 1860, iii, v, xix.

85. Heyne 1814, 125–26, 164–65.

86. Wise 1860, xix.

87. Heyne 1814, 125.

88. Martin, ed., 1838, 1:139; 3:141–42.

89. Twining 1832, 332–34. The indigenous technique of removing eye cataracts was also favorably reported: Breton 1826.

90. Twining 1832, 123, 132.

91. Martin 1837, 60.

92. Haines, n.d., 15–16; cf. Wise 1883, 69–76, for a critical account of *hakim*s.

93. *IMG* 1867, 2:17–18, 23; cf. Irvine 1848.

94. Hume 1977; *IMG* 1868, 3:87.

95. In addition to numerous articles in the *IMG* from 1866 to the 1890s, see Dutt 1877; Sheriff 1891; Koman 1921.

96. Annesley 1825, 45–46; Parkes 1846, x.

97. Dempster 1868, 19.

98. Harrison 1858, 37; Crawford 1914, 2:100–23, for the earlier history of the subordinate medical service.

99. *Centenary of Medical College, Bengal* 1935, 3–7; Bala 1987.

100. Gupta 1976, 369–70.

101. Of the first eleven graduates from the Calcutta Medical College in 1839, five were Kayasthas and four Vaidyas: the other two were a Christian and a Brahmin: Crawford 1914, 2:440.

102. Cited in Kopf 1969, 184.

103. *Centenary of Medical College, Bengal* 1935, 7–9; Crawford 1914, 2:434–35. For the debates of the period, see Stokes 1959, chap. 1; Rosselli 1974, 208–25.

104. Macaulay in de Bary 1968, 2:44–46.

105. Martin 1837, 60.

106. Haines, n.d., 34–35.

107. *Centenary of Medical College* 1835, 13.

CHAPTER 2

1. See Crawford 1914 and Harrison 1991 for the character and duties of the IMS.

2. A. Earle, Sec., Home (Med), 1 Sept. 1910, Home (Med), 37–55, notes, Dec. 1910, NAI.

3. Ramasubban 1982; 1984; 1988.

4. India's cantonments, which evolved from tented encampments to become permanent military bases for both European and Indian troops by the late eighteenth century, were located outside the main towns. This facilitated their segregated or enclavist nature. Nilsson 1968, 76–79.

5. Martin 1837, 155.

6. Alexander Tulloch, cited by Martin in *Report of the Commissioners Appointed to Inquire into the Organization of the Indian Army* (C. 2515), 1859, 167.

7. *Royal Commission on the Sanitary State of the Army* (C. 3184), 1863, xvii. McNeill (1979, 261) notes that in the Crimean War of 1854–56 ten times as many British soldiers died of dysentery as from Russian arms; in the Boer War of 1899–1902 five times the number of British troops perished from disease as from enemy action.

8. Geddes 1846, 74.

9. Ibid. For contrasting views, see MacGregor 1843, 8–9; Swinson and Scott, eds., 1968, 155. Lieutenant Richard Burton's view of the Bombay Army's Medical Board was typically acerbic: "a committee of ancient gentlemen who never will think you sufficiently near death to meet your wishes" (i.e., to be discharged or given sick leave). Burton 1851, 4.

10. Geddes 1846, v.

11. For the importance of statistics to the medical literature of the early nineteenth century, see Flynn 1965, 26–29; Carlson 1984, chap. 5; Cassedy 1984.

12. Rogers's editorial note to Kellie 1839.

13. Cantlie 1974, vol. 2, chap. 4.

14. Cook 1914, 2:1–22; *Royal Commission on the Sanitary State of the Army in India.*

15. Ewart 1859, 6, 10. With the passing of the Company, the issue of European settlement in India was again in the forefront (see Arnold 1983); but the prevalence of disease was one of the strongest arguments made against it.

16. Ewart 1859, 86–124.

17. Ibid., 125–46.

18. Ibid., 147–63.

19. *Report of the Commissioners Appointed to Inquire into the Cholera Epidemic of 1861 in Northern India* 1862, ii, 6, 248–50, 254. For further discussion of cholera and the army, see chapter 4 below.

20. Ewart 1859, 22.

21. Ibid., 44; cf. Moore 1867, 174; Chevers 1886, 4. Surprisingly, Curtin (1989) does not consider this factor in explaining high levels of British troop mortality in early nineteenth-century India.

22. Cook 1914, 2:19; Balfour and Scott 1924, 127–28; Cantlie 1974, 2:206.

23. Leith 1864, 11; Moore 1867, 173–74.

24. Ewart 1859, 14, 30, 152.

25. Ibid., 138–39.

26. *Sanitary State of the Army*, xix.

27. Ewart 1859, 2.

28. Ibid., 153. For a soldier's view of this disparity, see Douglas 1865, 3–4.

29. *Sanitary State of the Army*, xvi; for miasma as an explanation for sickness in jails, see Mouat 1856, 35–37; 1868, 44.

30. For the nature and significance of these developments, see Parkes 1864; Curtin 1989.

31. Klein 1973; Davis 1951, 36–37.

32. *Organization of the Indian Army*, 168. See also Martin 1837, 153–58; Riley 1987.

33. Parkes 1864, 554; Dempster 1868, 140.

34. Ewart 1859, 49; cf. Strong 1837 for an even more destructive approach to a "malarial" environment.

35. Murray 1856, 3; 1869, 6; India, *Rules Regarding the Measures to Be Adopted on the Outbreak of Cholera or Appearance of Smallpox* 1870.

36. Martin 1856, 114; cf. Martin, "Suggestions for promoting the health and efficiency of the British troops serving in the East Indies," *Organization of the Indian Army*, 167–69.

37. Parkes 1864, 555.

38. *India SCAR 1870*, 3; *1894*, 47.

39. Parkes 1864, 555–56.

40. E.g., at Murree in the 1880s: see Home (San), 82, May 1889, NAI.

41. E.g., Martin 1856, 218.

42. Martin 1837, 162.

43. Martin 1856, 300. Soldiers' own attitudes toward drink were quite varied. See Ryder 1854, 11–12, 23–24; Swinson and Scott, eds., 1968, 24, 28–29, 32–34, 146; Laverack, n.d., 182–83.

44. *Minutes of Evidence Taken before the Select Committee on the Affairs of the East India Company*, V, 10, 138; Geddes 1846, 15–16; BC, F/4/709, 19275, IOL.

45. Bngl Mil Cons, 1 May 1819, BC, F/4/643, 17790, IOL; see also Martin 1837, 164; Mackinnon 1848, 23.

46. Martin 1837, 165.

47. Geddes 1846, 16.

48. *Sanitary State of the Army*, 375.

49. Ibid., 375; Ewart 1859, chap. 4.

50. Manson 1898, 343–49; Rogers and Megaw 1930, 117.

51. *India SCAR 1895*, 45; *1910*, 16–17.

52. *Sanitary State of the Army*, 103.

53. *India SCAR 1880*, 25; *1895*, 47, 65.

54. Md Mil Cons, 1810, BC, F/4/379: 9435, IOL.

55. Ingledew to Physician-General, Md, 23 Sept. 1808, BC, F/4/345, 8031, IOL.

56. *India SCAR 1890*, 57.

57. See Ballhatchet 1980, chap. 1, for these and similar arguments.

58. Md Med Board Procs, 30 Apr. 1810, BC, F/4/379, 9435, IOL; Johnson 1813, 105.

59. Ballhatchet 1980, chap. 1. The term "lock hospital" is said to derive from "lazar (leper) hospital" as in Southwark in London, though "lock" aptly suggests the degree of confinement involved in these institutions in India.

60. One surgeon wittily observed, "During the period of the mercurial

mania, how common an event was destruction of the nasal and palatine bones; and the men who were then said to have suffered in the wars of Venus, probably suffered more from the wars of Mercury." Clark 1839, 390.

61. Brown 1887, 80–97.

62. Cited in *IMG* 1883, 18:102.

63. Ibid.

64. C. Macaulay, Sec, Bngl Mun to Home, 4 Jan. 1888, Home (San), 106, June 1888, NAI.

65. For this agitation, see Ballhatchet 1980, chap. 2.

66. Sec, Mil, 9 May 1889, Legis, 7–83, notes, Oct. 1889, NAI.

67. *India SCAR 1900*, 24–25; *1910*, 17.

68. Ibid., 17; *1913*, 22.

69. *India SCAR 1895*, 36; "Annual Returns," *India SCAR 1910*, 34.

70. Ewart 1880, 263–76.

71. *India SCAR 1890*, 39. Typhoid was not, of course, unknown in Britain at the time: see Smith 1990, 244–49.

72. Ranking 1869; Gordon 1878; Fayrer 1882; Hewlett 1883.

73. See King 1976, chap. 5; Spitzer 1968; Swanson 1977, for social and health segregation.

74. *India SCAR 1894*, 31.

75. *India SCAR 1890*, 33.

76. *India SCAR 1910*, 10–15; *1913*, 6; Home (San) 180–82, Aug. 1910, NAI.

77. Balfour and Scott 1924, 49.

78. *India SCAR 1913*, 5, 35; Rogers and Megaw 1930, 514.

79. Martin 1856, 217.

80. *India SCAR 1895*, 59, 62, 67.

81. *Affairs of the East India Company*, 5:15.

82. Murray 1839, 9–11, 17.

83. India, *The Army in India and Its Evolution* 1924: 120–21.

84. *Sanitary State of the Army*, 377–78; *Cholera 1861*, 220. For conditions in the Bengal Army in the first half of the century, see Barat 1962.

85. Brown 1887, 84.

86. *India SCAR 1890*, 71, 79; *1894*, 63–67; *1918*, 31. In 1918 a much larger percentage of Europeans than Indians was hospitalized with influenza (21.95: 13.68), but only half as many died of the disease (0.88: 1.52). For an earlier period, see Malcolmson 1835a; MacGregor 1843.

87. E.g., at Vishakhapatnam in August 1877: Colr, Vishakhapatnam, to Sec, Rev, 21 Aug. 1877, Md GO 2377, Rev (Famine), 17 Oct. 1877, IOL.

88. *India SCAR 1895*, 75–85.

89. Mason 1974, 237–38; Cassels 1987, 7–9, 94–95.

90. Nightingale was as skeptical about caste "prejudices" as she was about climate, suspecting that both were used to excuse official inertia. *Sanitary State of the Army*, 368.

91. Ibid., xxiii.

92. Murray 1839, 49.

93. Bengal, *Report of the Small-pox Commissioners* 1850, 75; *Bmb VR 1869–70*, xii. On vaccination, see chapter 3.

94. Martin 1856, 220.

95. Bingley and Nicholls 1897, 42; Bingley 1918, 75.

96. Bhardwaj 1975, 611.

97. *Army in India* 1924, 117.

98. *Sanitary State of the Army*, 371.

99. Great Britain, *Report on Measures Adopted for Sanitary Improvements in India up to the End of 1867*, 1–2.

100. Cited in Parkes 1864, 562–63; Cook 1914, 2:1, 33, 52. For Lawrence's guarded response, see Cook 1914, 2:158–59.

101. India, *Report of the Committee on Prison Discipline* 1838.

102. Hutchinson 1835, 3–7.

103. Hutchinson 1845, 205–6.

104. These developments should be seen against the background of changes in the criminal law in the early period of colonial rule. See Fisch 1983.

105. Lyons 1872, 253.

106. Cruikshank 1876, 1, 10–13. "The medical administration is the most important of all matters affecting jail management," *Rules for the Superintendence and Manaqement of Jails in the Province of Assam* 1898, 1:224.

107. Mouat 1856, 107.

108. Tinker 1974, 163–64.

109. Mouat 1856, 37, 41.

110. *Report of the Indian Jails Committee* 1920, 2:174.

111. Ibid., 2:11.

112. Ibid., 2:34–35, 50. See also Cardew 1891, 12–17.

113. For further discussion of the prison as a site of colonial control, see Arnold, forthcoming.

114. Jameson 1820, 321; Strong 1837.

115. *Sanitary Improvements 1867*, 71.

116. *Committee on Prison Discipline*, 9.

117. *India SCAR 1880*, 67; 1914, 124; India, *Report of the Indian Jail Conference* 1877, 22, 125.

118. Wiehe 1865, 45; Howell 1868, 124.

119. *Indian Jail Conference* 1877, 20–21. For the connections between food shortages and crime, see Arnold 1979.

120. *IMG* 1893, 28:293; cf. table 6.

121. *India SCAR 1880*, 83

122. *Indian Jails Committee* 1920, 2:42, 44.

123. *Indian SCAR 1910*, 87; *1913*, 61.

124. Cf. Sim 1990; Arnold forthcoming.

125. E.g., Stevens 1901; articles on TB and malaria in *IMG*, 35, Sept. and Oct. 1900; for dysentery, Home (San), 4–17, Sept. 1906, NAI; and malaria, see Home (San), 189–231, May 1910, NAI.

126. Parkes 1846, x.

127. Hodge 1867, appendix 400.

128. Mouat 1856, 43.

129. Hodge 1867, 87.

130. Home (Jails), 21–22, Nov. 1912, NAI.

131. Macrae 1894; R. Harvey, "Note on anti-plague inoculations," Home (San), 76, May 1898, NAI.

132. Home (Jails), 11, Jan. 1910, NAI.

133. Yang 1987. See also *Committee on Prison Discipline*, 30–34.

134. Arnold, forthcoming.

135. Jud letter to Bngl, 12 Aug. 1846, cited in Banerjee 1963, 339.

136. Mouat 1856, 76–77.

137. Leith 1851–52: 114–27.

138. Bengal, *Alimentary Articles in Bengal* 1863; Cornish 1863; Wiehe 1865.

139. *Committee on Prison Discipline*, 31–35; *Indian Jails Conference* 1877.

140. Mouat 1856, 87–88, 105–6; 1868, 16; Wilson 1874, 13–14.

141. E.g., T. R. Lewis, "A memorandum on the dietaries of labouring prisoners in Indian jails," *India SCAR 1880*, 153–206.

142. For the use of jail-based standards of diet and labor and the controversy that arose between W. R. Cornish, sanitary commissioner, Madras, and Sir William Temple on behalf of the Government of India, see Geddes 1874, 143–44; Cornish to Chief Sec, Md, 13 Mar. 1877, Md SC Procs, Mar. 1877, IOL.

143. McCay 1912, 188.

144. Ibid., 135, 190. McCay's recommended dietaries were subsequently introduced, despite opposition from local governments as well as prisoners: see Home (Jails), 17–24, Jan. 1914, NAI; Home (Jails), 18–25, Mar. 1918, NAI.

CHAPTER 3

1. *NWP VR 1866–67*, 4; Charles 1870, 1; James 1909, 1.

2. James 1909, 50. For smallpox generally, see Dixon 1962, Hopkins 1983.

3. *Bngl VR 1872*, 7.

4. James 1909, 64–67.

5. Quoted in ibid., 49.

6. Mohammad, ed., 1972, 142.

7. Md GO 2951, Education and Pub Health, 14 Oct. 1946, IOL; *Annual Report of the Director-General of Health Services 1947* 1:60.

8. Wadley 1980; Banerji 1972, 123; Bang 1973, 82.

9. Crooke 1896, 118–23; Caldwell 1887; cf. Nicholas 1981; Wadley 1980.

10. Crooke 1896, 122; Enthoven 1924, 262–65.

11. Wise 1883, 343–44.

12. Babb 1975, 126; cf. Misra 1969, 138–39.

13. *Bngl VR 1893–96*, xxiv; cf. Wise 1883, 87, 344.

14. Crooke 1896, 118; Babb 1975, 129; Wadley 1980, 35; Enthoven 1924, 263–64.

15. Crooke 1910, 285–86.

16. Wise 1883, 344.

17. Ibid.

18. *Missionary Register* 1836, 465; *Bngl VR 1869*, xxi. In southern India the goddess Mariamma had some but not all of the properties of Sitala as a smallpox deity: Djurfeldt and Lindberg 1975, 116–17, 139–41.

19. Jolly 1977, 9, 113–16; Nicholas 1981, 25–27.

20. Jolly 1977, 49–52; Zimmer 1948.

21. Deb 1831, 418–19; cf. Wise 1860, 233–34; Jolly 1977, 113.

22. Bengal, *Report of the Small-pox Commissioners* 1850, lxx.

23. Holwell 1767, 16–17. Holwell's account is reprinted, with an earlier description by Coult, in Dharampal 1971.

24. Holwell 1767, 14, 17–18, 24. For recent views on variolation and its consequences, see Razzell 1977; Hopkins 1983.

25. Holwell 1767, 19.

26. Ibid., 20.

27. Deb 1831, 417. For a description of variolation in northern, India, see *NWP VR 1869–70*, 21–22.

28. *Bngl VR 1869*, 2; *Bngl VR 1872–3*, 100–1.

29. Shoolbred 1804, 77; *Bngl VR 1872*, xiv–xv; K. McLeod, 20 Sept. 1872, Home (Pub), 156, Mar. 1873, NAI; *NWP VR 1866–7*, 6; *Bmb VR 1865*, viii–ix; *Bmb VR 1867*, xix; *Bmb VR 1870–71*, 28.

30. Davis 1978; *Bmb VR 1874–5*, 30.

31. *NWP VR 1869–70*, 23; *NWP VR 1870–71*, 14; *Bngl VR 1871*, 9; McLeod, 20 Sept. 1872, Home (Pub), 156, Mar. 1873, NAI; *Bngl VR 1872–3*, 100–1.

32. Deb 1831, 416.

33. *Small-pox Commissioners* 1850, 35; Wise 1883, 249, 349–50; *Bngl VR 1872*, 56.

34. O'Malley 1907, 71; Martin, ed., 1838, 1:139–40; 2:484, 508; *NWP VR 1872–3*, 31; Md BoR Procs, 20 Jan. 1801, BC F/4/96/1953, IOL; Md Jdl Cons, 26 May 1812, BC F/4/382/9625, IOL.

35. *Small-pox Commissioners* 1850, 37; *Bngl VR 1867–8*, 4; *NWP VR 1871–2*, 25.

36. Martin, ed., 1838, 2:691.

37. *NWP VR 1872–73*, 31.

38. James 1909, 10; McLeod, 20 Nov. 1872, Home (Pub), 156, Mar. 1873, NAI.

39. O'Malley 1907, 72.

40. Rogers and Megaw (1930, 515) remark, "Smallpox is now essentially a tropical disease."

41. Morehead 1856, 1:317–19; cf. *Small-pox Commissioners* 1850, 23.

42. Holwell 1767, 4; James 1909, 47; Shoolbred 1804, 94.

43. James 1909, 20.

44. *Small-pox Commissioners* 1850, 20–22; Morehead 1856, 1:320.

45. *Bngl VR 1869*, 3; *Small-pox Commissioners* 1850, 24.

46. Isaac Newton, Superintendent-General of Vaccination to Sec, Pnjb, n.d., Home (Pub), 245, Apr. 1872, NAI; Dy SC, Central Dt, to SC, Bmb, 17 July 1893, Bmb Gen, 1, 706, MSA.

47. Archibald Seton, Agent, Bareilly, to Sec, Secret and Pol, 9 June 1805, and Seton to Judge, Bareilly, 7 June 1805, Bngl Cons, 4 Oct. 1805, BC F/4/198/4452, IOL.

48. Bowers 1981, 24.

49. Minute, 18 June 1805, BC F/4/201/4544, IOL.

50. Md Pub Cons, 19 Jan. 1803, BC F/4/153/2613, IOL; Shoolbred 1804, 82.

51. Shoolbred 1805, 25; David White, Sec, Med Board, Bmb, 14 Nov. 1811, Bmb Pub Cons, 29 Jan. 1812, and J. M. Keate, Judge, Kaira Dt, to Chief Sec, Bmb, 4 Dec. 1812, Bmb Pub Cons, 12 Feb. 1812, BC F/4/429/10518, IOL.

52. Cameron 1831, 397–98; James 1909, 22

53. Shoolbred 1804, 26.

54. Cameron 1831, 387–88.

55. Stewart 1844, 9.

56. *NWP SCAR 1878*, 30.

57. Cameron 1831, 387.

58. *Small-pox Commissioners* 1850, 54.

59. Ibid., 66.

60. Shoolbred 1804, 2–4.

61. Martin, ed., 1838, 2:691; 3:484.

62. *Bngl VR 1869*, 1–11; Wise to Comr, Dacca Div, 14 Sept. 1871, Home (Pub), 366, Feb. 1872, NAI. Planck, the NWP Sanitary Commissioner, also believed that "inoculation is justifiable so long as vaccination cannot be enforced" (*NWP SCAR 1869*, 5).

63. MacLeod 1967; but cf. *Bmb VR 1858–9*, vii; *Md SCAR 1884*, 21.

64. Bowers 1981, 22.

65. James 1909, 37; *Bmb VR 1867*, xxi.

66. *Small-pox Commissioners* 1850, 50–53; *NWP SCAR 1876*, 28; *NWP VR 1895–6*, 14.

67. *Aryajanapriyam* (Madras), 8 Sept. 1891, Md NNR; *Bmb VR 1871–2*, xv.

68. Great Britain, *Report on Measures Adopted for Sanitary Improvements in India 1868*, 137.

69. James 1909, 27, 37–38.

70. *Bmb VR 1889–90*, 36; *Bmb VR 1911–14*, 3; *Bngl VR 1915–16*, 3.

71. James 1909, 76; Rogers 1926, 5.

72. *NWP VR 1876*, 29; *UP VR 1908–11*, 1.

73. *Bngl VR 1873*, ii–iii; *Bngl VR 1899–1902*, 2.

74. *Bngl VR 1867–8*, 13; *NWP VR 1869–70*, 2; *Bngl VR 1896–9*, 10.

75. Dyson, 30 June 1893, Bngl, Mun (San), 3, July 1894, WBSA.

76. *Bmb VR 1870–71*, 89; *Bmb VR 1874–5*, 19; *Bmb VR 1890–91*, 5; Bowers 1981, 23.

77. Major C. A. McMahon, Hissar Dt, to Sec, Pnjb, 2 Dec. 1871, Home (Pub), 246, Apr. 1872, NAI.

78. Avadh VR, 1872–3, Home (Pub), 495, July 1873, NAI; Martin, ed., 1838, 2:691.

79. *Small-pox Commissioners* 1850, lxviii, lxxii; *Bmb VR 1867*, 10; *NWP VR 1872–3*, 29.

80. *Bmb VR 1905–6*, 1; *Md VR 1889–90*, 5; *Report of the Health Survey and Development Committee* 1946, 1:47.

81. Shoolbred 1805, 24; *Bngl VR 1872–3*, 31.

82. Comr, Jullundur Div, to Sec, Pnjb, 10 Oct. 1871, Home (Pub), 246, Apr. 1872, NAI.

83. Bngl to CoD, 19 Mar. 1805, BC F/4/186/3906, IOL; *Bngl VR 1867–8*, 2; *Bngl VR 1869*, xix, xliv; *Bngl VR 1877*, 10; *Bmb VR 1858–9*, 25; *NWP VR 1870–71*, 11.

84. Christison, n.d., 9; *Bngl VR 1896*, xxvi; *Bmb VR 1865*, 2; *NWP VR 1873–4*, 21; Home (Pol), 246, Apr. 1872, NAI.

85. *Bngl VR 1872*, 45; *NWP VR 1872–3*, 32; *Gazetteer of the Bombay Presidency*, vol. 18, no. 1 (1885): 224–45. That increasing acceptance of vaccination did not lead to a loss of faith in Sitala is evident from recent anthropological studies, e.g., Babb 1975; Wadley 1980.

86. *NWP VR 1873–4*, 30; Yule and Burnell 1985, 919. Cf. use of the term "Devi doctor" in Ratnagiri, *Bmb VR 1869–70*, 24.

87. *Bngl VR 1877*, 7; *Bngl VR 1873*, 18; *Bngl VR 1878–9*, 25; *Bngl VR 1893–6*: xxiv–xxviii; Butter 1839, 169.

88. *Bngl VR 1867–8*, 5; CoD to Bngl, 6 Apr. 1808, BC F/4/297/6889, IOL; CoD to Bngl, 3 Sept. 1813, BC F/4/446/10749, IOL.

89. James 1909, 21.

90. Morehead 1856, 1:322–23; *Bmb VR 1858–9*, iv–v; India, *Papers on Vaccination in India* 1851, 17.

91. *NWP VR 1871–2*, 4; *Md SCAR 1884*, 113.

92. Supt, Hissar Div, to Sec, Pnjb, 2 Dec. 1871, Home (Pub), 246, Apr. 1872, NAI.

93. BC F/4/186/3906, IOL; *Small-pox Commissioners*, 28–29, 35, xxii; *Bngl VR 1870*, 3.

94. *Bngl VR 1873*, 1; James 1909, 31.

95. *NWP VR 1872–3*, 13, 32; *Bngl VR 1872*, 21.

96. Charles, 8 July 1871, and Powell to Dy Inspector-General of Hospitals, 8 July 1871, San Procs, 8, Mar. 1872, IOL.

97. J. Reid to Shoolbred, 13 June 1805, BC F/4/186/3906, IOL; Bmb to CoD, 14 Oct. 1813, BC F/4/429/10518, IOL.

98. *NWP VR 1872–3*, 11; *NWP SCAR 1879*, 35, 39.

99. *NWP VR 1878*, 20A.

100. *NWP VR 1877*, 41; *NWP VR 1878*, 24A.

101. *Bngl VR 1873*, 2–3.

102. *Bngl VR 1893–6*, xxiv–xxviii.

103. *Bmb VR 1867*, 19; *NWP VR 1872–3*, 14, 27; *Bngl VR 1873*, 4; *Bngl VR 1888–9*, 3; *Annual Report of the Calcutta Corporation 1898–9*, 2:39–40.

104. James 1909: 14; McLeod, 20 Mar. 1872, Home (Pub), 156, Mar. 1873, NAI.

105. Cuningham to Under Sec, Agriculture, Revenue and Commerce, 25 Sept. 1872, Home (Pub), 151, Nov. 1872, NAI.

106. Strachey, 3 Oct. 1872, ibid.

107. Legis, 12, Apr. 1865, NAI.

108. James 1909, 14.

109. Dalal 1930, 2:69–77.

110. Home (Jud), 89, Feb. 1890, NAI; Gidumal 1888, 222.

111. Legis, 95, 151, Aug. 1880, NAI. Sayyid Ahmad Khan's speeches are also printed in Mohammad, ed., 1972, 138–48. For his career and views generally, see Malik 1980.

112. Legis, 88–167, Aug. 1880, NAI.

113. Home (Pub), 246, Apr. 1872, NAI; see also discussion of compulsory vaccination in Bombay Presidency in Bmb Gen, 1, 706, 1894, MSA.

114. James 1909, 33; *Annual Report of the Director-General of Health Services 1950*, 53.

115. *Bmb VR 1895–6*, 22; *Md VR 1893–4*, 5.

116. *Md VR 1898–9*, 2; James 1909, 100.

117. E.g., *Bngl VR 1869*, xiii, and i of government review.

CHAPTER 4

1. The political and social impact of cholera epidemics on nineteenth-century Europe and North America has been widely discussed: see Durey 1979; McGrew 1965; Rosenberg 1962.

2. Steuart and Philipps 1819, i.

3. Annesley 1825, xv.

4. Anon. 1831, 613.

5. A. Stewart, "Circular to superintending surgeons," 3 Aug. 1818, BC F/4/595/14376, IOL. For a modern clinical account of cholera, see Barua and Burrows, eds., 1974, 129.

6. F. J. Mouat, 1858, cited in Tinker 1974, 141.

7. Scriven 1863, 14.

8. Rogers 1928, 8.

9. Moreau de Jonnès 1831, 76, 84.

10. Anon. 1831, 614; Fabre and Chailan 1835, 10.

11. Jameson 1820, 27, 170–75. For Calcutta, see also Bngl to CoD, 22 July 1818, BC F/4/610/15058, IOL.

12. Macnamara 1870, 25; Sec, Med Board to CS, Bombay, 13 Sept. 1819, Bmb Pub Procs, 29 Sept. 1819, IOL.

13. Scot 1824, 43–49; Colr, Cuddapah, to BoR, Md, 20 Sept. 1819, Md BoR Procs, 30 Sept. 1819, IOL.

14. Scot 1824, 29.

15. Jameson 1820, iii, 170, 183.

16. Kennedy 1846, 88.

17. Rogers 1928, 28, 37; *Md SCAR 1877*, lxiii.

18. Pollitzer 1959; Arnold 1989.

19. Kennedy 1827, v–vi.

20. Young 1831, 63. In the cholera year of 1877, 65 Europeans died of the disease in the Madras Presidency, equal to 4.4 per 1,000 of the European population; among Indians the equivalent rate was 12.2 (*Md SCAR 1887*, lxvii). By 1900 Europeans were said no longer to dread cholera (Giles 1904, 131–32).

21. Jameson 1820, 110–11.

22. Steuart and Philipps 1819, xxxi; Scot 1824, 167.

23. J. M. Cuningham, SC, to Sec, India, 13 June 1871, San Procs, 2, 1 July 1871, IOL. For the continuing association of cholera with Calcutta, see Pollitzer 1959, 94; Banerjee and Hazra 1974, 5.

24. *Bmb SCAR 1877*, 170; *Md SCAR 1877*, lxiii.

25. Rogers 1928, 32.

26. Madras, *Review of the Madras Famine, 1876–78* 1881, 125; *Md SCAR 1880*, 12. However, many recorded cases of cholera may in fact have been "famine diarrhea" (W. R. Cornish in *Md SCAR 1877*, xxv).

27. Ibid., xxv–xxvi; cf. Post 1990.

28. J. Kellie, "Remarks on the Cause of Epidemic Cholera," in Rogers, ed., 1848, 232, 235.

29. Jameson 1820, 12–17.

30. Roberts 1897, 1:185; Rotton 1858, 199–219; Wise 1894.

31. "History of the cholera epidemic of 1867 in northern India," V/25/840/1A, IOL, pp. 319–20.

32. India, *Report of the Commissioners Appointed to Inquire into the Cholera Epidemic of 1861 in Northern India*, 63.

33. Sleeman 1844, 1:211–12; Crooke 1896, 1:138–40.

34. Scot 1824, 237.

35. Clough 1899, 90–94.

36. Moreau de Jonnès 1831, 114. For other interpretations linking cholera to British invasion and interference, see Enthoven 1924, 258. As this and other sources make clear, British rule was only one, if a particularly common, explanation given for the cholera epidemics.

37. Macnamara 1876, 34–36; Hora 1933, 1–4; Basu 1963, 25–28, 195–98 (with thanks to Gautam Bhadra for these references).

38. MacPherson 1872, 6, 115; Steuart and Philipps 1819, xxvii.

39. E.g., Opler 1963, 35; Beals 1976, 195–96; Hardiman 1987.

40. Keith, Calcutta, to LMS, London, 1 Jan. 1818, LMS Archive, SOAS, London.

41. Kennedy 1846, ix–x.

42. J. Babington, Criminal Judge, Northern Konkan, to CS, Bmb, 10 Jan. 1820; petition from the "Christian Coolies of Chendnee," 28 Sept. 1818, BC F/4/768/20874, IOL.

43. F. A. Oakes, Colr, Guntur, to BoR, 31 May 1819, Md BoR Procs, 7 June 1819, IOL; Colr, Cuddapah, to BoR, 14 Apr. 1820, Md BoR Procs, 24 Apr. 1820, IOL.

44. BoR to CS, Md, 17 Apr. 1820, Md BoR Procs, 17 Apr. 1820, IOL; Md BoR Procs, 25 May 1820, IOL.

45. Kennedy 1827, x–xii.

46. Keith to LMS, 1 Jan. 1818, LMS Archive.

47. The ways in which Muslims responded to cholera epidemics are less well documented, but see Thurston 1912, 119–20; North-Western Provinces, *Reports on Cholera in the Meerut, Rohilcund and Ajmere Divisions in the Year 1856*, 11.

48. Whitehead 1921, 37–39, citing J. F. Richards, 1920. See also Weir 1886; Fawcett 1890.

49. Crooke 1896, 1:141–43, 166–70; *Gazetteer of the Bombay Presidency*, vol. 9, part 1, 1910: 414–15; Francis 1907, 75.

50. Crooke 1896, 1:170; Abbott 1932, 112; Haikerwal 1934, 66–67.

51. Guha 1983, 238–46. See also Dunlop 1858, 24–26; Sen 1957, 398–400.

52. Mgt, Agra, to Comr, NWP, 27 Apr. 1860, NWP Jud Procs, 29 May 1860, IOL.

53. Comr, Agra, to Sec, NWP, 10 May 1860, ibid.

54. J. Babington, Judge, and S. Marriott, Mgt, Northern Konkan, to CS, Bmb, 15 Aug. 1818, Bmb Pub Procs, 26 Aug. 1818, IOL.

55. Minute, 21 Aug. 1818, ibid.

56. *Reports on Cholera, 1856*, 28–29; Crooke 1896, 1:141.

57. R. Tytler to Mgt, Jessore, 23 Aug. 1817, BC F/4/610/15058, IOL; Scot 1824, 203; Steuart and Philipps 1819, xlii. Cf. Curtis 1807, 81, 125.

58. Jameson 1820, 205–6; Smith 1861, 72–74.

59. Undated "Instructions" sent by Sec, Bngl Med Board, to Sec, Bngl, 20 Sept. 1817, BC, F/4/610/15058, IOL.

60. Tamil address of Maha Ganapati Sastri and Ramakrishna Sastri, 19 Oct. 1818; Sec, Md, to Med Board, 5 Nov. 1818; Sec, Med Board, to CS, Md, 6 Nov. 1818, Md Pub Procs, 10 Nov. 1818, IOL.

61. Jameson 1820, 243–44.

62. *Reports on Cholera, 1856*, 10–11; Murray 1856, 9.

63. Judge, Southern Konkan, to CS, Bmb, 19 May 1820, Bmb Pub Procs, 24 May 1820, IOL; *Reports on Cholera, 1856*, 11.

64. Steuart and Philipps 1819, xxxviii; Scot 1824, 203; cf. Howard-Jones 1972, 373–95. But some surgeons bled Indian patients for cholera, e.g., Hutchinson 1832, 135–76.

65. Sec, Med Board, to CS, Bmb, 22 Apr. 1819, Bmb Pub Procs, 28 Apr. 1819: Colr, Guntur, to BoR, 21 Oct. 1823, Md BoR Procs, 27 Oct. 1823, IOL.

66. Md Med Board to Madras, 31 May 1819, Md Pub Procs, 11 June 1819, IOL.

67. Sec, Bngl, to Mgt, Murshidabad, 25 Nov. 1817, BC F/4/610/15058, IOL.

68. Chapman in Rogers, ed., 1848, 207.

69. Scot 1849, 116; cf. Martin 1856, 350–51.

70. John Murray, "Report on the Hurdwar cholera of 1867," in Madras, *Report Regarding the Control of Pilgrimages in the Madras Presidency* 1868, appendix B; Malleson 1868. More recent medical assessments have tended to endorse the importance of Hindu fairs and festivals in cholera epidemics. See Lal 1937; Banerjea 1951; Pollitzer 1959.

71. Jameson 1820, xvi–xvii; Steuart and Philipps 1819, 151.

72. Moreau de Jonnès 1831, 143–45, 179.

73. Buchanan 1812, 22–28.

74. Ingram 1956, 35–53; Cassels 1987.

75. *Missionary Register 1828*, 560.

76. Buckley to Civil Asst Surgeon, Cuttack, 28 Nov. 1867, Home (Pub), 164, 1 Jan. 1870, NAI.

77. Conférence Sanitaire Internationale 1866, 21. On cholera, the hajj, and the international sanitary conferences, see Howard-Jones 1975; Roff 1982.

78. Smith 1868, part 2, 5, 8.

79. Ibid., part 2, 11–12.

80. Ibid., part 2, 36.

81. Cornish 1871, 150.

82. Hunter 1872, 1:145, 156, 166–67.

83. India, *Proceedings of the International Sanitary Conference Opened at Constantinople on the 13th February 1866*, 8.

84. Malleson 1868; Home (Pub), 163–240, 1 Jan. 1870, NAI.

85. *Report of Cholera Committee* 1868; *Control of Pilgrimages in Madras*.

86. Home (Pub), 163–240, 1 Jan. 1870, NAI.

87. Hunter 1872, 1:157–58.

88. Ibid., 165.

89. Smith 1868, part 4, 7.

90. *Control of Pilgrimages in Madras*, 40.

91. Under-Sec's note, 28 May 1868, Home (Pub), 163–240, 1 Jan. 1870, NAI.

92. For the local administration of north Indian pilgrimage sites in the late nineteenth-century, see Prior 1990, 180–226.

93. Cuningham 1884, 24; cf. Maclean 1824; White 1837.

94. Christie 1828, 97; Corbyn 1832, 110; but for a contagionist view, see Hutchinson 1832.

95. Jameson 1820, 27, 87.

96. Murray, "Report on the Hurdwar cholera of 1867."

97. For the controversy between Cuningham and de Renzy, see San Procs, 4–7, Feb. 1872, IOL; San Procs, 12–13, Feb. 1875, NAI; Klein 1980, 39–40. Rogers (1928, 12) thought the most charitable view that could be taken of Cuningham was that "he considered it his duty to support in every way possible the political views of the Government of India."

98. Cuningham 1884, 23.

99. *Lancet* 1874 1:482–83.

100. Cuningham, n.d., 21, 23.

101. Bryden 1869, 91–92, 243. An obituary of Bryden commented on his "too lively powers of generalization." "He found pathology and etiology in his numbers, and drew from them inferences which, to his mind, possessed all the reality of objective existences whereas they were but subjective creations—often mere figures of speech." *IMG* 1881, 16:23.

102. Cornish 1871, 1–4; Rogers 1928, 58, 83.

103. Cuningham to Under Sec, 21 Dec. 1871, San Procs, 5, Feb. 1872, IOL.

104. Lewis and Cunningham 1878, 115.

105. Bellew 1885, v.

106. Cuningham, notes, 21 July and 1 Sept. 1884, Home (San), 16–30, Oct. 1884, NAI; Cuningham 1884, 108–21.

107. Fayrer to Under SoS for India, 19 May 1884, Home (San), 21, Oct. 1884, NAI; Klein and Gibbes 1885. For the gradual and partial acceptance of Koch's bacillus theory, see Harrison 1991, 177–82.

108. "It is no longer theory to suppose that climatic factors have a definite relationship with the incidence of cholera in India" (Russell and Sundarajan in *India HCAR 1928*, 59). Cf. King in *Md SCAR 1893*, 61–62; Rogers 1928, 4.

109. Rogers 1928, 6.

110. *NWP SCAR 1892*, 29; Memorial of the "General orthodox Hindu meeting," Lahore, 15 July 1892, Home (Pub), 109, Aug. 1892, NAI; Sec, British Indian Association, to Sec, Home, 18 June 1892, Home (Pub), 25, Dec. 1892, NAI. For this episode, see also Prior 1990, 203–16.

111. Roberts 1897, 1:443.

112. Roberts, 2 Oct. 1892, and Lansdowne 5 Oct. 1892, Home (Jud), 94, Jan. 1893, NAI.

113. Sec, Home, to Sec, Bmb, 24 July 1905, Home (San), 320, July 1905, NAI.

114. Martin 1856, 340.

115. Rogers 1957, 1193.

116. Haffkine 1895; Rice, 20 Oct. 1893, Home (San), 21, Dec. 1893, NAI; see also the notes to Home (Med), 10, Apr. 1900, NAI.

117. *India HCAR 1930*, 1:91.

118. Banerjea 1951, 32–33.

CHAPTER 5

1. Klein 1973, 639.

2. Ibid., 639–43; Davis 1951, 36–52; Mills 1988, 1–40.

3. For mortality in Bombay, see Klein 1986, 725–54.

4. *India HCAR 1929*, 1:69. For the epidemiology of plague in India, see Hirst 1953.

5. Crooke 1926, 118. Whitehead 1921 contains photographs of a shrine to a "Plague-Amma" ("Mother") at Bangalore (plates XI, XII).

6. Bmb to Bngl, 1 Oct. 1896, Mun (Med), 32, Feb. 1897, WBSA.

7. Snow 1897, 1–6, 11–12, 15; Couchman 1897, 5ff.

8. Legis, 37–46, Feb. 1897, NAI.

9. Couchman 1897, 5, 17; Gatacre 1897, 3.

10. Catanach 1988, 151–52.

11. Sir John Woodburn, procs of Governor-General's Council, 4 Feb. 1897, Legis, 37–46, appendix 23, Feb. 1897, NAI. The viceroy, Elgin, in a letter to the secretary of state for India, Lord Hamilton, 10 Feb. 1897, also referred to "the fear that foreign powers might introduce regulations and re- strictions disastrous to the commerce of the country" among his reasons for the Epidemic Diseases Act: Home (San), 75, Feb. 1897, NAI.

12. Couchman 1897, 33–34; Howard-Jones 1975, 78–80.

13. The "mahamari" reported in Kumaon between the 1820s and 1850s was probably typhus rather than plague; but the "Pali plague" of the 1830s in Rajasthan might well have been bubonic plague: Renny 1851; Stiven 1854; Adams 1899, 230–31.

14. Report of Pune Municipality, 2 June 1897, Bmb, Gen, 70, 908, 1898, MSA.

15. Lt.-Governor, Bngl, in Governor-General's Council, 4 Feb. 1897, Legis, 37–46, appendix 23, Feb. 1897, NAI.

16. Snow 1897, 5.

17. Ibid., 5; Morris 1965, 55.

18. J. Neild Cook, health officer, Calcutta, "Report on plague in Calcutta, 31 August 1898," *Report of the Epidemics of Plague in Calcutta* 1900: 10–11.

19. Snow 1897, 7.

20. Resol, 10 Oct. 1896, Bngl, Mun (Med), 68, Feb. 1897, WBSA; R. Harvey's note on plague administration, 18 Apr. 1898, Home 784, Aug. 1898, NAI.

21. Couchman 1897, 24. Only seven deaths among "pure Europeans" were reported between November 1896 and April 1898, but there were 18 among "domiciled Europeans" (perhaps here including Anglo-Indians): Campbell 1898, 105.

22. Catanach 1988, 156.

23. Woodburn, in Governor-General's Council, 4 Feb. 1897, appendix 23, Legis, 37–46, Feb. 1897, NAI; Cleghorn, note, 2 Feb. 1897, Home (San), 65, Feb. 1897, NAI.

24. Resol, 10 Oct. 1896, Bngl, Mun (Med), 68, Feb. 1897, WBSA.

25. Undated report by W. C. Rand, in *Supplement to the Account of Plague Administration in the Bombay Presidency from September 1896 till May 1897*, 2–3; Catanach 1988, 153.

26. Bngl, Mun (Med), 115, Feb, 1897, WBSA.

27. Cook, "Report on plague in Calcutta," 10; Bngl, Mun (Med), 121, Feb. 1897, WBSA.

28. Cf. Arnold, ed., 1988.

29. India, *The Etiology and Epidemiology of Plague: A Summary of the Work of the Plague Commission* 1908, 2, 81–83; Catanach 1988, 163.

30. Gatacre 1897, 51.

31. Nathan 1898, 1:40.

32. Campbell 1898, 52.

33. *Mahratta*, 30 Dec. 1896. For the role of the press in government policy, see Paul 1979, chap. 5.

34. *Bangavasi*, 27 Feb. 1897, Bngl *NNR*.

35. *Mahratta*, 27 June 1897, 3; cf. *Hitavadi*, 12 Feb. 1897, Bngl *NNR*.

36. *Gujarati*, 18 Apr. 1897, Bmb *NNR*.

37. Snow 1897, 74.

38. *Gujarati*, 18 Apr. 1897, Bmb *NNR*; *Dnyan Prakash*, 19 Apr. 1897, Bmb *NNR*.

39. *Mahratta*, 21 Nov. 1897, Bmb *NNR*.

40. Gatacre 1897, 51.

41. *Kesari*, 6 Apr. 1897, Bmb *NNR*; *Mahratta*, 23 May 1897, 5.

42. Gatacre 1897, 14.

43. Mukherjee to Sec, Mun, 3 Oct. 1896, Bngl, Mun (Med), 40 Feb. 1896, WBSA.

44. Gatacre 1897, 14.

45. *Prabakar*, 30 Oct. 1896; *Kaiser-e-Hind*, 1 Nov. 1896, Bmb *NNR*.

46. Campbell 1898, 23–24; *Vartahar*, 23 Mar. 1898, Bmb *NNR*.

47. Home (Pub), 291–302, June 1900, NAI; *Hindustan*, 15 Apr. 1900, NWP *NNR*.

48. *Kalapataru*, 24 Oct. 1897, Bmb *NNR*. The standard procedure for male passengers was for them to "open their body clothing, and a Medical Officer feels each man's chest with both hands, which enables him to detect any increase of temperature. The superficial glands in the neck, arm-pits, and groins are then examined. The tongue and eyes are looked at." If a high temperature or enlarged or tender glands were detected, the traveler was sent for a more thorough examination: Home (San), 250, July 1900, NAI.

49. *Gurakhi*, 19 Feb. 1897, Bmb *NNR*; also *Bangavasi*, 27 Feb. 1897, Bngl *NNR*.

50. *Nizam-ul-Mulk*, 16 Apr. 1900, NWP *NNR*. At Kalyan, 3,320 plague suspects had been removed from trains up to the end of December 1898, of whom 234 were later found to have plague. In Bengal 1.8 million travelers were examined in the same period, and of these 41,854 were detained: Home (San), 250, July 1900, NAI.

51. *Champion*, 18 July 1897; *Dnyan Prakash* 19 Apr. 1897; *Sudharak*, 10 May 1897, Bmb *NNR*.

52. *Vartahar*, 10 Jan. 1898, Bmb *NNR*.

53. *Dnyan Prakash*, 15 Mar. 1897, Bmb *NNR*.

54. *Bombay Samachar*, 12 May 1897, Bmb *NNR*; *Hitavadi*, 13 May 1898, Bngl *NNR*.

55. *Dnyan Prakash*, 15 Mar. 1897; *Kesari*, 6 Apr. 1897, Bmb *NNR*. Rand's committee, by contrast, found it "a matter of great satisfaction" that "no credible complaint that the modesty of a woman had been intentionally insulted was ever made either to themselves or to the officers under whom the troops worked": Rand in *Supplement to the Account of Plague Administration in the Bombay Presidency*, 34.

56. *Moda Vritt*, 15 July 1897; *Kesari*, 2 Feb. 1898, Bmb *NNR*.

57. Bngl, Mun (Med), 89, Feb. 1898, WBSA.

58. SoS to Bmb, 24 Aug. 1897, Home (San), 142, Sept. 1897, NAI. Surgeon-Major W. S. Reade, in urging that corpse inspection be adopted as the "sheet-anchor" of plague detection, could see nothing in it to "hurt the caste or susceptibilities of the various races of India": Bngl, Mun (Med), 2 Feb. 1898, WBSA.

59. Elgin to Governor, Bmb, 26 Aug. 1897, Home (San), 143, Sept. 1897, NAI; Campbell 1898, 23.

60. *Hitavadi*, 30 Oct. 1896, Bngl *NNR*.

61. *Mahratta*, 6 June 1897, 4.

62. Harvey, 21 June 1900, Home (San), 244–52, July 1900, NAI.

63. NWP resol, 27 Apr. 1898, Home (San), 521, May 1898, NAI.

64. *Praja Pokar*, 10 Mar. 1897; *Deshi Mitra*, 11 Mar. 1897, Bmb *NNR*.

65. Rand in *Supplement to the Account of Plague Administration in the Bombay Presidency*, 7; Gatacre 1897, 179–80; Campbell 1898, 56, 64.

66. *Vartanidhi*, 3 Mar. 1897; *Champion*, 21 Mar. 1897; *Ahmedabad Times*, 11 Apr. 1897; *Indian Spectator*, 20 May 1898, Bmb *NNR*.

67. *Hindustan*, 26 Apr. 1900, NWP *NNR*; Snow 1897, 4.

68. Cook, "Report on plague in Calcutta," 25.

69. *Civil and Military News*, 18 May 1898, Pnjb *NNR*; *Hitavadi*, 6 May 1898, Bngl *NNR*; Mgt, Howrah, to Comr, Burdwan, 5 May 1898, Bngl, Jud (Police), 14–16, Aug. 1898, WBSA.

70. Dy Comr to Comr, Delhi, 5 Mar. 1898, Home (San), 550, May 1898, NAI.

71. Home (San) (Plague), 16 July 1900, in San Despatches to London, 14, 26 July 1900, IOL. For a seminal discussion of rumor in India, see Guha 1983, 251–77.

72. NWP resol, 15 May 1900, Home (Pub), 298, June 1900, NAI.

73. *Poona Vaibhar*, 21 Feb. 1897, Bmb *NNR*. Famine was widespread in western India at the time.

74. *Hindustan*, 26 Apr. 1900, NWP *NNR*.

75. Wilkinson 1904a, 71.

76. *Mahratta*, 20 Dec. 1896, 1, 3.

77. Snow 1897, 15.

78. *Kaiser-e-Hind*, 1 Nov. 1896, Bmb *NNR*.

79. Crooke linked *momiai* with the Arabic *mumiya*, an embalmed body (hence the English "mummy") and *mum*, meaning "wax." In India the term connoted a magical balm thought to cure wounds and to make the user invulnerable: Crooke 1926, 111–12. I am grateful to David Hardiman for drawing my attention to this and the following sources.

80. Enthoven, preface to ibid., 2.

81. Lely 1906, 29.

82. Maconochie 1926, 83.

83. *Indian Spectator*, 1 Nov. 1896, Bmb *NNR*.

84. *Tohfah-i-Hind*, 20 Apr. 1900, NWP *NNR*; Wilkinson 1904a, 71; Cook, "Report on plague in Calcutta," 14.

85. *Bangavasi*, 14 May 1898; Cook, "Report on plague in Calcutta," 14, 23–25.

86. *Prayag Samachar*, 8 May 1899, NWP *NNR*.

87. *Aftab-i-Punjab*, 9 May 1898, Pnjb *NNR*; Wilkinson 1904a, 28; Maconochie 1926, 208.

88. Wilkinson 1904a, 28.

89. Cook, "Report on plague in Calcutta," 25; cf. Catanach 1983, 224–26.

90. *Mahratta*, 23 Jan. 1898, 1; Lely 1906, 29.

91. Home (San) (Plague), 16 July 1900, San Despatches, 14, 26 July 1900, IOL.

92. Cook, "Report on plague in Calcutta," 23.

93. Home (San), 543–50, May 1898, NAI; *Patiala Akhbar*, 21 Jan. 1898, Pnjb *NNR*.

94. *Prayag Samachar*, 20 Apr. 1899; *Liberal* (Azamgarh), 24 Sept. 1899; *Oudh Akhbar* (Lucknow), 30 Oct. 1899, NWP *NNR*.

95. *Hindustan*, 8 Apr. 1899, NWP *NNR*.

96. NWP resol, 15 May 1900, Home (Pub), 298, June 1900, NAI.

97. Cook, "Report on plague in Calcutta," 10.

98. *Poona Vaibhar*, 21 Feb. 1897, Bmb *NNR*.

99. Mgt, Howrah, to Comr, Burdwan, 5 May 1898, Bngl, Jud (Police), 14 Aug. 1898, WBSA; Cook, "Report on plague in Calcutta," 23–25.

100. *Mahratta*, 28 Mar. 1897, 3.

101. *Kaiser-e-Hind*, 1 Nov. 1896; *Kalpataru*, 3 Mar. 1897; *Indian Spectator*, 7 Mar. 1897; *Gurakhi*, 4 Feb. 1898; *Dhureen*, 9 Mar. 1898, Bmb *NNR*.

102. *Hitavadi*, 13 May 1898, Bngl *NNR*.

103. *Basumati*, 12 May 1898, Bmb *NNR*.

104. *Mahratta*, 5 Mar. 1898, Bmb *NNR*.

105. Gatacre 1898, 223–31. For the attitude of the European press in India, see *Mahratta*, 11 Apr. 1897, 6.

106. Nathan 1898, 1:436.

107. Wilkinson 1904a, 5. Cf. Catanach 1984: 183–92.

108. For events in Pune in 1896–97, see Cashman 1975, 113; Catanach 1987, 198–215; Karandikar, n.d., 134–70; Parvate 1958: 82–91.

109. Bmb resol, 26 June 1885, Bmb Gen, 91, 332, 1885, MSA.

110. Lamb to Spence, 3 May 1897, Bmb, Gen, 70, 908, 1898, MSA.

111. Spence, 7 May 1897, and note (by CS?), 18 May 1897, ibid.

112. Rand in *Supplement to the Account of Plague Administration in the Bombay Presidency*, 7, 12–14.

113. *Mahratta*, 14 Mar. 1897, 1, 3. The other members were Surgeon-Captain W. W. O. Beveridge and Lt.-Col. C. R. Phillips.

114. Lamb, 28 Feb. 1897; Rand in *Supplement to the Account of Plague Administration in the Bombay Presidency*, 3.

115. Rand, ibid., 7.

116. *Annual Report of Poona City Municipality, 1896–97*, 25.

117. For Barry's report and Lamb's endorsement, see Bmb, Gen, 70, 908, 1898, MSA.

118. Lamb to Spence, 18 June 1897, and memos by Spence, 21 June 1897, and C. Ollivant, 19 Sept. 1898, ibid.

119. *Mahratta*, 31 Oct. 1897; *Kesari*, 2 Nov. 1897; *Moda Vritt*, 4 Nov. 1897, Bmb *NNR*.

120. Furedy 1978, 77–78, 81. See H. H. Risley, to Sec, Home, 2 Nov. 1897, KW II to Home (San), 197–205, Dec. 1897, NAI.

121. Resol, 3 Feb. 1898, Home, 300, Feb, 1898, NAI.

122. *Aftab-i-Punjab*, 9 May 1898, Pnjb *NNR*. For the various riots, see: Home (San), 294, May 1898, NAI; Mun (Med), 14–16, Aug. 1898, WBSA; Home (San), 177–82, Dec. 1898, NAI; Home (San), 720–24, Jan. 1899, NAI; Prior 1990, 216–24.

123. E.g., at Pune on 2 Apr. 1897 (*Mahratta*, 4 Apr. 1897) and Bombay in Mar. 1897 (*Muslim Herald*, 24 Mar. 1897), Bmb *NNR*.

124. Elgin, 14 June 1897, Home (San), 483–90, July 1897, NAI.

125. Home (San), 553, May 1898, NAI; *Akhbar-i-Am*, 9 Feb. 1898, Pnjb *NNR*.

126. Home (San), 554, May 1898, NAI.

127. Surgeon-Major Bannerman, Dy SC, Md, 12 Apr. 1898, Home, (San), 812, Aug. 1898, NAI.

128. MacDonnell to Elgin, 29 Apr. 1898, Home, 777–813, KW V, Aug. 1898, NAI.

129. Harvey's note, 18 Apr. 1898, Home, 784, ibid.

130. Haffkine, "Report on bacteriology of plague," 1 Oct. 1897, in Snow 1897, 40; see also Haffkine to Government of India, 21 June 1898, Home (San), 766, Aug. 1898, NAI.

131. Harvey, note, 5 July 1898, Home (San), 766–71, Aug. 1898. On Haffkine's Indian career, see Lutzker, n.d., 11–19.

132. J. P. Hewett, Sec, Home, to CSs, etc., 19 Aug. 1898, Home (San), 804, Aug. 1898, NAI; Sec, Bngl, to Sec, Home, 9 Mar. 1900, Home (San), 13, Apr. 1900, NAI; Wilkinson 1904b, 6–7; *Punjab Plague Manual, 1909*, 1.

133. Wilkinson 1904b, 10–12; Home (San), 51–64, Jan. 1905, NAI; Home (San), 151–62, Dec. 1906, NAI; Home (San), 165–71, Jan. 1908, NAI; Catanach 1988, 159–61.

134. Campbell 1898, 24.

135. Comr, Delhi, to Sec, Pnjb, 7 Mar. 1898, Home (San), 549, May 1898, NAI.

136. MacDonnell, 1 Apr. 1898, Home (San), 173, Apr. 1898, NAI; Mac-Donnell to Viceroy, 16 Apr. 1900, Home (Pub), 293, June 1900, NAI; Campbell 1898, 54–55.

137. *Kesari*, 28 Sept. 1897, Bmb *NNR*.

138. *Mahratta*, 26 Nov. 1897, Bmb *NNR*.

139. Elgin to SoS, 25 Aug. 1898, Home, 809, Aug. 1898, NAI.

140. *Administrative Report of the Commissioners of Calcutta for 1898–99*, 1:13. (See *Annual Administration Reports of the Corporation* in bibliography.)

141. Great Britain, *The Indian Plague Commission, 1898–99* (Cd 139), 1900. For the setting up of the commission and the official reception of its report, see notes to Home, 777–813, Aug. 1898, NAI; Home (San), 244–52, July 1900, NAI.

142. *Etiology and Epidemiology of Plague*, i.

143. Catanach 1988, 165–66, Hirst 1953.

144. It could be argued that some of these changes were in the pipeline anyway: Harrison 1990, 19–40. But plague was undoubtedly an important accelerator and facilitator.

145. Snow 1897, 16; Campbell 1898, 60, 137.

146. *Gazetteer of Bombay City and Island* 1910, 3:186ff. For the effects of plague operations on vaccination and hospital admissions, see *India SCAR 1899*, 143; Cook, "Report on plague in Calcutta," 23.

147. India, *Proceedings of the First All-India Sanitary Conference* 1912, 1–2.

CHAPTER 6

1. Bates 1975, 352. For the ancestry of the term *hegemony* and Gramsci's use of it, see Anderson 1976–77, 5–78.

2. Femia 1975, 31.

3. Buci-Glucksmann 1980, 110; 1982, 119.

4. Gramsci 1971, 12.

5. Ibid., 170, 263.

6. Ibid., 263.

7. The phrase "limited raj" belongs to Yang 1989, but cf. Frykenberg 1965. For an extended discussion of hegemony in India, which concludes that colonialism was characterized by a failure of hegemony, see Guha 1989. The concept of hegemony as "ideological domination" is also effectively discussed in Scott 1985, 314ff.

8. Lovett 1899, 2:223; Hacker 1887, 54.

9. Barnes 1903. For an example of such medical proselytizing among women in Punjab in the 1880s, see Greenfield 1886, and for the "cultural imperialism" of the zenana missions, Forbes 1986.

10. Quoted in Grant 1894, 1:ciii–civ. Harvey spoke in similar terms in his presidential address to the Indian Medical Congress at Calcutta in 1894: *IMG* 1895, 30:1–6.

11. Tinker 1968, 73, 287–89.

12. Gangulee 1939, 145–46.

13. Crawford 1914, 2:391–432. For Bombay, see *Gazetteer of Bombay City and Island* 1910, 3:181–84.

14. Bengal, *Report of the Committee for the Establishment of a Fever Hospital . . . in Calcutta* 1840, 35, 46; Auckland to Martin, 24 May 1836, ibid., appendix B, 6.

15. Auckland to Martin, 24 May 1836, ibid., appendix B, 6.

16. J. R. Martin, 29 Apr. 1837, D. Stewart, 1 May 1837, ibid., appendix C, xciii–iv, xcvi.

17. *The Imperial Gazetteer of India* 1907, 4:462.

18. *MARCD 1852*, 4; *1860*, 4; *MARCHD 1891*, 3, 7.

19. *MARCHD 1900*. For continuing deficiencies in rural health care after 1914, see Muraleedharan 1987.

20. *MARCD 1855*, 6; *MARCHD 1900*, 6.

21. David Hare to J. C. Sutherland, 9 Mar. 1837, *Report of the Committee for the Establishment of a Fever Hospital*, appendix B, 16. For low-caste servants sent by European employers, see Ramcomul Sen, 8 May 1837, ibid., civ, and, in Bombay's hospitals, Morehead 1856, 1:13.

22. *MARCD 1866*, 22.

23. *MARCD 1852*, 12; *1855*, 62; *1863*, 22, 27.

24. *MARCD 1861*, 64.

25. *MARCD 1852*, 14.

26. Day 1902, 250.

27. *MARCHD 1880*, 8.

28. *MARCD 1852*, 23.

29. *MARCD 1868–9*, 69.

30. *MARCD 1853*, 1.

31. *MARCD 1856*, 2.

32. *MARCD 1857*, vii.

33. *MARCD 1858*, 79.

34. Ibid., 110, 160.

35. Balfour and Young 1929, 124–25.

36. Clark 1773, 41–42.

37. Twining 1835, 1:27, 2:437–38.

38. Moore 1877, viii, ix.

39. Mill 1858, 1:309, 311.

40. Nair 1990.

41. In 1919 one-quarter of all infant mortality in the United Provinces was attributed to tetanus: *UP SCAR 1919*, 5. On TB, see Kailas Chunder Bose, "Tuberculosis," in India, *Proceedings of the First All-India Sanitary Conference 1911*, 133–6.

42. *DFAR 1890*, 112.
43. Billington 1895, 2.
44. Cited in Jaggi 1979, 143. Cf. Mayo 1927.
45. *MARCD 1858*, 37; Ranking 1868.
46. *DFAR 1890*, 197.
47. *Administration Report of the Corporation of Madras Health Department 1913*, 28.
48. Ibid., 34.
49. *MARCHD 1891*, 8, 13.
50. *MARCHD 1900*, 186; *DFAR 1890*, 130.
51. Home (Pub), 50, 9 July 1870, NAI; Balfour and Young 1929, 13, 129.
52. Home (Med), 91–97, Oct. 1888, NAI; *DFAR 1895*, 77–78.
53. *DFAR 1910*, 61–62.
54. India, Home (Med), 124–48, Sept. 1914, NAI; Balfour and Young 1929, 130–31, 139.
55. Ibid., 128; Blackham cited in Jaggi 1979, 143.
56. *IMG* Oct. 1875, 274–75; July 1882, 184.
57. Scharlieb 1924.
58. Hoggan 1882.
59. Kittredge 1889, 3.
60. Ibid., 11.
61. Lutzker 1973; Blake 1990.
62. Kittredge 1889, 29–30.
63. *DFAR 1890*, 8.
64. Engels, forthcoming. For a more balanced account, see Balfour and Young 1929.
65. *DFAR 1895*, 267; *Report of the Bengal Branch of the Dufferin Fund 1900*, 10.
66. *DFAR 1907*, 28.
67. *IMG*, Apr. 1899, 134.
68. *DFAR 1890*, 8.
69. *DFAR 1895*, 269, 282.
70. *DFAR 1890*, 16; *1895*, 86; *1910*, 8–9.
71. *DFAR 1895*, 277.
72. For the debates and issues of the period, see Heimsath 1964; Engels 1983.
73. Lutzker 1973, 193.
74. *DFAR 1890*, 15; see the *NNRs* of the period for Bombay, e.g., *Mahratta*, 10 Apr. 1886, *Subodh Patrika* 4 Apr. 1886; *Jame Jamshed*, 21 Aug. 1886.
75. Engels, forthcoming.
76. GO 1490, Md, Local and Mun (Plague), 2 Dec. 1898, TNA; *NNRs* Bombay and Bengal, Feb.–Mar. 1897; *Mahratta*, 17 Oct. 1897.
77. Bngl Mun (Med), 13–138, Feb. 1897, WBSA; Home (San), 197–205, Dec. 1897, NAI .

78. *DFAR 1890*, 19, 21, 71–78; *1895*, 13, 160, 354–56.

79. *DFAR 1928*, 84.

80. Dufferin to SoS, 11 Sept. 1886, Home (Med), 85, Sept. 1886, NAI.

81. Home (Med), 39–42, Feb. 1912, NAI; *DFAR 1911*, 2–5.

82. *DFAR 1928*, 85–86.

83. Borthwick 1984, 164.

84. *Imperial Gazetteer of India* 1907, 4:461–62.

85. GO 983, Med, 9 July 1861, *MARCD 1859*, i; *1865*, 8–9; GO 610, Pub, 1 Sept., 1892, *MARCHD 1891*, 1.

86. Hemingway 1906, 157–58.

87. *DFAR 1890*, 28–29.

88. *DFAR 1895*, 52.

89. For princely patronage, see *DFAR 1890*, 13–14; cf. Hutchins 1967, chap. 8.

90. By 1900 the net was being cast more widely: for instance, the patrons and management committee of the Madras Caste and Gosha Hospital included not only the Prince of Arcot and Nawab Begum of Carnatic but also lawyers, judges, and other members of the new urban elite: *Report of the Victoria Hospital for Caste and Gosha Women, Madras, 1900*. The appeal for Calcutta's School of Tropical Medicine, launched in 1914, ranged even more widely across princes, zamindars, the urban middle class, and European business houses: Bengal, *An Appeal on Behalf of the Calcutta School of Tropical Medicine and Hygiene and the Carmichael Hospital for Tropical Diseases*, 9–10.

91. *Gazetteer of Bombay City and Island* 1910, 3:188; Home (Med), 64–85, Sept. 1886, NAI; *DFAR 1890*, 53.

92. Pitale 1870, 168.

93. *Gazetteer of Bombay City and Island* 1910, 3:137, 188–91. For an earlier tradition of Parsi "gifting," see White 1991.

94. *Bmb VR 1869–70*, xix; *1875–6*, 7–8.

95. Bannerman 1900, 2, 13; Snow 1897, 16. Cf. Klein 1988, 729.

96. Pitale 1870, 313–14.

97. *Gazetteer of Bombay City and Island* 1910, 3:184, 193.

98. Ibid., 197; Campbell 1898, 55.

99. *Gazetteer of Bombay City and Island* 1910, 3:186.

100. Tilak's attitude toward Western medicine was somewhat equivocal. His papers published articles on recent scientific discoveries—such as Yersin's discovery of the plague bacillus—but in a review of a book on Ayurvedic medicine he called for "a judicious combination" of the Western and Indian systems: *Mahratta*, 14 Feb. 1897.

101. Ibid., 11 Apr. 1897.

102. *Kesari*, 28 Sept. 1897, Bmb *NNR*.

103. E.g., *Kaiser-e-Hind*, 1 Nov. 1896; *Kalpataru*, 3 Mar. 1897; *Dhureen*, 9 Mar. 1898 (Bmb *NNR*); *Hitavadi*, 13 May 1898; *Basumati*, 12 May 1898 (Bngl *NNR*).

104. Gillion 1969, 136.

105. Tinker 1968, 73; Oldenburg 1984, 99.

106. In addition to Gillion and Oldenburg, see Harrison 1980, 166–95; Goode 1916.

107. Harrison 1980, 176–77.

108. Tinker 1968, 44–45.

109. *IMG* 1895, 30:465–67.

110. Gokhale 1920, 98–99; Tinker 1968, 280.

111. Tinker, 70.

112. Ibid., 51.

113. For Nair, see Pillai 1920; Nair (1968).

114. Proceedings of the Council of the Corporation of Madras: meetings of 28 Apr., 28 Aug., 25 Sept., and 30 Oct., 1905.

115. Ibid., for 26 Mar., 16 Oct., 20 Nov., 1906.

116. Ibid., for 4 May 1909, pp. 5–8.

117. Ibid., for 4 May 1909, pp. 13–14.

118. Jeffery 1988b, 171.

119. E.g., Bonarjee 1899; Rudolph and Rudolph 1967, 161–68.

120. Cited in Lutzker 1973, 198.

121. Cited in *Indian Medical Record*, 1890, 1:249.

122. Ibid. (Dec. 1890), 328–32.

123. Quoted in Heimsath 1964, 152.

124. Cited in ibid., 167.

125. Gokhale 1920, 929, 932–33.

126. India, *Proceedings of the Second All-India Sanitary Conference* 1913, 2:514–23. For a later but remarkably similar critique by a leading Indian scientist, see P. C. Ray 1935, vol. 2, chaps. 7 and 11 ("Emasculation and demartialisation of the Indian people under British rule").

127. Vivekananda 1910, 1213.

128. Ibid., 1214, 1226.

129. Gandhi 1945, 26.

130. Parekh 1989, 9, 63.

131. Brown 1989, 37, 40, 43.

132. On white attitudes in South Africa, see Swanson 1977; Parekh 1989, 144.

133. Gandhi 1938, 44–45.

134. Ibid., 58–59.

135. *IMG* 1887, 22:9.

Glossary

ayah	nursemaid
Ayurveda	Hindu system of medicine
bhadralok	"respectable" middle class in Bengal
dai	Indian midwife
devi	goddess
ghura	earthenware pot
hakim	Yunani practitioner
kaviraj	Ayurvedic practitioner (in Bengal)
lakh	100,000
mela	fair, festival
puja	worship
raiyatwari	a land revenue system based on individual peasant proprietors (*raiyat*s)
sastra	Hindu religious text
sati	immolation of Hindu widow on her husband's funeral pyre
sirkar	government
thagi	crime committed by a Thag (or Thug)
tika	mark
tikadar	inoculator ("mark-maker")
vaidya	Ayurvedic practitioner
Yunani	Muslim system of medicine
zamindar	landholder
zenana	women's quarters

Bibliography

ARCHIVES

India Office Library and Records, London
Board's Collections
Bombay Public Proceedings
Madras Board of Revenue Proceedings
Madras Revenue Proceedings
Madras Sanitary Commissioner's Proceedings
Madras Public Proceedings
North-Western Provinces Judicial Proceedings
Sanitary Despatches from India
Native Newspaper Reports (Bengal, Bombay, Madras, North-Western
    Provinces/United Provinces, Punjab)

School of Oriental and African Studies, London
London Missionary Society Archive

National Archives of India, New Delhi
Home
Home (Jails)
Home (Judicial)
Home (Medical)
Home (Public)
Home (Sanitary)
Home (Sanitary) (Plague)
Legislative
Sanitary Proceedings

Nehru Memorial Library, New Delhi
Mahratta (microfilm)

Maharashtra State Archives, Bombay
Bombay General

Tamil Nadu Archives, Madras
Madras Local and Municipal (Plague)

Madras Corporation
Proceedings of the Corporation Council

West Bengal State Archives, Calcutta
Bengal Judicial (Police)
Bengal Municipal (Medical)
Bengal Municipal (Sanitary)

OFFICIAL REPORTS AND PUBLICATIONS

Great Britain
The Indian Plague Commission, 1898–99. 1900. (Cd. 139).
Minutes of Evidence Taken before the Select Committee on the Affairs of the East India Company. 1832. (C. 735). Vol. V: Military.
Report of the Commissioners Appointed to Inquire into the Organization of the Indian Army. 1859. (C. 2515).
Report on Measures Adopted for Sanitary Improvements in India up to the End of 1867. 1868.
Report on Measures Adopted for Sanitary Improvements in India during the Year 1868, and up to the Month of June 1869. 1869. (C. 5319).
Royal Commission on the Sanitary State of the Army in India. 1863. (C. 3184). Vol. I: Minutes of Evidence.

India
The Army in India and Its Evolution. 1924. Calcutta: Superintendent of Government Printing.
The Etiology and Epidemiology of Plague: A Summary of the Work of the Plague Commission. 1908. Calcutta: Superintendent of Government Printing.
The Imperial Gazetteer of India. 1907. Oxford: Clarendon Press.
Leprosy in India: Reports of the Leprosy Commission in India, 1890–91. 1893. Calcutta: Superintendent of Government Printing.
Papers on Vaccination in India. 1851. Calcutta: Military Orphan Press.
Proceedings of the First All-India Sanitary Conference Held at Bombay on 13th and 14th November 1911. 1912. Calcutta: Superintendent of Government Printing.
Proceedings of the International Sanitary Conference Opened at Constantinople on the 13th February 1866. 1868. Calcutta: Superintendent of Government Printing.
Proceedings of the Second All-India Sanitary Conference Held at Madras, November 11th to 16th, 1912. 1913. Simla: Government Central Branch Press.

Report of the Commissioners Appointed to Inquire into the Cholera Epidemic of 1861 in Northern India. 1862. Calcutta.

Report of the Committee on Prison Discipline. 1838. Calcutta: Baptist Mission Press.

Report of the Health Survey and Development Committee. 1946. 4 vols. Delhi: Manager of Publications.

Report of the Indian Jails Committee, 1919–20. 1920. 5 vols. Calcutta: Superintendent, Government Central Press.

Report of the Indian Jail Conference. 1877. Calcutta: Home Secretariat Press.

Rules Regarding the Measures to Be Adopted on the Outbreak of Cholera or Appearance of Smallpox. 1870.

Assam

Rules for the Superintendence and Management of Jails in the Province of Assam. 1899. 2 vols. Calcutta: Superintendent of Government Printing.

Bengal

An Appeal on Behalf of the Calcutta School of Tropical Medicine and Hygiene and the Carmichael Hospital for Tropical Diseases. 1920. Calcutta: Bengal Secretariat Press.

Report by Civil Medical Officers on the Nature, Growth and Mode of Preparation of the Various Alimentary Articles Consumed as Food by the Industrial and Laboring Population in the Several Districts of Bengal, North-Western Provinces, Punjab, Oude and British Burmah. 1863. Calcutta: Home Secretariat Press.

Report of the Committee for the Establishment of a Fever Hospital, and for Inquiring into Local Management and Taxation in Calcutta. 1840. Calcutta: Bishop's College Press.

Report of the Epidemics of Plague in Calcutta During the Years 1898–99, 1899–1900 up to 30th June 1900. 1900. Calcutta: Municipal Press.

Report of the Small-pox Commissioners. 1850. Calcutta: Military Orphan Press.

Bombay

Gazetteer of Bombay City and Island. Vol. 3. 1910. Bombay: Times Press.

Gazetteer of the Bombay Presidency. Vol. 9, part I: Gujarat *Population, Hindus*. 1910: Government Central Press.

Gazetteer of the Bombay Presidency. Vol. 18, part I: Poona. 1885. Bombay: Government Central Press.

Supplement to the Account of Plague Administration in the Bombay Presidency from September 1896 till May 1897.

Madras

Medical Reports Selected by the Medical Board. 1855. Madras: Christian Knowledge Society's Press.

Report of Cholera Committee. 1868. Madras: Gantz Bros.
Report Regarding the Control of Pilgrimages in the Madras Presidency. 1868. Madras: Gantz Bros.
Review of the Madras Famine, 1876–1878. 1881. Madras: Government Press.

North-Western Provinces (United Provinces)

Reports on Cholera in the Meerut, Rohilcund and Ajmere Divisions in the Year 1856. 1857. Agra: Secundra Orphan Press.

Punjab

Punjab Plague Manual, 1909. 1909. Lahore: Punjab Government Press.

ADMINISTRATION REPORTS

Annual Administration Reports of the Dufferin Fund.
Annual Administration Reports of the Sanitary Commissioners and Health Commissioners. (India, Bengal, Bombay, Madras, North-Western Provinces).
Annual Reports of the Madras Dispensaries and Civil Hospitals.
Annual Vaccination Reports (Bengal, Bombay, Madras, North-Western Provinces).
Annual Administration Reports of the Corporation (Calcutta, Madras, Pune).
Annual Reports of the Corporation Health Officers (Calcutta, Madras).
Reports of the Victoria Hospital for Caste and Gosha Women, Madras.

SERIALS

British Medical Journal
Indian Medical Gazette
Indian Medical Record
Lancet
Madras Quarterly Medical Journal
Missionary Register
Transactions of the Medical and Physical Society of Bombay
Transactions of the Medical and Physical Society of Calcutta

WORKS THROUGH 1947

Abbott, J. 1932. *The Keys of Power: A Study of Indian Ritual and Belief.* London: Methuen.
Adams, Archibald. 1899. *The Western Rajputana States: A Medico-Topographical and General Account of Marwar, Sirohi, Jaisalmir.* London: Army and Navy Stores.
Ainslie, Whitelaw. 1826. *Materia Indica; or, some Account of Those Articles Which Are Employed by the Hindoos, and Other Eastern Nations, in Their Medicine, Arts, and Agriculture.* 2 vols. London: Brown and Green.

Anon. 1831. "The Asiatic Cholera." *Fraser's Magazine* 19:613–25.

Annesley, James. 1825. *Sketches of the Most Prevalent Diseases of India.* London: Underwood.

————. 1828. *Researches into the Causes, Nature, and Treatment of the Most Prevalent Diseases of India, and of Warm Climates Generally.* 2 vols. London: Longman, Rees, Orme, Brown and Green.

Balfour, Andrew. 1925. "Some British and American Pioneers in Tropical Medicine and Hygiene." *Transactions of the Royal Society of Tropical Medicine and Hygiene* 19:189–229.

Balfour, Andrew, and Henry Harold Scott. *Health Problems of the Empire: Past, Present and Future.* London: Collins.

Balfour, Margaret I., and Ruth Young. 1929. *The Work of Medical Women in India.* London: Oxford University Press.

Ballingall, George. 1818. *Practical Observations on Fever, Dysentery, and Liver Complaints as They Occur Amongst the European Troops in India.* Edinburgh: Brown and Constable.

Bannerman, W. B. 1900. *Statistics of Inoculations with Haffkine's Anti-Plague Vaccine, 1897–1900.* Bombay: Government Central Press.

Barnes, Irene H. 1903. *Behind the Purdah: The Story of C.E.Z.M.S. Work in India,* London: Marshall Brothers (first published 1897).

Bellew, H. W. 1885. *The History of Cholera from 1862 to 1881.* London: Trubner and Co.

Billington, Mary Frances. 1895. *Women in India.* London: Chapman and Hall.

Bingley, A. H. 1918. *Handbooks for the Indian Army: Jats, Gujars, and Ahirs.* Calcutta: Superintendent of Government Printing, India.

Bingley, A. H., and A. Nicholls. 1897. *Caste Handbooks for the Indian Army: Brahmans.* Simla: Government Central Printing Office.

Bonarjee, P. D. 1899. *A Handbook of the Fighting Races of India* (reprinted New Delhi: Asian Publication Services, 1975).

Breton, P. 1826. "On the Native Mode of Couching." *Transactions of the Medical and Physical Society of Calcutta* 2:341–82.

Brown, D. Blair. 1887. "The Pros and Cons of the Contagious Diseases Act as Applied to India." *Transactions of the Medical and Physical Society of Bombay,* n.s., 11:80–97.

Bryden, James L. 1869. *Epidemic Cholera in the Bengal Presidency: A Report on the Cholera of 1866–68, and Its Relations to the Cholera of Previous Epidemics.* Calcutta: Superintendent of Government Printing.

Buchanan, Claudius. 1812. *Christian Researches in Asia.* 5th ed. London: Caldwell and Davies.

Burton, Richard F. 1851. *Goa and the Blue Mountains, or, Six Months on Sick Leave.* London: Bentley.

Butter, Donald. 1839. *Outlines of the Topography and Statistics of the Southern Districts of Oudh and of the Cantonment of Sultanpur-Oudh.* Calcutta: Huttmann.

Caldwell, R. 1887. "On Demonology in Southern India." *Journal of the Anthropological Society of Bombay* 1:91–105.

Cameron, W. 1831. "On Vaccination in Bengal." *Transactions of the Medical and Physical Society of Calcutta* 5:385–421.

Campbell, James MacNabb. 1898. *Report of the Bombay Plague Committee on the Plague in Bombay, 1st July 1897 to the 30th April 1898.* Bombay: "Times of India" Steam Press.

Cardew, A. G. 1891. *Report on Jail Administration in Madras.* Madras: Government Press.

Centenary of Medical College, Bengal, 1835–1934. 1935. Calcutta: Centenary Volume Sub-Committee.

Centenary Review of the Asiatic Society of Bengal from 1784 to 1883. 1885. Calcutta: Thacker, Spink and Co.

Charles, T. Edmondston. 1870. *Popular Information on Small-pox, Inoculation and Vaccination.* Calcutta: Bengal Secretariat Press.

Chevers, Norman. 1886. *A Commentary on the Diseases of India.* London: Churchill.

Christie, Alexander Turnbull. 1828. *Observations on the Nature and Treatment of Cholera.* Edinburgh: Maclachlan and Stewart.

Christison, A. n.d. *Report on the Vaccine Operations in the Agra Division, 1858–59.*

Clark, John. 1773. *Observations on the Diseases in Long Voyages to Hot Countries and Particularly on Those Which Prevail in the East Indies.* London: Wilson and Nicol.

Clark, John. 1839. "Report on Syphilis in H. M. 13th Light Dragoons." *Madras Quarterly Medical Journal* 1:370–410.

Clough, Emma Rauschenbusch. 1899. *While Sewing Sandals, or, Tales of a Telugu Pariah Tribe.* London: Hodder and Stoughton.

Conférence Sanitaire Internationale. 1866. *Rapport sur les Questions du Programme Relatives a l'Origine, a l'Endémicité, a la Transmissibilité et a la Propagation du Choléra.* Constantinople: Imprimerie Centrale.

Cook, Edward. 1914. *The Life of Florence Nightingale.* 2 vols. London: Macmillan.

Corbyn, Frederick. 1832. *A Treatise on the Epidemic Cholera as It Has Prevailed in India.* Calcutta: Thacker and Co.

Cornish, W. R. 1863. *Reports on the Nature of the Food of the Inhabitants of the Madras Presidency.* Madras: Government Press.

————. 1871. *Cholera in Southern India: A Record of the Progress of Cholera in 1870 and Resume of the Records of Former Epidemic Invasions of the Madras Presidency.* Madras: Government Gazette Press.

Couchman, M. E. 1897. *Account of the Plague Administration in the Bombay Presidency, from September 1896 till May 1897.* Bombay: Government Central Press.

Crawford, D. G. 1914. *A History of the Indian Medical Service, 1600–1913.* 2 vols. London: Thacker and Co.

————. 1930. *Roll of the Indian Medical Service, 1615–1930.* London: Thacker and Co.

Crooke, William. 1896. *The Popular Religion and Folklore of Northern India.* 2 vols. (2d ed., reprinted Delhi: Munshiram Manoharlal, 1968).

————. 1910. "Religious Songs from Northern India." *Indian Antiquary* 39:268–87.

————. 1926. *The Popular Religion and Folklore of Northern India.* 3d ed. London: Oxford University Press.

Cruikshank, J. 1876. *A Manual of Jail Rules for the Superintendence and Management of Jails in the Bombay Presidency.* Bombay: Government Central Press.

Cuningham, J. M. n.d. *Report on the Cholera Epidemic of 1879 in Northern India with Special Reference to the Supposed Influence of the Hurdwar Fair.*

————. 1884. *Cholera: What Can the State Do to Prevent It?* Calcutta: Superintendent of Government Printing, India.

Curtis, Charles. 1807. *An Account of the Diseases of India, as They Appeared in the English Fleet, and in the Naval Hospital, in Madras in 1782 and 1783.* Edinburgh: Laing.

Dalal, R. D. 1930. *Manual of Vaccination for the Bombay Presidency.* 2 vols. Bombay: Government Central Press.

Day, Lal Behari. 1902. *Bengal Peasant Life.* London: Macmillan.

Deb, Randha Kanta. 1831. "Account of the Tikadars." *Transactions of the Medical and Physical Society of Calcutta* 5:416–18.

Dempster, T. E. 1868. *The Prevalence of Organic Disease of the Spleen as a Test for Detecting Malarious Localities in Hot Climates.* Calcutta: Superintendent of Government Printing.

Douglas, William. 1865. *Soldiering in Sunshine and Storm.* Edinburgh: Black.

Drury, Heber. 1873. *The Useful Plants of India with Notices of Their Chief Value in Commerce, Medicine and the Arts.* 2d ed. London: Allen.

Dubois, Abbé J. A. 1905. *Hindu Manners, Customs and Ceremonies.* 3d ed. London: Clarendon Press.

Dunlop, Robert Henry Wallace. 1858. *Service and Adventure with the Khakee Ressalah, or Meerut Volunteer Horse, during the Mutinies of 1857–58.* London: Bentley.

Dutt, Udoy Chand. 1877. *The Materia Medica of the Hindus, Compiled from Sanskrit Medical Works.* Calcutta: Thacker, Spink and Co.

Elliot, J. 1863. *Report on Epidemic Remittent and Intermittent Fever Occurring in Parts of Burdwan and Nuddea Divisions.* Calcutta: Bengal Secretariat Office.

Enthoven, R. E. 1924. *The Folklore of Bombay.* Oxford: Clarendon Press.

Ewart, Joseph. 1859. *A Digest of the Vital Statistics of the European and Native Armies in India.* London: Smith, Elder and Co.

————. 1880. "Enteric Fever in India, with Some Observations on Its Probable Etiology in That Country." *Epidemiology Society of London: Papers on Continued Fever*. London.

Fabre, Augustin, and Fortuné Chailan. 1835. *Histoire de choléra-morbus asiatique*. Marseilles: Marins Olive.

Fawcett, F. 1890. "On Some Festivals to Village Goddesses." *Journal of the Anthropological Society of Bombay* 2:261–82.

Fayrer, Joseph. 1882. *On the Climate and Fevers of India*. London: Churchill.

———. 1897. *Sir James Ranald Martin*. London: Innes and Co.

Francis, W. 1907. *Madras District Gazetteers: Vizagapatam*. Madras: Government Press.

Gandhi, M. K. 1938. *Hind Swaraj or Indian Home Rule*. Ahmadabad: Navajivan Publishing House.

———. 1945. *Autobiography, or, the Story of My Experiments with Truth*. Ahmadabad: Navajivan Publishing House.

Gangulee, N. 1939. *Health and Nutrition in India*. London: Faber and Faber.

Gatacre, W. F. 1897. *Report on the Bubonic Plague in Bombay, 1896–97*. Bombay: "Times of India" Steam Press.

Geddes, J. C. *Administrative Experience Recorded in Former Famines*. 1874. Calcutta: Bengal Secretariat Press.

Geddes, William. 1846. *Clinical Illustrations of the Diseases of India*. London: Smith, Elder and Co.

Gidumal, Dayaram. 1888. *The Life and Life-Work of Behramji M. Malabari*. Bombay: Education Society's Press.

Giles, C. M. 1904. *Climate and Health in Hot Countries and the Outlines of Tropical Climatology*. London: Bale, Sons and Danielson.

Gokhale, G. K. 1920. *Speeches of Gopal Krishna Gokhale*. 3d ed. Madras: Natesan.

Goode, S. W. 1916. *Municipal Calcutta: Its Institutions in Their Origin and Growth* (reprinted Calcutta: Bibhash Gupta, 1986).

Gordon, C. A. 1878. *Report on Typhoid or Enteric Fever in Relation to British Troops in the Madras Command*. Madras: Government Press.

Grant, A. E. 1894. *The Indian Manual of Hygiene*. 2 vols. Madras: Higginbotham and Co.

Greenfield, M. Rose. 1886. *Five Years in Ludhiana*. London: Partridge and Co.

Hacker, J. H. 1887. *Memoirs of Thomas Smith Thomson*. London: Religious Tract Society.

Haffkine, W. M. 1895. *Anti-Cholera Inoculation*. Calcutta: Thacker, Spink and Co.

Haikerwal, Bejoy Shankar. 1934. *Economic and Social Aspects of Crime in India*. London: Allen and Unwin.

Haines, Hermann A. n.d. *Memorial of the Life and Work of Charles Morehead*. London: Allen.

Harrison, James. 1858. "The Origins and Progress of the Bengal Medical College." *Indian Annals of Medical Science* 5:37–54.

Hemingway, F. R. 1906. *Madras District Gazetteers: Tanjore*. Madras: Government Press.

Hewlett, T. G. 1883. *Report on Enteric Fever*.

Heyne, Benjamin. 1814. *Tracts, Historical and Statistical, on India: With Journals of Several Tours Through Various Parts of the Peninsula*. London: Baldwin.

Hirsch, August. 1883. *Handbuch der Historisch-Geographischen Pathologie*. 3 vols. Stuttgart: Enke.

Hodge, George Alexander. 1867. *The Bengal Jail Manual*. Calcutta: Smith.

Hoggan, Frances Elizabeth. 1882. "Medical Women for India." *Contemporary Review* 42:267–75.

Holwell, J. Z. 1767. *An Account of the Manner of Inoculating for the Small Pox in the East Indies*. London: Becket and de Hondt.

Hora, Sunder Lal. 1993. "Worship of the Deities Ola, Jhola and Bon Bibi in Lower Bengal." *Journal of the Asiatic Society of Bengal* n.s. 29: 1–4.

Howell, A. P. 1868. *Note on Jails and Jail Discipline in India, 1867–68*. Calcutta: Superintendent of Government Printing.

Hunter, W. W. 1872. *Orissa*. 2 vols. London: Smith, Elder and Co.

Hunter, William. 1804. *An Essay on the Diseases Incident to Indian Seamen, or Lascars, on Long Voyages*. Calcutta: East India Company's Press.

Hutchinson, James. 1832. *Observations on Cholera Asphyxia*. Calcutta: Baptist Mission Press.

———. 1835. *A Report on the Medical Management of the Native Jails*. Calcutta: Thacker and Co.

———. 1845. *Observations on the General and Medical Management of Indian Jails and on Some of the Principal Diseases Which Infest Them*. Calcutta: Huttmann.

Irvine, R. H. 1848. *A Short Account of the Materia Medica of Patna*. Calcutta: Military Orphan Press.

James, S. P. 1909. *Small-pox and Vaccination in British India*. Calcutta: Thacker, Spink and Co.

Jameson, James. 1820. *Report on the Epidemick Cholera Morbus, as It Visited the Territories Subject to the Presidency of Bengal in the Years 1817, 1818, and 1819*. Calcutta: Government Gazette Press.

Johnson, James. 1813. *The Influence of Tropical Climates, More Especially the Climate of India, on European Constitutions*. London: Stockdale.

Kellie, James. 1839. "On the Prevention of Army Disease in Goomsur." *Madras Quarterly Medical Journal*. 1:273–76.

Kennedy, R. H. 1827. *Notes on the Epidemic Cholera*. Calcutta: Baptist Mission Press.

———. 1846. *Notes on the Epidemic Cholera*. 2d ed. London: Smith, Elder and Co.

Kittredge, G. A. 1889. *A Short History of the "Medical Women for India" Fund of Bombay*. Bombay: Education Society's Press.

Klein, E., and Heneage Gibbes. 1885. *Cholera: Inquiry by Doctors Klein and*

Gibbes, and Transactions of a Committee Convened by the Secretary of State for India in Council, 1885.

Koman, M. C. 1921. *Report of the Investigation of Indigenous Drugs.* Madras: Government Press.

Lal, R. B. 1937. "Fairs and Festivals in India." *Indian Medical Gazette* 72:96–101.

Laverack, Alfred. n.d. *A Methodist Soldier in the Indian Army.* London: Longley.

Leith, A. H. 1851–52. "A Contribution to Dietetics." *Transactions of the Medical and Physical Society of Bombay* n.s. 1:114–27.

———. 1864. *Report on the General Sanitary Condition of the Bombay Army.* Bombay: Education Society's Press.

Lely, F. S. P. 1906. *Suggestions for the Better Governing of India.* London: Rivers.

Lewis, T. R., and D. D. Cunningham. 1878. *Cholera in Relation to Certain Physical Phenomena.* Calcutta: Superintendent of Government Printing.

Lind, James. 1808. *An Essay on Diseases Incidental to Europeans in Hot Climates.* London: Becket and de Hondt.

Lovett, Richard. 1899. *The History of the London Missionary Society, 1795–1895.* 2 vols. London: Frowde.

Lyons, R. T. 1872. *A Treatise on Relapsing Fever or Famine Fever.* London: King.

McCay, D. 1912. *Investigations into the Jail Dietaries of the United Provinces with Some Observations on the Influence of Dietary on the Physical Development and Well-Being of the People of the United Provinces.* Calcutta: Superintendent of Government Printing.

MacGregor, W. L. 1843. *Practical Observations on the Principal Diseases Affecting the Health of the European and Native Soldiers in the North-Western Provinces of India.* Calcutta: Thacker and Co.

Mackinnon, Kenneth. 1848. *A Treatise on the Public Health, Climate, Hygiene and Prevailing Diseases of Bengal and the North-West Provinces.* Kanpur: Cawnpore Press.

Maclean, Charles. 1824. *Evils of Quarantine Laws, and Non-Existence of Pestilential Contagion.* London: Underwood.

M'Clelland, John. 1859. *Sketch of the Medical Topography, or Climate and Soils, of Bengal and the N.-W. Provinces.* London: Churchill.

Macnamara, C. 1870. *A Treatise on Asiatic Cholera.* London: Churchill.

———. 1876. *A History of Asiatic Cholera.* London: Macmillan.

Macnamara, F. N. 1880. *Climate and Medical Topography in Their Relations to the Disease Distribution of the Himalayan and Sub-Himalayan Districts of British India.* London: Longmans, Green and Co.

Maconochie, Evan. 1926. *Life in the Indian Civil Service.* London: Chapman and Hall.

MacPherson, John. 1872. *Annals of Cholera from the Earliest Periods to the Year 1817.* London: Ranken and Co.

Macrae, R. 1894. "Cholera and Preventive Inoculation in Gaya Jail." *Indian Medical Gazette* 29:334–38.

Malcolmson, John Grant. 1835a. *A Practical Essay on the History and Treatment of Beriberi.* Madras: Vepery Mission Press.

———. 1835b. *Observations on Some Forms of Rheumatism Prevailing in India.* Madras: Vepery Mission Press.

Malleson, G. B. 1868. *Report on the Cholera Epidemic of 1867 in Northern India.* Calcutta.

Manson, Patrick. 1898. *Tropical Diseases: A Manual of the Diseases of Warm Climates.* London: Cassell and Co.

Martin, James Ranald. 1837. *Notes on the Medical Topography of Calcutta.* Calcutta: Huttmann.

———. 1856. *The Influence of Tropical Climates on European Constitutions.* London: Churchill.

Martin, Montgomery, ed. 1838. *The History, Antiquities, Topography and Statistics of Eastern India.* 3 vols. London: Allen.

Mayo, Katherine. 1927. *Mother India.* London: Cape.

Mill, James. 1858. *The History of British India.* 5th ed. London: Madden.

Mittra, Peary Chand. 1880. *Life of Dewan Ramcomul Sen.* Calcutta: Bose and Co.

Moore, W. J. 1867. "Results of Sanitation in India." *Indian Medical Gazette* 2:173–76.

———. 1877. *A Manual of Family Medicine for India.* 2d ed. London: Churchill.

Moreau de Jonnès, Alexandre. 1831. *Rapport au conseil supérior de santé sur le choléra-morbus pestilentiel.* Paris: Cosson.

Morehead, Charles. 1856. *Clinical Researches on Disease in India.* 2 vols. London: Longman, Brown, Green, and Longman.

Mouat, F. J. 1856. *Report on Jails Visited and Inspected in Bengal, Behar, and Arracan.* Calcutta: Military Orphan Press.

———. 1868. *Report on the Statistics of the Prisons of the Lower Provinces of the Bengal Presidency for 1861, 1862, 1863 1864, and 1865.* Calcutta: Alipore Jail Press.

Mukhopadhyaya, Girindranath. 1923. *History of Indian Medicine from the Earliest Ages to the Present Time.* 2 vols. Calcutta: University of Calcutta.

Murray, John. 1839. *On the Topography of Meerutt.* Calcutta: Huttmann.

———. 1856. *Report on the Attack of Cholera in the Central Prison at Agra in 1856.* Agra: Secundra Orphan Press.

———. 1869. *Report on the Treatment of Epidemic Cholera.* Calcutta: Superintendent of Government Printing.

Nathan, R. 1898. *The Plague in Northern India, 1896, 1897.* 2 vols. Simla: Government Central Printing Office.

O'Malley, L. S. S. 1907. *Bengal District Gazetteers: Balasore.* Calcutta: Bengal Secretariat Book Depot.

O'Shaughnessy, W. B. 1844. *The Bengal Pharmacopoeia and General Con-*

spectus of Medical Plants Arranged According to the Natural and Therapeutic Systems. Calcutta: Bishop's College Press.

Parkes, E. A. 1846. *Remarks on the Dysentery and Hepatitis of India.* London: Longman, Brown, Green and Longman.

———. 1864. *A Manual of Practical Hygiene.* London: Churchill.

Pillai, Somasundaram. 1920. *Dr. T. M. Nair, M.D.* Madras: A.K.V. Press.

Pitale, Balkrishna Nilaji. 1870. *The Speeches and Addresses of Sir H. B. E. Frere.* Bombay.

Playfair, George. 1833. *The Taleef Shereef, or Indian Materia Medica.* Calcutta: Medical and Physical Society of Calcutta.

Ranken, James. 1838. *Report on the Malignant Fever Called the Pali Plague Which Prevailed in Some Parts of Rajpootana Since the Month of July 1836.* Calcutta: Huttmann.

Rankine, Robert. 1839. *Notes on the Medical Topography of the District of Sarun.* Calcutta: Huttmann.

Ranking, J. L. 1868. *Report of the Lying-in Hospital and Dispensary for Women and Children, Madras.* Madras: Government Press.

———. 1869. *Report upon Prevalence of Typhoid Fever at Bangalore.*

———. n.d. *Report on Military Sanitation in the Presidency of Madras.* Madras: Government Press.

Ray, Prafulla Chandra. 1935. *Life and Experiences of a Bengali Chemist.* 2 vols. Calcutta: Chuckervertty, Chatterjee and Co.

Renny, C. 1851. *Medical Report on the Mahamurree in Gurhwal in 1849–50.* Agra: Secundra Orphan Press.

Roberts, Lord. 1897. *Forty-one Years in India: From Subaltern to Commander-in-Chief.* 2 vols. London: Bentley and Son.

Rogers, Leonard. 1926. *Small-pox and Climate in India: Forecasting of Epidemics.* London: HMSO.

———. 1928. *The Incidence and Spread of Cholera in India: Forecasting and Control of Epidemics.* Calcutta: Thacker, Spink and Co.

Rogers, Leonard, and John W. D. Megaw. 1930. *Tropical Medicine.* London: Churchill.

Rogers, Samuel, ed. 1848. *Reports on Asiatic Cholera in Regiments of the Madras Army from 1828 to 1844.* London: Richardson.

Ross, Ronald. 1923. *Memoirs.* London: Murray.

Rotton, John Edward Wharton. 1858. *The Chaplain's Narrative of the Siege of Delhi from the Outbreak at Meerut to the Capture of Delhi.* London: Smith, Elder and Co.

Russell, A. J. H., and E. R. Sundarajan. 1928. *The Epidemiology of Cholera in India.* Calcutta: Thacker, Spink and Co.

Ryder, John. 1854. *Four Years' Service in India.* 2d ed. Leicester: Thompson and Son.

Scharlieb, Mary. 1924. *Reminiscences.* London: Williams and Norgate.

Scot, William. 1824. *Report of the Epidemic Cholera as It Has Appeared in the Territories Subject to the Presidency of Fort St George.* Madras: Asylum Press. 2d ed., 1849. Edinburgh: Blackwood and Sons.

Scriven, J. B. 1863. *Report on Epidemic Cholera in the Punjab and Its Dependencies during 1862.* Lahore: Government Press.

Sheriff, Mohideen. 1891. *Materia Medica of Madras.* 2 vols. Madras: Government Press.

Shoolbred, John. 1804. *Report on the Progress of Vaccine Inoculation in Bengal, 1802–3.* Calcutta: East India Company's Press.

———. 1805. *Report on the State and Progress of Vaccine Inoculation in Bengal during the Year 1804.* Calcutta: East India Company's Press.

Sleeman, W. H. 1844. *Rambles and Recollections of an Indian Official.* 2 vols. London: Hatchard.

Smith, David B. 1861. *Report on Epidemic Cholera as It Prevailed in the City of Delhi, at Goorgaon, and the Surrounding Districts, During the Rainy Season of 1861.* Lahore: Government Press.

———. 1868. *Report on Pilgrimage to Juggernauth in 1868.* Calcutta: Lewis.

Snow, P. C. H. 1897. *Report on the Outbreak of Bubonic Plague in Bombay, 1896–97.* Bombay: "Times of India" Steam Press.

Steuart, R. and B. Philipps. 1819. *Reports on the Epidemic Cholera Which Has Raged Throughout Hindostan and the Peninsula of India Since August 1817.* Bombay: Government of Bombay.

Stevens, C. R. 1901. *Report of an Epidemic of Cerebro-Spinal Fever Occurring in Bhagalpur Central Jail in 1899–1900.* Calcutta: Bengal Secretariat Press.

Stewart, Duncan. 1844. *Report on Small-pox in Calcutta, 1833–34, 1837–38, 1843–44.* Calcutta: Huttmann.

Stiven, W. S. 1855. *Report on the Epidemic in the Moradababad District in 1854.* Agra: Secundra Orphan Press.

Strong, F. P. 1837. *Extracts from the Topography and Vital Statistics of Calcutta.* Calcutta.

Taylor, James. 1840. *A Sketch of the Topography and Statistics of Dacca.* Calcutta: Huttmann.

Thacker's Indian Directory. 1890. Calcutta: Thacker, Spink and Co.

Thacker's Indian Directory. 1900. Calcutta: Thacker, Spink and Co.

Thurston, Edgar. 1912. *Omens and Superstitions of Southern India.* London: Unwin.

Turner, J. A., and B. K. Goldsmith. 1917. *Sanitation in India.* 2d ed. Bombay: Times of India.

Twining, William. 1832. *Clinical Illustrations of the More Important Diseases of Bengal with the Results of an Enquiry into Their Pathology and Treatment.* Calcutta: Baptist Mission Press. 2d ed., 1835. 2 vols. Calcutta: Mission Press.

Vivekananda, Swami. 1910. *The Complete Works of the Swami Vivekananda.* Vol. 5. Almora: Advaita Ashram.

Waring, Edward John. 1860. *Pharmacopoeia of India.* London: Allen and Co.

———. 1897. *Remarks on the Uses of Some of the Bazaar Medicines and Common Medical Plants of India.* 5th ed. London: Churchill.

Weir, T. S. 1886. "Note on Sacrifices in India as a Means of Averting Epidemics." *Journal of the Anthropological Society of Bombay* 1:35–36.

White, W. 1837. *The Evils of Quarantine Laws*. London: Wilson.

Whitehead, Henry. 1921. *The Village Gods of South India*. 2d ed. Calcutta: Association Press.

Wiehe, C. G. 1865. *Journal of a Tour of Inspection of the Principal Jails in India Made by the Inspector General of Prisons, Bombay Presidency*. Bombay: Education Society's Press.

Wilkinson, E. 1904a. *Report on Plague in the Punjab from October 1st, 1901, to September 30th, 1902*. Lahore: Punjab Government Gazette.

———. 1904b. *Report on Plague and Inoculation in the Punjab from October 1st, 1902, to September 30th, 1903*. Lahore: Government Press.

Wilson, H. H. 1825. "Kushta, or Leprosy, as Known to the Hindus." *Transactions of the Medical and Physical Society of Calcutta* 1:1–44.

Wilson, W. J. 1874. *Memorandum on the Progress of the Jail Department in the Madras Presidency from 1865 to 1874*. Madras: Government Press.

Wise, James. 1883. *Notes on the Races, Castes, and Trades of Eastern India*. London: Harrison.

———. 1894. *The Diary of a Medical Officer During the Great Indian Mutiny of 1857*. Cork: Guy and Co.

Wise, T. A. 1860. *Commentary on the Hindu System of Medicine*. 2d ed. London: Trubner and Co.

Young, H. 1831. *Remarks on the Cholera Morbus*. Smith, Elder and Co.

WORKS AFTER 1947

Anderson, Perry. 1976–77. "The Antimonies of Antonio Gramsci." *New Left Review* 100:5–78.

Archer, Mildred. 1980. *Early Views of India: The Picturesque Journeys of Thomas and William Daniell, 1786–1794*. London: Thames and Hudson.

Archer, Mildred, and Ronald Lightbrown. 1982. *India Observed: India as Viewed by British Artists, 1760–1860*. London: Victoria and Albert Museum.

Arnold, David. 1979. "Dacoity and Rural Crime in Madras, 1860–1940." *Journal of Peasant Studies* 6:140–67.

———. 1983. "White Colonization and Labour in Nineteenth-Century India." *Journal of Imperial and Commonwealth History*. 11:133–58.

———. 1986. *Police Power and Colonial Rule: Madras, 1859–1947*. Delhi: Oxford University Press.

———. 1987. "Touching the Body: Perspectives on the Indian Plague, 1896–1900." In *Subaltern Studies V*, edited by Ranajit Guha. Delhi: Oxford University Press.

———. 1989. "Cholera Mortality in British India, 1817–1947." In *India's Historical Demography: Studies in Famine, Disease and Society*, edited by Tim Dyson. London: Curzon Press.

——. n.d. "The Colonial Prison: Penology and Medicine in Nineteenth-Century India." Forthcoming.

——, ed. 1988. *Imperial Medicine and Indigenous Societies*. Manchester: Manchester University Press.

Babb, Lawrence A. 1975. *The Divine Hierarchy: Popular Hinduism in Central India*. New York: Columbia University Press.

Bala, Poonam. 1987. "State and Indigenous Medicine in Nineteenth and Twentieth-Century Bengal, 1800–1947." Ph.D. thesis, University of Edinburgh.

Ballhatchet, Kenneth. 1980. *Race, Sex and Class under the Raj: Imperial Attitudes and Policies and Their Critics, 1793–1905*. London: Weidenfeld and Nicolson.

Banerjea, A. C. 1951. "Note on Cholera in the United Provinces." *Indian Journal of Medical Research* 39:17–40.

Banerjee, Bireswar, and Jayatri Hazra. 1974. *Geoecology of Cholera in West Bengal: A Study in Medical Geography*. Calcutta: Hazra.

Banerjee, Tapas Kumar. 1963. *Background to Indian Criminal Law*. Bombay: Orient Longmans.

Banerji, Amiya Kumar. 1972. *West Bengal District Gazetteers: Howrah*. Calcutta: Government of West Bengal.

Bang, B. G. 1973. "Current Concepts of the Smallpox Goddess Sitala in Parts of West Bengal." *Man in India* 53:79–104.

Barat, Amiya. 1962. *The Bengal Native Infantry: Its Organization and Discipline, 1796–1852*. Calcutta: Mukhopadyay.

Barua, Dhiman, and William Burrows, eds. 1974. *Cholera*. Philadelphia: Saunders.

Basalla, George. 1967. "The Spread of Western Science." *Science* 156:611–22.

Basu, Gopendrakrishna. 1963. *Banglar Loukik Devata* (Folk gods of Bengal). Calcutta: Dey's Publishing House.

Bates, Thomas R. 1975. "Gramsci and the Theory of Hegemony." *Journal of the History of Ideas* 36:351–66.

Beals, A. R. 1976. "Strategies of Resort to Curers in South India." In *Asian Medical Systems: A Comparative Study*, edited by Charles Leslie. Berkeley: University of California Press.

Bhardwaj, Surinder M. 1975. "Attitude towards Different Systems of Medicine: A Survey of Four Villages in the Punjab in India." *Social Science and Medicine* 9:603–12.

——. 1981. "Homoeopathy in India." In *The Social and Cultural Context of Medicine in India*, edited by Giri Raj Gupta. New Delhi: Vikas Publishing House.

Blake, Catriona. 1990. *The Charge of the Parasols: Women's Entry to the Medical Profession*. London: The Women's Press.

Borthwick, Meredith. 1984. *The Changing Role of Women in Bengal, 1849–1905*. Princeton: Princeton University Press.

Bowers, John Z. 1981. "The Odyssey of Smallpox Vaccination." *Bulletin of the History of Medicine* 55:17–33.

Brown, Judith M. 1989. *Gandhi: Prisoner of Hope.* New Haven: Yale University Press.

Buci-Glucksmann, Christine. 1980. *Gramsci and the State.* London: Lawrence and Wishart.

———. 1982. "Hegemony and Consent." In *Approaches to Gramsci*, edited by Anne Showstack Sassoon. London: Writers and Readers.

Cantlie, Neil. 1974. *A History of the Army Medical Department.* 2 vols. Edinburgh: Churchill Livingstone.

Carlson, Dennis G. 1984. *African Fever: A Study of British Science, Technology, and Politics in West Africa, 1787–1864.* Canton, Mass.: Science History Publications.

Cashman, R. I. 1975. *The Myth of the Lokamanya: Tilak and Mass Politics in Maharashtra.* Berkeley: University of California Press.

Cassedy, James H. 1984. *American Medicine and Statistical Thinking, 1800–1860.* Cambridge: Harvard University Press.

Cassels, Nancy Gardner. 1987. *Religion and Pilgrim Tax under the Company Raj.* Delhi: Manohar.

Catanach, I. J. 1983. "Plague and the Indian Village." In *Rural India: Land, Power and Society under British Rule*, edited by P. G. Robb. London: Curzon Press.

———. 1984. "'Fatalism'?: Indian Responses to Plague and Other Crises." *Asian Profile* 12:183–92.

———. 1987. "Poona Politicians and the Plague." In *Struggling and Ruling: The Indian National Congress, 1885–1985*, edited by Jim Masselos. London: Oriental University Press.

———. 1988. "Plague and the Tensions of Empire: India, 1896–1918." In *Imperial Medicine and Indigenous Societies*, edited by David Arnold. Manchester: Manchester University Press.

Curtin, Philip D. 1964. *The Image of Africa: British Ideas and Action, 1780–1850.* Madison: University of Wisconsin Press.

———. 1989. *Death by Migration: Europe's Encounter with the Tropical World in the Nineteenth Century.* Cambridge: Cambridge University Press.

Davis, C. 1978. "Variolation in the Rajasthan Desert." *Indian Journal of Public Health* 22:134–39.

Davis, Kingsley. 1951. *The Population of Indian and Pakistan.* Princeton: Princeton University Press.

de Bary, William Theodore. 1968. *Sources of Indian Tradition.* New York: Columbia University Press.

de Figueiredo, John M. 1984. "Ayurvedic Medicine in Goa, According to European Sources in the Sixteenth and Seventeenth Centuries." *Bulletin of the History of Medicine* 58:225–35.

Dharampal. 1971. *Indian Science and Technology in the Eighteenth Century: Some Contemporary European Accounts.* Delhi: Impex Indica.

Dixon, C. W. 1962. *Smallpox*. London: Churchill.

Djurfeldt, Goran, and Staffan Lindberg. 1975. *Pills Against Poverty: A Study of the Introduction of Western Medicine in a Tamil Village*. London: Curzon Press.

Doyal, Lesley. 1979. *The Political Economy of Health*. London: Pluto Press.

Durey, Michael. 1979. *The Return of the Plague: British Society and the Cholera, 1831–2*. Dublin: Gill and Macmillan.

Engels, Dagmar. 1983. "The Age of Consent Act of 1891: Colonial Ideology in Bengal." *South Asia Research* 3:107–31.

———. n.d. *Beyond Purdah*. Forthcoming.

Fanon, Frantz. 1970. *A Dying Colonialism*. Harmondsworth: Penguin Books.

Femia, Joseph. 1975. "Hegemony and Consciousness in the Thought of Antonio Gramsci." *Political Studies* 23: 29–48.

Fisch, Jorg. 1983. *Cheap Lives and Dear Limbs: The British Transformation of the Bengal Criminal Law, 1769–1817*. Wiesbaden: Steiner.

Flynn, M. W. 1965. "Introduction" to Edwin Chadwick, *Report on the Sanitary Condition of the Labouring Population of Great Britain*. Edinburgh: University Press.

Forbes, Geraldine. 1986. "In Search of the 'Pure Heathen': Missionary Women in Nineteenth-Century India." *Economic and Political Weekly* 21: WS 2–8.

Foucault, Michel. 1976. *The Birth of the Clinic*. London: Tavistock Publications.

———. 1979. *Discipline and Punish: The Birth of the Prison*. Harmondsworth: Penguin Books.

———. 1980. *Power/Knowledge: Selected Interviews and Other Writings, 1972–1977*. Brighton: Harvester Press.

Frykenberg, Robert Eric. 1965. *Guntur District, 1788–1848: A History of Local Influence and Central Authority in South India*. Oxford: Clarendon Press.

Furedy, Chris. 1978. "Lord Curzon and the Reform of the Calcutta Corporation 1899: A Case Study in Imperial Decision-making." *South Asia* n.s. 1:75–89.

Gillion, Kenneth L. 1969. *Ahmedabad: A Study in Indian Urban History*. Canberra: Australian National University Press.

Gramsci, Antonio. 1971. *Selections from Prison Notebooks*. London: Lawrence and Wishart.

Guerra, Francisco. 1963. "Medical Colonization of the New World." *Medical History* 7:147–54.

Guha, Ranajit. 1963. *A Rule of Property for Bengal: An Essay on the Idea of Permanent Settlement*. Paris: Mouton and Co.

———. 1983. *Elementary Aspects of Peasant Insurgency in Colonial India*. Delhi: Oxford University Press.

———. 1989. "Dominance without Hegemony and Its Historiography." In *Subaltern Studies VI*, edited by Ranajit Guha. Delhi: Oxford University Press.

Gupta, Brahmananda. 1976. "Indigenous Medicine in Nineteenth- and Twentieth-Century Bengal." In *Asian Medical Systems: A Comparative Study*, edited by Charles Leslie. Berkeley: University of California Press.

Hardiman, David. 1987. *The Coming of the Devi: Adivasi Assertion in Western India*. Delhi: Oxford University Press.

Harrison, J. B. 1980. "Allahabad: A Sanitary History." In *The City in South Asia*, edited by K. Ballhatchet and J. B. Harrison. London: Curzon Press.

Harrison, Mark. 1990. "Towards a Sanitary Utopia? Professional Visions and Public Health in India, 1880–1914." *South Asia Research* 10:19–40.

———. 1991. "Public Health and Medical Research in India, c. 1860–1914." D.Phil. thesis, Oxford University.

Headrick, Daniel R. 1981. *The Tools of Empire: Technology and European Imperialism in the Nineteenth Century*. New York: Oxford University Press.

Hegel, G. W. F. 1956. *The Philosophy of History*. New York: Dover Publications.

Heimsath, Charles H. 1964. *Indian Nationalism and Hindu Social Reform*. Princeton: Princeton University Press.

Hirst, L. Fabian. 1953. *The Conquest of Plague: A Study of the Evolution of Epidemiology*. Oxford: Clarendon Press.

Hopkins, Donald R. 1983. *Princes and Peasants: Smallpox in History*. Chicago: University of Chicago Press.

Howard-Jones, Norman. 1972. "Cholera Therapy in the Nineteenth Century." *Journal of the History of Medicine* 27:373–95.

———. 1975. *The Scientific Background of the International Sanitary Conferences, 1851–1938*. Geneva: WHO.

Hume, John C. 1977. "Rival Traditions: Western Medicine and Yunan-i Tibb in the Punjab, 1849–1889." *Bulletin of the History of Medicine* 51:214–31.

Hutchins, Francis G. 1967. *The Illusion of Permanence: British Imperialism in India*. Princeton: Princeton University Press.

Ingram, Kenneth. 1956. *Reformers in India, 1793–1833: An Account of the Work of Christian Missionaries on Behalf of Social Reform*. Cambridge: Cambridge University Press.

Jaggi, O. P. 1979. *History of Science, Technology and Medicine in India, XIII: Western Medicine in India: Medical Education and Research*. Delhi: Atma Ram and Sons.

Jeffery, Roger. 1988a. *The Politics of Health in India*. Berkeley: University of California Press.

———. 1988b. "Doctors and Congress: The Role of Medical Men and Medical Politics in Indian Nationalism." In *The Indian National Congress and the Political Economy of India, 1885–1985*, edited by Mike Shepperdson and Colin Simmons. Aldershot: Avebury.

Jolly, Julius. 1977. *Indian Medicine*. 2d ed. Delhi: Munshiram Manoharlal.

Jordanova, Ludmila. 1989. *Sexual Visions: Images of Gender in Science and Medicine between the Eighteenth and Twentieth Centuries*. Hemel Hempstead: Harvester Wheatsheaf.

Karandikar, S. L. n.d. *Lokamanya Bal Gangadhar Tilak: The Hercules and Prometheus of Modern India*. Pune: Author.

King, Anthony D. 1976. *Colonial Urban Development: Culture, Social Power and Environment*. London: Routledge and Kegan Paul.

Klein, Ira. 1973. "Death in India." *Journal of Asian Studies* 32: 639–59.

———. 1980. "Cholera Therapy and Treatment in Nineteenth Century India." *Journal of Indian History* 58:35–51.

———. 1986. "Urban Development and Death: Bombay City, 1870–1914." *Modern Asian Studies* 20:725–54.

———. 1988. "Plague, Policy and Popular Unrest in British India." *Modern Asian Studies* 22:723–55.

Kopf, David. 1969. *British Orientalism and the Bengal Renaissance: The Dynamics of Indian Modernization, 1773–1835*. Berkeley: University of California Press.

Kuhn, Thomas S. 1970. *The Structure of Scientific Revolutions*. 2d ed. Chicago: University of Chicago Press.

Learmonth, Andrew. 1988. *Disease Ecology: An Introduction*. Oxford: Blackwell.

Leslie, Charles. 1974. "The Modernization of Asian Medical Systems." In *Rethinking Modernization: Anthropological Perspectives*, edited by John J. Poggie and Robert N. Lynch. Westport, Conn.: Greenwood Press.

———, ed. 1976. *Asian Medical Systems: A Comparative Analysis*. Berkeley: University of California Press.

Livingstone, David N. 1987. "Human Acclimatization: Perspectives on a Contested Field of Enquiry in Science, Medicine and Geography." *History of Science* 15:359–94.

Lutzker, Edythe. 1973. *Edith Pechey-Phipson, M.D.: The Story of England's Foremost Pioneering Woman Doctor*. New York: Exposition Press.

———. n.d. "Waldemar Mordecai Haffkine." In *Haffkine Institute Platinum Jubilee Commemoration Volume, 1899–1974*. Bombay: Haffkine Institute.

McGrew, Roderick E. 1965. *Russia and the Cholera, 1823–1832*. Madison: University of Wisconsin Press.

MacLeod, Roy M. 1967. "The Frustration of State Medicine, 1880–1899." *Medical History* 11:15–40.

McNeill, William H. 1979. *Plagues and Peoples*. Harmondsworth: Penguin Books.

Malik, Hafeez. 1980. *Sir Sayyid Ahmad Khan and Muslim Modernization in India and Pakistan*. New York: Columbia University Press.

Marriott, McKim. 1955. "Western Medicine in a Village of Northern India." In *Health, Culture and Community: Case Studies of Public Reactions to Health Programs*, edited by Benjamin D. Paul. New York: Sage Foundation.

Marshall, P. J., and Glyndwr Williams. 1982. *The Great Map of Mankind: British Perceptions of the World in the Age of Enlightenment*. London: Dent.

Mason, Philip. 1974. *A Matter of Honour: An Account of the Indian Army, Its Officers and Men.* London: Cape.

Mills, I. D. 1988. "The 1918–19 Influenza Pandemic: The Indian Experience." *Indian Economic and Social History Review* 23: 1–40.

Misra, Babagrahi. 1969. "Sitala: The Small-pox Goddess of India." *Asian Folklore Studies* 28:133–41.

Mohammad, Shan, ed. 1972. *Writings and Speeches of Sir Syed Ahmad Khan.* Bombay: Nachiketa Publications.

Morris, Morris D. 1965. *The Emergence of an Industrial Labor Force in India: A Study of the Bombay Cotton Mills, 1854–1947.* Berkeley: University of California Press.

Muraleedharan, V. R. 1987. "Rural Health Care in Madras Presidency, 1919–39." *Indian Economic and Social History Review* 24:323–34.

Nair, Janaki. 1990. "Uncovering the Zenana: Visions of Indian Womanhood in Englishwomen's Writings, 1813–1940." *Journal of Women's History* 2:8–34.

Nair, A. A. 1968. "Dr T. M. Nair: A Liberator of the Masses." In *Justice Party Golden Jubilee Souvenir, 1968.* Madras: Justice Party.

Nandy, Ashis. 1983. *The Intimate Enemy: Loss and Recovery of Self under Colonialism.* Delhi: Oxford University Press.

Neelameghan, A. 1963. *Development of Medical Societies and Medical Periodicals in India, 1780 to 1920.* Calcutta: Indian Association of Special Libraries and Information Centres.

Nicholas, Ralph W. 1981. "The Goddess Sitala and Epidemic Smallpox in Bengal." *Journal of Asian Studies* 41:21–44.

Nilsson, Sten. 1968. *European Architecture in India, 1750–1850.* London: Faber and Faber.

Oldenburg, Veena Talwar. 1984. *The Making of Colonial Lucknow, 1856–1877.* Princeton: Princeton University Press.

Opler, Morris. 1963. "The Cultural Definition of Illness in Village India." *Human Organization* 22:32–35.

Parekh, Bhikhu. 1989. *Gandhi's Political Philosophy: A Critical Examination.* Basingstoke: Macmillan.

Parvate, T. V. 1958. *Bal Gangadhar Tilak: A Narrative and Interpretive Review of His Life, Career and Contemporary Events.* Ahmadabad: Navajivan Publishing House.

Patterson, T. J. S. 1987. "The Relationship of Indian and European Practitioners of Medicine from the Sixteenth Century." In *Studies on Indian Medical History*, edited by G. Jan Meulenbeld and Dominik Wujastyk. Groningen: Forsten.

Paul, S. N. 1979. *Public Opinion and British Rule: A Study of the Influence of Indian Public Opinion on British Administration and Bureaucracy, 1899–1914.* New Delhi: Metropolitan Book Co.

Pelling, Margaret. 1978. *Cholera, Fever and English Medicine, 1825–1865.* Oxford: Oxford University Press.

Pollitzer, R. 1959. *Cholera.* Geneva: WHO.

Post, John D. 1990. "Nutritional Status and Mortality in Eighteenth-Century Europe." In *Hunger in History: Food Shortage, Poverty and Deprivation*, edited by Lucile F. Newman. Cambridge, Mass.: Blackwell.

Prior, Katherine. 1990. "The British Administration of Hinduism in North India, 1780–1900." Ph.D. thesis, University of Cambridge.

Ramasubban, Radhika. 1982. *Public Health and Medical Research in India: Their Origins under the Impact of British Colonial Policy.* Stockholm: SAREC.

———. 1984. "The Development of Health Policy in India." In *India's Demography: Essays on the Contemporary Population*, edited by Tim Dyson and Nigel Crook. Delhi: South Asia Publishers.

———. 1988. "Imperial Health in British India, 1857–1900." In *Disease, Medicine and Empire: Perspectives on Western Medicine and the Experience of European Expansion*, edited by Roy MacLeod and Milton Lewis. London: Routledge.

Razzell, Peter. 1977. *The Conquest of Smallpox: The Impact of Inoculation on Smallpox Mortality in Eighteenth Century Britain.* Firle: Caliban Books.

Riley, James C. 1987. *The Eighteenth-Century Campaign to Avoid Disease.* Basingstoke: Macmillan.

Roff, William R. 1982. "Sanitation and Security: The Imperial powers and the Nineteenth Century Hajj." In *Arabian Studies VI*, edited by R. B. Serjeant and R. L. Bidwell. London: Scorpion Communications.

Rogers, Leonard. 1957. "Thirty Years' Research on the Control of Cholera Epidemics." *British Medical Journal* 2:1193–97.

Rosenberg, Charles E. 1962. *The Cholera Years: The United States in 1832, 1849, and 1866.* Chicago: University of Chicago Press.

Rosselli, John. 1974. *Lord William Bentinck: The Making of a Liberal Imperialist, 1774–1839.* London: Chatto and Windus.

Rudolph, Lloyd I., and Susanne Hoeber Rudolph. 1967. *The Modernity of Tradition: Political Development in India.* Chicago: University of Chicago Press.

Russell, Paul F. 1955. *Man's Mastery of Malaria.* London: Oxford University Press.

Said, Edward W. 1978. *Orientalism.* London: Routledge and Kegan Paul.

Scott, James C. 1985. *Weapons of the Weak: Everyday Forms of Peasant Resistance.* New Haven: Yale University Press.

Sen, A. K. 1980. "Famine Mortality: A Study of the Bengal Famine of 1943." In *Peasants in History: Essays in Honour of Daniel Thorner*, edited by E. J. Hobsbawm, et al. Calcutta: Oxford University Press.

Sen, Surendra Nath. 1957. *Eighteen Fifty-Seven.* Delhi: Government of India Publications Division.

Sheridan, Richard B. 1985. *Doctors and Slaves: A Medical and Demographic History of Slavery in the British West Indies, 1680–1834.* Cambridge: Cambridge University Press.

Sim, Joe. 1990. *Medical Power in Prisons: The Prison Medical Service in England, 1774–1989.* Milton Keynes: Open University Press.

Smith, F. B. 1990. *The People's Health 1830–1910*. London: Weidenfeld and Nicolson.

Sontag, Susan. 1983. *Illness as Metaphor*. Harmondsworth: Penguin Books.

Spitzer, Leo. 1968. "The Mosquito and Segregation in Sierra Leone." *Canadian Journal of African Studies* 2:49–61.

Stokes, Eric. 1959. *The English Utilitarians and India*. Oxford: Oxford University Press.

Swanson, Maynard W. 1977. "The Sanitation Syndrome: Bubonic Plague and Urban Native Policy in Cape Colony, 1900–1909." *Journal of African History* 18:387–410.

Swinson, Arthur, and Donald Scott, eds. 1968. *The Memoirs of Private Waterfield*. London: Cassel.

Tinker, Hugh. 1968. *The Foundations of Local Self-Government in India, Pakistan and Burma*. London: Pall Mall Press.

———. 1974. *A New System of Slavery: The Export of Indian Labour Overseas, 1830–1920*. London: Oxford Unversity Press.

Turshen, Meredeth. 1984. *The Political Ecology of Disease in Tanzania*. New Brunswick: Rutgers University Press.

Vaughan, Megan. 1991. *Curing Their Ills: Colonial Power and African Illness*. Oxford: Polity Press.

Vicziany, Marika. 1986. "Imperialism, Botany and Statistics in early Nineteenth-Century India: The Surveys of Francis Buchanan (1762–1829). *Modern Asian Studies* 20:625–60.

Wadley, Susan S. 1980. "Sitala: The Cool One." *Asian Folklore Studies* 39:33–62.

White, David L. 1991. "From Crisis to Community Definition: The Dynamics of Eighteenth-Century Parsi Philanthropy." *Modern Asian Studies* 25:303–20.

Wilson, H. H. 1979. *The Art of War and Medical and Surgical Sciences of Hindus*. Delhi: Nag Publishers.

Yang, Anand A. 1985. "Dangerous Castes and Tribes: The Criminal Tribes Act and the Magahiya Doms of Northeast India." In *Crime and Criminality in British India*, edited by A. A. Yang. Tucson: University of Arizona Press.

———. 1987. "Disciplining 'Natives': Prisons and Prisoners in Early Nineteenth Century India." *South Asia* 10:29–45.

———. 1989. *The Limited Raj: Agrarian Relations in Colonial India, Saran District, 1793–1920*. Berkeley: University of California Press.

Yule, Henry, and A. C. Burnell. 1985. *Hobson-Jobson: A Glossary of Colloquial Anglo-Indian Words and Phrases*. London: Routledge and Kegan Paul.

Zimmer, H. R. 1948. *Hindu Medicine*. Baltimore: Johns Hopkins.

Zimmermann, Francis. 1987. *The Jungle and the Aroma of Meats: An Ecological Theme in Hindu Medicine*. Berkeley: University of California Press.

Index

Compositor: Asco Trade Typesetting Ltd., Hong Kong
Text: Times Roman
Display: Gill Sans
Printer and Binder: BookCrafters

HISTORY/ASIAN STUDIES/MEDICINE

Colonizing the Body

State Medicine and Epidemic Disease in Nineteenth-Century India
David Arnold

In this innovative analysis of medicine and disease in colonial India, David Arnold explores the vital role of the state in medical and public health activities, arguing that these activities were a critical site of interaction and conflict between the British authorities and their Indian subjects.

By combining the study of an increasingly authoritative medical discourse with an account of the practical constraints and political consequences of medical interventionism, Arnold demonstrates that Western medicine as practiced in India was not simply transferred from West to East, from metropole to colony, but was also fashioned in response to local needs and Indian conditions.

Arnold focuses on three major epidemic diseases—smallpox, cholera, and plague—to illustrate the varied forms and impact of medical interventionism and mark the principal stages of emerging public health policy. He examines such colonial enclaves as the army and the jails, where colonial medicine seemed most powerful, as well as the nature of popular resistance and the contrasting character of indigenous medical beliefs and practitioners. As part of a dominant environmentalist and Orientalist paradigm, he argues, Western medicine became a critical battleground between the colonized and the colonizers, but also prepared the way for a later nationalist hegemony.

By emphasizing the colonial dimension of medicine, *Colonizing the Body* makes a major contribution to the social history of medicine and to the developing literature on the body. Through an in-depth discussion of medical texts and practices, it highlights the centrality of the body to political authority in British India and shows how medicine both influenced and articulated the intrinsic nature and contradictions of colonial rule.

DAVID ARNOLD is Professor of South Asian History at the School of Oriental and African Studies, University of London.

9 780520 082953   90000

ISBN 0-520-08295-8

UNIVERSITY OF
CALIFORNIA PRESS

Berkeley 94720